Case Studies in Pediatrics

Case Studies in Pediatrics

Editor: Veronica Kelly

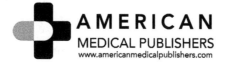

AMERICAN
MEDICAL PUBLISHERS
www.americanmedicalpublishers.com

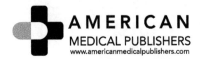

Cataloging-in-Publication Data

Case studies in pediatrics / edited by Veronica Kelly.
  p. cm.
Includes bibliographical references and index.
ISBN 979-8-88740-614-5
1. Pediatrics. 2. Children--Diseases. 3. Children--Diseases--Case studies.
4. Children--Health and hygiene. I. Kelly, Veronica.
RJ47.3 .P43 2023
618.92--dc23

American Medical Publishers,
41 Flatbush Avenue,
1st Floor, New York,
NY 11217, USA

ISBN 979-8-88740-614-5 (Hardback)

Contents

                Resumed with Multidisciplinary Care...193
                Diana Simão Raimundo, Carolina Figueiredo, Ana Raposo and
                Bernardo Dias Pereira

            Permissions

            List of Contributors

            Index

Preface

Pediatrics is a branch of medicine that focuses on the medical care of infants, children, and adolescents. It addresses their unique physical, emotional and developmental needs. Pediatric care spans a wide range of medical services, including preventive care, routine check-ups, immunizations, diagnosis, and treatment of acute and chronic illnesses. Pediatrics also plays an important role in assessing and managing the physical and mental well-being of children, monitoring their growth and development, and providing guidance to parents or caregivers. The disorders and medical conditions which are treated within pediatrics range from common childhood illnesses like respiratory infections and ear infections to chronic conditions such as asthma, allergies, diabetes, and behavioral disorders. This book includes some of the vital pieces of works being conducted across the world, on various topics which fall under the umbrella of pediatrics. Those in search of information to further their knowledge will be greatly assisted by it.

This book is a result of research of several months to collate the most relevant data in the field.

When I was approached with the idea of this book and the proposal to edit it, I was overwhelmed. It gave me an opportunity to reach out to all those who share a common interest with me in this field. I had 3 main parameters for editing this text:

1. Accuracy – The data and information provided in this book should be up-to-date and valuable to the readers.

2. Structure – The data must be presented in a structured format for easy understanding and better grasping of the readers.

3. Universal Approach – This book not only targets students but also experts and innovators in the field, thus my aim was to present topics which are of use to all.

Thus, it took me a couple of months to finish the editing of this book.

I would like to make a special mention of my publisher who considered me worthy of this opportunity and also supported me throughout the editing process. I would also like to thank the editing team at the back-end who extended their help whenever required.

Editor

Screening Children with a Family History of Central Congenital Hypoventilation Syndrome

Hina Emanuel,[1] Kimberly Rennie,[1] Kelly Macdonald,[2] Aravind Yadav ⓘ,[1] and Ricardo A. Mosquera ⓘ[1]

[1]Department of Pediatrics, The University of Texas Health Science Center at Houston, McGovern Medical School, Houston, TX, USA
[2]University of Houston, Texas Institute for Measurement, Evaluation, and Statistics, Department of Psychology, Houston, TX, USA

Correspondence should be addressed to Ricardo A. Mosquera; ricardo.a.mosquera@uth.tmc.edu

Academic Editor: Ashraf T. Soliman

Congenital central hypoventilation syndrome (CCHS) is a rare genetic disorder of an autonomic nervous disorder that affects breathing. It is characterized by respiratory insufficiency secondary to insensitivity to hypoxemia and hypercarbia, particularly during sleep leading to persistent apnea. We report four individuals across two generations harboring heterozygous 25 poly-alanine repeats mutations (PARMs) in PHOX2B with a varying degree of phenotypic clinical manifestations. Two family members who reported to be "asymptomatic" were subsequently diagnosed with CCHS, based on genetic testing, obtained because of their family history. Genetic studies in the family including a mother and three offsprings revealed in-frame five amino acid PARMs of PHOX2B consistent with CCHS in addition to full clinical assessment. All affected individuals had evidence of hypercapnia on blood gas analysis with PCO_2 in the range of 32–70 (mean; 61). Nocturnal polysomnogram revealed evidence of hypoventilation in two individuals (1 offspring and mother) with the end-tidal CO_2 median of 54. Magnetic resonance imaging of brain revealed no abnormalities in the brain stem. There was no evidence of cor pulmonale on echocardiograms in all individuals. Neuro-psychological testing was conducted on all four patients; two patients (mother and 1 offspring) had normal results, while the other two offspring exhibited some impairments on neuropsychological testing. This case series emphasizes the importance of screening first-degree relatives of individuals with confirmed CCHS to minimize complications associated with long-term ventilatory impairment. It also suggests that some patients with CCHS should undergo neuropsychological evaluations to assess for cognitive weaknesses secondary to their CCHS.

1. Introduction

Congenital central hypoventilation syndrome (CCHS) is also known as Ondine's curse and is an autosomal dominant disease with an estimated incidence of one per 200,000 live births. CCHS is characterized by respiratory insufficiency, dysregulation of ventilatory hemostasis during nonrapid eye movement (NREM) leading to alveolar hypoventilation, and arterial hypoxemia in settings of normal lung mechanics. CCHS is diagnosed in the absence of primary neuromuscular, metabolic, infectious, pulmonary, or cardiac diseases or brainstem lesion [1]. The disease-defining gene for CCHS

is the paired-like homeobox 2B gene (PHOX2B). Mutations in PHOX2B are responsible for CCHS. Polyalanine repeat mutations (PARMs) in PHOX2B account for more than 90% of CCHS cases. The majority of PARMs are considered to arise *de novo*, and about 10% of the mutations are inherited mostly from asymptomatic parents with somatic mosaicism and rarely from affected parents [2,3].

We present the case of a family with a mother and three offsprings from different biological fathers with identical polyalanine repeat mutations of PHOX2B with varying degree of penetrance, expressivity, and, henceforth, clinical manifestations. We highlight discord in phenotypic and genotypic expression among the family of a mother and three offsprings and importance of screening first-degree relatives to identify CCHS in individuals with no overt symptoms.

2. Methods

The identification of CCHS in a family of two siblings prompted evaluation of the rest of the family members for CCHS. We performed genetic testing to confirm diagnosis of CCHS in all family members. Individuals with confirmed genetic testing for CCHS underwent complete clinical assessment. Complete clinical assessment included overnight polysomnogram using standard protocol in the mother and two siblings, neuropsychological evaluation using valid standardized scales which was conducted by a licensed neuropsychologist, and a cardiological assessment by using an electrocardiograph and echocardiograph.

All individuals ($n = 4$, age; range, 1–31 years) had PHOX2B sequence analysis carried out, which showed heterozygous p. Ala241 (25) polyalanine repeats, the Epworth Sleepiness Scale (ESS) score between 4 and 5, normal brain MRI, echocardiogram with no cor pulmonale, and full-scale intelligence quotient (FSIQ) and showed average intellectual functioning for proband's brother (106) and proband's mother (94), significant impairment in cognitive, language, and motor development (70) for proband's sister, below average intellectual functioning (83) for proband, and a mean PCO_2 of 61 mmHg for all four individuals (See Table 1, Figure 1).

3. Clinical Details

The proband is a 7-year-old child of Hispanic background who was born at 39 weeks of gestation via normal vaginal spontaneous delivery and had apnea briefly after birth, requiring invasive mechanical ventilation for a week. He was successfully weaned to room air with no recurrence of an apneic event during the neonatal period; however, he was readmitted with acute respiratory failure with hypoxemia and hypercarbia, PCO_2 max 68 (Table 1, Figure 1), and apneas at five weeks of age, requiring invasive positive pressure ventilation. Infectious, metabolic, cardiac, pulmonary, and brain stem lesion disorders were ruled out. Nocturnal polysomnogram (NPSG) was not performed at the time of diagnosis; however, subsequent polysomnogram performed on positive pressure ventilation (SIMV pressure control; rate 15, pressure control 13, pressure support 15, PEEP 5) revealed an apnea hypopnea index (AHI) of zero per hour, transcutaneous CO_2 in the range of 30–40's, and average baseline oxygen saturations of 99% on room air (Table 1). Prolonged QT interval was evident on the electrocardiogram. The echocardiogram reported minimal tricuspid regurgitation with no right ventricular strain (Table 1). Chest radiographs reported no lung parenchymal pathology, and magnetic resonance imaging (MRI) ruled out brain stem disorders (Table 1). PHOX2B sequence analysis revealed heterozygous 25 polyalanine repeat mutations which confirmed the diagnosis of CCHS (Table 1). A tracheostomy tube was placed for long-term ventilatory support. He was eventually weaned to room air during a day at one year of age with continued nocturnal ventilatory respiratory support. Neuropsychological testing indicated below-average intellectual functioning. The proband met criteria for a diagnosis of attention deficit hyperactivity disorder (Table 1).

The proband's 12-month-old maternal half-sister was born at 40 weeks of gestation via normal vaginal delivery. She was discharged home on room air 2 days after birth. She was readmitted with multiple episodes of apnea and respiratory failure with hypoxemia and hypercapnia at seven days of life requiring invasive ventilation and eventually tracheostomy placement for long-term ventilatory support. Infectious, cardiological, neurological, and primary pulmonary etiologies were ruled out. No pathological rhythm abnormalities were identified on the electrocardiogram. NPSG was not performed at the time of diagnosis although blood gases showed hypercapnia; PCO_2 max 70 (Table 1, Figure 1). Echocardiography showed normal heart structures (Table 1). MRI revealed no intracranial or brain stem pathology. Due to high degree of clinical suspicion of CCHS in settings of siblings with CCHS, PHOX2B genetic analysis was sent. PHOX2B sequence analysis revealed heterozygous p. Ala24.1(25) polyalanine repeats which confirmed diagnosis of CCHS (Table 1). Neuropsychological testing for this patient indicated significant impairment in her cognitive, language, and motor development (Table 1). Screening for socioemotional and behavioral disorders was negative.

The case of two siblings with CCHS prompted screening of other family members, which included the mother and the 10-year-old brother. In addition to routine screening as part of standard care of CCHS, we included clinical assessment to inquire about the symptoms of CO_2 narcosis, autonomic dysregulation, day-time sleepiness, anxiety, and depression. There was no evidence of clinical manifestations of autonomic dysregulation in other family members. The proband's 10-year-old full brother was born at 36 weeks of gestation via normal vaginal delivery with a medical history significant for episodes of apnea in settings of respiratory syncytial virus but otherwise have been unremarkable from pulmonary standpoint. PHOX2B analysis was performed at 10 years of age for screening in settings of the family history of CCHS. PHOX2B sequence analysis showed identical PHOX2B mutation 25 polyalanine repeats (Table 1). Blood gas showed a PCO_2 of 58 (Table 1, Figure 1). NPSG revealed an apnea hypopnea index (AHI) of 3.4/hr, obstructive AHI of 3.4/hr, central AHI of 0.2/hr, and REM supine AHI of 0.2/hr (Table 1). End-tidal CO_2 averaged 56 during NREM sleep, with a maximum value of 66, and remained above 50, 79% of total sleep time (TST). Average oxygen saturation remained 94% during TST (Table 1). EES was reported as 4/24 (Table 1). The echocardiogram showed small PDA, trivial pulmonary, and tricuspid regurgitation with no right ventricular strain. No pathological rhythm variants on the electrocardiogram were identified. MRI of the brain revealed no evidence of brain stem disorders. No ophthalmological, neurological, or gastrointestinal problems were observed. Neuropsychological testing indicated intact intellectual

TABLE 1: Baseline characteristics of the study population.

Case	Age (years)	PHOX2B	PCO₂ (maximum)	ESS*	AHI/hr**	O₂ sat*** (average)	MRI brain	ECHO (cor pulmonale)	FSIQ******
Proband	7	p. Ala24.1(25)	67	4	0****	99%	Normal	Negative	83
Proband's sister	1	p. Ala24.1(25)	70	N/A*****	N/A	97%	Normal	Negative	70
Proband's brother	10	p. Ala24.1(25)	56	4	3.4	94%	Normal	Negative	106
Proband's mother	31	p. Ala24.1(25)	53	5	12.6	94%	N/A	Negative	94

*Epworth sleepiness scale. **Apnea hypopnea index. ***Oxygen saturation on room air. ****NPSG performed on respiratory support with resultant AHI of 0/hr. *****Data not available at time of this writing. ******Full-scale IQ as measured by the Wechsler scale of intelligence for children-fifth edition for the proband and the proband's brother and the Wechsler adult intelligence scale of intelligence-fourth edition for the proband's mother. For the proband's sister, the score reflects the patient's performance on the cognitive development portion of the Bayley scales of infant development-third edition. Scores falling between 85 and 115 are within the normal limits.

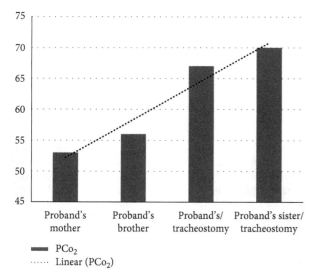

FIGURE 1: PCO₂ in index case and first-degree relatives except the father with and without tracheostomy.

functioning, and no concerns regarding socioemotional and behavioral functioning were identified (Table 1).

The proband's mother had PHOX2B sequence analysis carried out at thirty years of age. Results of PHOX2B analysis showed heterozygous p. Ala241(25) polyalanine repeats (Table 1). She reported early morning headaches and fatigue upon awakening. She did not have cardiological, ophthalmological, and neurological evaluation performed at the time of this writing. A blood PCO₂ of 54 was observed (Table 1, Figure 1). Nocturnal polysomnogram showed a total sleep efficiency of 87% with a TST of 400 mins, AHI index of 12.6/hr, recorded average oxygen saturation of 94%, and end-tidal CO₂ averaged 52 torr during entire sleep and >50 torr for 60% of TST. The ESS score was reported as 5/24 (Table 1). Results of the mother's neuropsychological testing indicated intact intellectual functioning (Table 1).

4. Discussion

This family demonstrates a novel *PHOX2B* p. Ala24.1(25) gene in four individuals across two generations with highly

variable penetrance ranging from respiratory failure during the neonatal period to later age with hypoventilation while asleep. Our study emphasizes the importance of screening of parents and at-risk siblings with subtle clinical findings through genetic analysis to identify PHOX2B pathogenic variant. In addition, given the rarity of disease, varied clinical manifestation, and lack of experience of medical professionals as evidenced by the previous literature, this study seeks to increase awareness of CCHS diagnosis, clinical manifestation, and long-term outcomes [4,5]. Through incorporation of questions pertaining to sleep, neurocognitive functioning, and general well-being, this study highlights the importance of comprehensive evaluation of CCHS including NPSG, evaluation of breathing while awake, echocardiogram, Holter monitoring and screening for neurocristopathies, and neuropsychological evaluation. Our case study highlights the importance of screening of at-risk asymptomatic family members through screening questions and a pertinent medical history followed by genetic testing. Genetic testing should not be limited to parents alone but should be extended to all family members at risk for CCHS. Had it not been for screening, the proband's 10-year-old brother and the mother would have remained undetected.

A mutation in the *PHOX2B* gene is a requisite to diagnosis of CCHS. PHOX2B is involved in the regulation of the autonomic nervous system and respiratory control neurons. The majority (>90%) of PHOX2B mutations are heterozygous for an in-frame triplet duplication PARMs with the resultant genotype of 24–33 alanine repeats [6]. The CCHS phenotype has not been associated with any degree of somatic mosaicism so far, suggesting a germline origin for most PARMs in affected CCHS patients, which is consistent with our case series. De novo PHOX2B pathogenic variant accounts for most of the cases of CCHS with remaining cases of CCHS transmitted from affected parents with some degree of mosaicism, germline or somatic in PHOX2B variant with 50%, or a lower chance of acquiring pathogenic variant. The presence of the same PHOX2B mutation in parent-offspring supports an autosomal mode of inheritance. Our case series presents the identical PHOX2B mutation with varying degrees of penetrance and the time of onset which could be secondary to gene modifiers [7,8].

The evaluation of parents, children, and at-risks siblings of individuals with CCHS depends on the pathogenic variant identified in the proband. Our study emphasizes the importance of screening first-degree relatives of an individual in a stepwise approach [9–11], prenatal testing, and genetic counseling to make informed medical and personal decisions. The PHOX2B screening test (fragment analysis) is performed if child has PARM or frame shift NPARM. PHOX2B mutation confirmed CCHS. If no mutation is identified, no further testing is advised; however, germline mosaicism cannot be ruled out. If the PHOX2B pathogenic variant is identified, there is a risk of transmitting mutation in pregnancy and warrants prenatal testing as the risk to the sibs is 50% if the proband's parent is affected, risk is 50% or lower if the proband's affected parent has mosaicism for the PHOX2 pathogenic variant, and even if the proband's parents are unaffected, there still remains risk to the proband's siblings due to mosaicism. Once the pathogenic variant is identified, genetic counseling can be offered to individuals at risk for CCHS to make informed decisions, prenatal testing, and preimplantation genetic diagnosis and to discuss future outcomes for themselves and offsprings before pregnancy. Results of our neuropsychological testing suggest that cognitive deficits may be associated with medical severity of CCHS. Routine neuropsychological testing may be warranted, especially for patients with more severe forms of the disease.

In conclusion, this case series highlights the importance of screening at-risk family members of an individual with CCHS; so genetic counseling can be offered to at-risk individuals in regard to long-term health implications of CCHS. This case report emphasizes the need of validated tools to screen for specific sleep, neurocognitive, and general well-being questions pertaining to CCHS in family members of the affected individual. Further research is needed to provide insight into applicability and outcomes of screening tools in clinical practice. With early diagnosis and careful ventilatory management, the sequelae of hypoxia and morbidity should be minimized and long-term outcome improved.

References

[1] T. J. Moraes, I. MacLusky, D. Zielinski, and R. Amin, "Section 11: central hypoventilation, congenital and acquired," *Canadian Journal of Respiratory, Critical Care, and Sleep Medicine*, vol. 2, no. sup1, pp. 78–82, 2018.

[2] D. E. Weese-Mayer, E. M. Berry-Kravis, L. Zhou et al., "Idiopathic congenital central hypoventilation syndrome: analysis of genes pertinent to early autonomic nervous system embryologic development and identification of mutations in PHOX2b," *American Journal of Medical Genetics*, vol. 123A, no. 3, pp. 267–278, 2003.

[3] E. M. Berry-Kravis, L. Zhou, C. M. Rand, and D. E. Weese-Mayer, "Congenital central hypoventilation syndrome: PHOX2B mutations and phenotype," *American Journal of Respiratory and Critical Care Medicine*, vol. 174, no. 10, pp. 1139–1144, 2006.

[4] R. Kerbl, H. Litscher, H. M. Grubbauer et al., "Congenital central hypoventilation syndrome (Ondine's curse syndrome) in two siblings: delayed diagnosis and successful noninvasive treatment," *European Journal of Pediatrics*, vol. 155, no. 11, pp. 977–980, 1996.

[5] Idiopathic congenital central hypoventilation syndrome: diagnosis and management," *American Journal of Respiratory and Critical Care Medicine*, vol. 160, no. 1, pp. 368–373, 1999.

[6] D. Trochet, Y. Mathieu, L. C. D. Pontual et al., "In Vitrostudies of non poly alanine PHOX2B mutations argue against a loss-of-function mechanism for congenital central hypoventilation," *Human Mutation*, vol. 30, no. 2, pp. E421–E431, 2009.

[7] S. Parodi, M. P. Baglietto, A. P. Prato et al., "A novel missense mutation in thePHOX2B gene is associated with late onset central hypoventilation syndrome," *Pediatric Pulmonology*, vol. 43, no. 10, pp. 1036–1039, 2008.

[8] R. Amin, A. Riekstins, S. Al-Saleh, C. Massicotte, A. L. Coates, and I. MacLusky, "Presentation and treatment of monozygotic twins with congenital central hypoventilation syndrome," *Canadian Respiratory Journal*, vol. 18, no. 2, pp. 87–89, 2011.

[9] D. E. Weese-Mayer, E. M. Berry-Kravis, and L. Zhou, "Adult identified with congenital central hypoventilation syndrome-mutation inPHOX2bGene and late-onset CHS," *American Journal of Respiratory and Critical Care Medicine*, vol. 171, no. 1, p. 88, 2005.

[10] L. S. Doherty, J. L. Kiely, P. C. Deegan et al., "Late-onset central hypoventilation syndrome: a family genetic study," *European Respiratory Journal*, vol. 29, no. 2, pp. 312–316, 2006.

[11] D. E. Weese-Mayer, P. P. Patwari, C. M. Rand, A. M. Diedrich, N. L. Kuntz, and E. M. Berry-Kravis, "Congenital central hypoventilation syndrome (CCHS) and PHOX2B mutations," in *Primer on the Autonomic Nervous System*, D. Robertson, I. Biaggioni, G. Burnstock, P. A. Low, and J. F. R. Paton, Eds., pp. 445–450, Academic Press, Oxford, UK, 2012.

A Novel Mutation in the *EIF2B4* Gene Associated with Leukoencephalopathy with Vanishing White Matter

D. Hettiaracchchi ⓘ,[1] N. Neththikumara,[1] B. A. P. S. Pathirana,[1] A. Padeniya,[2] and V. H. W. Dissanayake ⓘ[1]

[1]Human Genetics Unit, Faculty of Medicine, University of Colombo, Colombo, Sri Lanka
[2]National Hospital of Sri Lanka, Colombo, Sri Lanka

Correspondence should be addressed to D. Hettiaracchchi; dinebine@gmail.com

Academic Editor: Ozgur Cogulu

1. Introduction

Leukoencephalopathy with vanishing white matter (VWM; MIM #603896) is an autosomal recessive disorder, characterized by childhood ataxia, spasticity, and variable optic atrophy. The course is chronic progressive with episodes of rapid deterioration, provoked by febrile illnesses, minor head trauma, or acute fright, with most patients succumbing to illness within few years of onset. Three forms of VWM has been described based on disease onset, which ranges from a subacute infantile form (onset age <1 year), an early childhood form (onset age 1–5 years), and a late-childhood/juvenile form (onset age 5–15 years) [1–3]. The diagnosis is based on clinical findings, characteristic MRI features indicative of vanishing of the cerebral white matter, and an identifiable pathogenic variant in one of the genes (*EIF2B1*, *EIF2B2*, *EIF2B3*, *EIF2B4*, and *EIF2B5*) encoding for the 5 subunits of eukaryotic translation initiation factor 2B (eIF2B), which is essential in all cells of the body for the initiation of translation of RNA into protein during protein synthesis and its regulation under different stress conditions such as fever [4, 5]. Its effect is predominantly seen on oligodendrocytes and astrocytes while there is sparing of other cell types [2].

2. Case Report

The proband is the only child of a 2nd degree consanguineous marriage of Sri Lankan origin. She was well up to 8 months when she developed a fever for one day, following which the child had acute developmental regression that lasted for 3 months accompanied with bilateral lower limb weakness and speech regression. The child then developed an upper respiratory tract infection, following which she was unresponsive for 30 minutes. The MRI scan showed marked hyperintense and subcortical white matter in T2 WI bilaterally with involvement of dentate nuclei and white matter tracts. Myelination was around 3 months, which corresponded to the current developmental age of the child. All biochemical parameters were within normal limits. The proband succumbed to illness at 18 months. She also had a first cousin with similar features who died at the age of 21 years (Figure 1).

3. Methods

3.1. Whole Exome Sequencing. DNA was extracted from the proband's whole blood leucocytes using Qiagen DNA extraction Mini KIT according to the manufacturer's protocol. Whole exome sequencing (WES) of the extracted DNA was performed on an Illumina® HiSeq 4000 Next Generation Sequencer using the SureSelect® Human All Exon V6 kit.

3.2. Bioinformatics Analysis. Data analysis was performed using an in-house-developed variant calling annotation pipeline. Paired-end Fastq files were aligned to the GrCh37 human reference sequence using BWA-MEM algorithm to produce SAM file. The SAM to BAM conversion, sorting, and

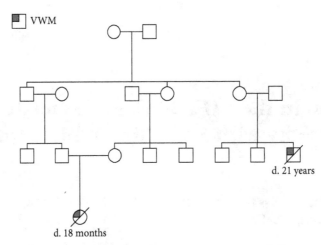

FIGURE 1: Pedigree chart of the proband with affected family members.

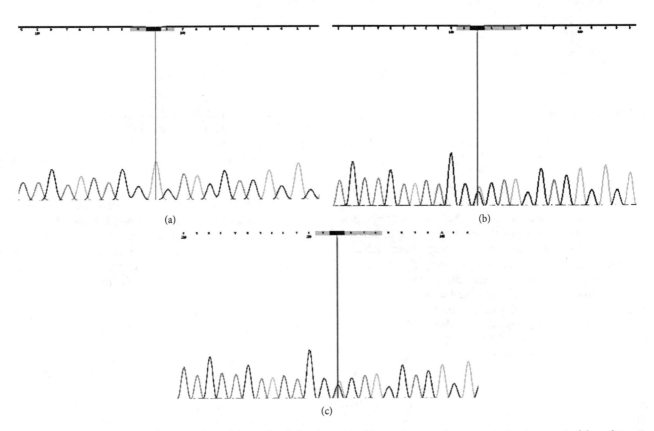

FIGURE 2: (a) Sanger sequence chromatogram of the proband showing a novel homozygous missense mutation in exon 5 of the eukaryotic translation initiation factor 2B subunit delta (*EIF2B4*) gene, ENST00000493344: c.614C>T [p.Pro205Leu] causing leukoencephalopathy with vanishing white matter (VWM). (b) Mother of the proband with a heterozygous mutation. (c) Father of the proband with a heterozygous mutation.

indexing were performed using SAM tools, and deduping of reads were performed using Picard tools. Variant discovery was performed using the Genome Analysis Tool Kit (GATK) Haplotype caller, followed by realigning of the deduped BAM around indels. Annotation of the resulted VCF file was performed using SNP-eff with Refseq, dbSNP, 1000 Genomes, Exome Variant Server, Exome Aggregation Consortium,

phastCons100way, ClinVar, and locus-specific databases. MutationTaster, SIFT, PolyPhen2, and Provean were used to in silico functional prediction. Reported benign variants resided in the genes causing VWM were filtered out using virtual gene panel. Remaining variants were further scrutinized considering their availability in public databases, their conservation, and their functional impact on the protein.

TABLE 1: Results of in silico mutation prediction analysis.

Algorithm	Prediction	Score
PolyPhen2[a]	Probably damaging (HumDiv- model)	0.998
PolyPhen2[a]	Probably damaging (HumVar- model)	0.980
Provean[b]	Deleterious	−4.92
SIFT[c]	Damaging	0.032
MutationTaster[d]	Disease causing	0.999

[a]http://genetics.bwh.harvard.edu/pph2; deleterious threshold >0.5. [b]http://provean.jcvi.org/index.php; score threshold is −2.5 for binary classification. [c]http://sift.jcvi.org/www/SIFT_chr_coords_submit.html threshold <0.05. [d]http://www.mutationtaster.org; scores range from 0.0 to 1.0.

4. Results

A novel missense mutation in exon 5 of the eukaryotic translation initiation factor 2B subunit delta gene (EIF2B4), ENST00000493344: c.614C>T| p.Pro205Leu was detected (read depth: 60x). The patient was a homozygote for the mutation. Mutation was also seen in the Sanger sequence chromatogram. (Figure 2) p.Pro205Leu was a novel mutation and therefore is absent in population genetic databases and clinical databases. It results in a nonconservative amino acid substitution, which impacts the physiochemical nature of the protein. This mutation resides in a highly conserved region among different species through out the evolution (phastCons100way_vertebrate score = 1). In silico prediction tools universally concluded that p.Pro205Leu has a deleterious effect (Table 1) on protein structure and function.

5. Discussion

Vanishing white matter disease (VWM) is autosomal recessive leukodystrophy linked to mutations in translation initiation factor 2B (eIF2B), and it is the only brain disease recognized to date, which involves this initiation factor. Reduction in eIF2B activity leads to a cascade of cellular events resulting in a sustained improper activation of the unfolded protein response and concomitant expression of proliferation, prosurvival, and proapoptotic downstream effectors. These events predispose VWM cells to stress-induced hyperreactive damage [6–8]. Even though the cellular consequences of EIF2B mutations on neural cells are unknown, cell cultures from the brain of an individual with VWM carrying mutations in subunit 5 of eIF2B (encoded by EIF2B5) have generated morphologically normal oligodendrocytes and abnormal astrocytes in vitro, suggesting that a deficiency in astrocyte function may contribute to the loss of white matter in VWM leukodystrophy [6].

The resulting pathological manifestations include increasing white matter rarefaction and cystic degeneration, oligodendrocytosis with highly characteristic foamy oligodendrocytes, meager astrogliosis with dysmorphic astrocytes, and loss of oligodendrocytes by apoptosis, but their exact pathophysiology is poorly understood [7, 9, 10]. Currently, treatment strategies involving neural stem cell transplantation are being explored, but their robust proliferative capacity coupled with difficulty to control their differentiation potential remains the main challenge for cell-based therapy, as these transplanted cells can potentially generate undesired neural cell types [11, 12]. Due to astrocytes being the predominantly affected cell type, transplantation of immature astrocytes might have a theoretical benefit.

The high incidence of low-frequency mutations limits rapid genetic confirmation of the disease, especially in cases of undiagnosed leukodystrophy [13, 14]. In our patient, the P205L was a novel mutation and therefore is absent in population genetic databases and clinical databases. It results in a nonconservative amino acid substitution, which impacts the physiochemical nature of the protein. We can conclude that all in silico tools predict a deleterious impact on protein function, hence giving rise to the phenotypic features of VWM leukodystrophy. By reporting this novel mutation, we wish to facilitate its early detection.

Additional Points

Key Clinical Message: Leukoencephalopathy with vanishing white matter is an autosomal recessive disorder characterized by childhood ataxia, spasticity, and variable optic atrophy. Pathological variants in one of the five genes encoding the five subunits of eukaryotic translation initiation factor eIF2B has been implicated. The authors report a novel homozygous variant in EIF2B4 gene.

Authors' Contributions

D. Hettiaracchchi, A. Padeniya, and V. H. W. Dissanayake were the clinicians looking after the patient. B. A. P. S. Pathirana performed laboratory testing. N. Neththikumara performed bioinformatics analysis. D. Hettiaracchchi wrote the first draft of the manuscript with contributions from all. All authors reviewed, modified, and approved the final version of the manuscript.

References

[1] M. S. van der Knaap, P. A. J. Leegwater, A. A. M. Könst et al., "Mutations in each of the five subunits of translation initiation factor eIF2B can cause leukoencephalopathy with vanishing white matter," *Annals of Neurology*, vol. 51, no. 2, pp. 264–270, 2002.

[2] M. S. van der Knaap, J. C. Pronk, and G. C. Scheper, "Vanishing white matter disease," *Lancet Neurology*, vol. 5, no. 5, pp. 413–423, 2006.

[3] P. A. J. Leegwater, J. C. Pronk, and M. S. van der Knaap, "Leukoencephalopathy with vanishing white matter: from magnetic resonance imaging pattern to five genes," *Journal of Child Neurology*, vol. 18, no. 9, pp. 639–645, 2003.

[4] O. Scali, C. Di Perri, and A. Federico, "The spectrum of mutations for the diagnosis of vanishing white matter disease," *Neurological Sciences*, vol. 27, no. 4, pp. 271–277, 2006.

[5] R. Schiffmann and O. Elroy-Stein, "Childhood ataxia with CNS hypomyelination/vanishing white matter disease—a common leukodystrophy caused by abnormal control of protein synthesis," *Molecular Genetics and Metabolism*, vol. 88, no. 1, pp. 7–15, 2006.

[6] J. Dietrich, M. Lacagnina, D. Gass et al., "EIF2B5 mutations compromise GFAP+ astrocyte generation in vanishing white

matter leukodystrophy," *Nature Medicine*, vol. 11, no. 3, pp. 277–283, 2005.

[7] M. Bugiani, I. Boor, J. M. Powers, G. C. Scheper, and M. S. van der Knaap, "Leukoencephalopathy with vanishing white matter: a review," *Journal of Neuropathology and Experimental Neurology*, vol. 69, no. 10, pp. 987–996, 2010.

[8] P. A. J. Leegwater, G. Vermeulen, and A. A. M. Könst, "Subunits of the translation initiation factor eIF2B are mutant in leukoencephalopathy with vanishing white matter," *Nature Genetics*, vol. 29, no. 4, pp. 383–388, 2001.

[9] M. S. van der Knaap, W. Kamphorst, P. G. Barth, C. L. Kraaijeveld, E. Gut, and J. Valk, "Phenotypic variation in leukoencephalopathy with vanishing white matter," *Neurology*, vol. 51, no. 2, pp. 540–547, 1998.

[10] B. van Kollenburg, J. van Dijk, J. Garbern et al., "Glia-specific activation of all pathways of the unfolded protein response in vanishing white matter disease," *Journal of Neuropathology and Experimental Neurology*, vol. 65, no. 7, pp. 707–715, 2006.

[11] M. Bugiani, I. Boor, B. van Kollenburg et al., "Defective glial maturation in vanishing white matter disease," *Journal of Neuropathology and Experimental Neurology*, vol. 70, no. 1, pp. 69–82, 2011.

[12] P. S. Leferink, N. Breeuwsma, M. Bugiani, M. S. van der Knaap, and V. M. Heine, "Affected astrocytes in the spinal cord of the leukodystrophy vanishing white matter," *Glia*, vol. 66, no. 4, pp. 862–873, 2018.

[13] J. Maletkovic, R. Schiffmann, J. R. Gorospe et al., "Genetic and clinical heterogeneity in eIF2B-related disorder," *Journal of Child Neurology*, vol. 23, no. 2, pp. 205–215, 2008.

[14] T. J. E. Muttikkal, D. R. Montealegre, and J. A. Matsumoto, "Enhancement of multiple cranial and spinal nerves in vanishing white matter: expanding the differential diagnosis," *Pediatric Radiology*, vol. 48, no. 3, pp. 437–442, 2018.

An Atypical Case of *Bartonella henselae* Osteomyelitis and Hepatic Disease

Dionna M. Mathews,[1] **Katie M. Vance** ⓘ**,**[2] **Pamela M. McMahon,**[2] **Catherine Boston,**[3] **and Michael T. Bolton** ⓘ[4]

[1]*Our Lady of the Lake Children's Hospital, Baton Rouge, LA, USA*
[2]*Division of Academic Affairs, Our Lady of the Lake Regional Medical Center, Baton Rouge, LA, USA*
[3]*Pediatric Hematology/Oncology, Our Lady of the Lake Children's Hospital/St. Jude Affiliate Baton Rouge, Baton Rouge, LA, USA*
[4]*Pediatric Infectious Diseases, Our Lady of the Lake Children's Hospital, Baton Rouge, LA, USA*

Correspondence should be addressed to Michael T. Bolton; michael.bolton@fmolhs.org

Academic Editor: Albert M. Li

Bartonella henselae is a Gram-negative bacterium and the causative agent of cat scratch disease (CSD). Atypical presentations of *B. henselae* that involve the musculoskeletal, hepatosplenic, cardiac, or neurologic systems are rare. In this case report, we describe a case of *B. henselae* osteomyelitis involving bilateral iliac bones complicated by hepatic lesions in a 12-year-old immunocompetent female patient. Although *B. henselae* is a rare cause of osteomyelitis, it should be considered when patients who present with fever, pain, and lymphadenopathy do not respond to routine osteomyelitis therapy.

1. Introduction

Bartonella henselae, a Gram-negative bacterium, is the causative agent of cat scratch disease (CSD) that typically involves the mononuclear phagocyte system and presents as local lymphadenopathy, often accompanied by fever [1]. *B. henselae* infections are thought to occur when a human is bitten or scratched by an infected cat [2–4] and may be transmitted by cat fleas or by an infected cat licking the nonintact skin of a human [5–7]. IgM is often elevated only briefly and is commonly normal during the course of the disease [8]. IgG titers greater than 1 : 256 are typically indicative of previous or active disease [6]. Children and teenagers make up approximately 80% of patients diagnosed with CSD [2]. Although infrequent, *B. henselae* can affect almost every organ system after hematogenous, lymphatic, or contiguous spread.

Bartonella osteomyelitis most frequently occurs in the spine. The pelvic girdle is the most common site of *Bartonella* osteomyelitis outside of the spine and occurs in 42% of all nonspinal cases [3]. *Bartonella* osteomyelitis typically presents as tenderness or pain in the affected area [4]. Magnetic resonance imaging (MRI) or radionuclide bone scanning is often used to diagnose osteomyelitis. Clinicians must rely on serologic testing, polymerase chain reaction testing (PCR), or Warthin–Starry silver staining to identify *B. henselae* as the causative organism because it does not grow in culture [3, 4]. We present a case of *B. henselae* osteomyelitis involving bilateral iliac bones complicated by hepatic lesions in an immunocompetent patient.

2. Case Presentation

A previously healthy 12-year-old female presented to the emergency department 4 days after completing a 3-day course of trimethoprim/sulfamethoxazole prescribed for a urinary tract infection. She complained of a 9-day history of fever and 3-day history of left hip pain associated with joint movement. The patient denied trauma, erythema, or swelling in the area of pain, but exposure history uncovered prolonged cat contact. Her initial exam revealed full range of motion of all extremities though she exhibited tenderness to

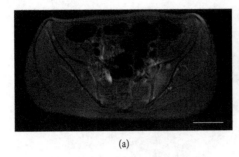
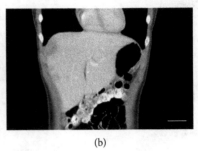

(a)   (b)

FIGURE 1: MRI and CT of patient's *Bartonella* bone and hepatic lesions. (a) An MRI obtained of the patient's pelvis shows small, scattered lesions throughout the iliac architecture. (b) A CT of the patient's abdomen shows hepatic lesions indicative of *B. henselae*. Bar, 5 cm.

palpation of her left hip. The remainder of the exam was unremarkable, including absence of any lymphadenopathy, bruising, erythema, or edema of the affected joint.

The patient's initial workup was significant for normocytic anemia (hemoglobin of 11.9 g/dL and hematocrit of 34.5%) and normal liver function tests. She was noted to have elevated inflammatory markers—an erythrocyte sedimentation rate greater than 120 mm/h and C-reactive protein of 68.6 mg/L. Urinalysis showed small amounts of leukocyte esterase and bacteria but only 0–5 white blood cells (WBCs). Urine and blood cultures were obtained and showed no bacterial growth.

An X-ray of the hip showed no acute abnormalities; however, a subsequent MRI showed a small left sacroiliac joint effusion with mild marrow edema that was concerning for infectious or inflammatory sacroiliitis (Figure 1(a)). Scattered small round lesions replaced bone marrow throughout the iliac architecture.

The patient was admitted with a working diagnosis of septic arthritis and received clindamycin intravenously. Joint fluid obtained via CT-guided aspiration revealed clear fluid with 15 WBCs, 200 red blood cells, and sterile cultures. Antibiotics were discontinued given that these findings were inconsistent with pyogenic arthritis, and she was improving clinically. Concern for possible leukemia based on the abnormal bony lesions led to an oncologic evaluation, including a chest X-ray, peripheral blood smear, and measurement of lactate dehydrogenase and uric acid, all of which were within normal limits.

Due to recrudesce of fever following the discontinuation of antibiotics, Epstein–Barr virus, cytomegalovirus, and *B. henselae* antibodies were measured. The patient's fever again declined without directed therapy, and she was discharged home with a diagnosis of transient synovitis.

The patient had intermittent low-grade fevers the week following her discharge. Her *B. henselae* titers were suggestive of recent infection (IgG > 1:1024, IgM negative). Due to known hepatic involvement of *B. henselae* in association with disseminated *Bartonella* disease, imaging (abdominal ultrasound followed by CT scan; Figure 1(b)) was performed and showed multiple liver lesions thought to be consistent with disseminated *B. henselae* infection. Cytopathology of the biopsied sample taken from the hepatic lesions revealed scars consistent with resolving *Bartonella*

liver lesions. While we observed inflammation, we did not observe the granulomatous inflammation that is a more classic sign of CSD. PCR of the lesions was negative for *B. henselae*. Further oncologic evaluations of the hepatic lesions were negative, as was a QuantiFERON–Gold test for tuberculosis.

The patient had clinical resolution after a 6-week azithromycin regimen. An MRI of the patient's pelvis at the end of therapy showed near complete resolution of the abnormalities in the iliac bones, which were fully resolved in an MRI obtained one year later. Furthermore, a CT of the patient's abdomen obtained at the end of therapy revealed that the liver lesions were decreasing in size, consistent with resolving infection. The patient's inflammatory markers also were normal.

3. Discussion

CSD often goes unrecognized due to nonspecific signs and symptoms and the disease's usual self-limiting natural course. Osteomyelitis caused by *B. henselae* is rare (observed in 0.1%–0.3% of CSD patients) but has long been recognized to occur in both immune compromised and immune competent patients [9, 10]. Although PCR is generally considered more sensitive for the diagnosis of *B. henselae* infection than is serology, its sensitivity is still not very good, with a reported range from 43% to 76% [4]. Indeed, we were unable to detect *B. henselae* from hepatic sampling via PCR. Insufficient fluid volume precluded testing on the joint sample, and blood was not sampled for PCR detection. The diagnosis of disseminated *B. henselae* was based on significantly elevated titers, radiographic findings, and epidemiologic history.

An oncologic process often is included in the differential diagnoses of patients who present with CSD, as *B. henselae* can produce osteolytic bone lesions that may be misdiagnosed as tumors [3, 4]. While an oncologic process was considered in the differential diagnosis of our patient's bony lesions, our patient's symptoms, combined with an unremarkable corroborative diagnostic evaluation and resolution, excluded a malignancy.

Bartonella osteomyelitis most commonly involves the axial skeleton, with several cases reported in the vertebrae, skull, sternum, ribs, and pelvis [1, 11, 12]. While Rozmanic et al.

documented vertebral and unilateral ilial involvement, our case involves bilateral iliac infection with hepatic lesions and concurrent lack of transaminitis of an immunocompetent child [13]. The pathogenesis of *Bartonella* osteomyelitis is not well understood. In most cases of *Bartonella* osteomyelitis, the bone lesion occurs at a distance from the involved lymph nodes, suggesting hematogenous or lymphatic spread of the infection [4, 10, 14]. *Bartonella* osteomyelitis usually presents subacutely in the axial skeleton, as we observed in our patient, unlike hematogenous osteomyelitis, which presents acutely and typically involves the appendicular skeleton [9].

CSD typically resolves within weeks to months regardless of antimicrobial therapy due to its self-limiting nature. However, studies show that various antibiotics have been used to treat the multitude of clinical manifestations produced by *B. henselae* [1]. A single clinical trial that showed mild-to-moderate hastening of initial recovery with azithromycin therapy supports its use as a first-line agent for lymphadenopathy [15]. However, azithromycin's efficacy in treating patients with atypical CSD, including patients with osteomyelitis and hepatosplenic involvement, has yet to be evaluated [4, 15–17]. Our patient's history of significant cat exposure, elevated anti-*B. henselae* IgG titer, and radiographic findings in bone and liver supported the diagnosis of CSD. We treated our patient with azithromycin given the severity of her symptoms and the evidence of multisystem involvement. After a prolonged course of therapy, she appears to have made a full recovery.

References

[1] K. Puri, A. J. Kreppel, and E. P. Schlaudecker, "*Bartonella* osteomyelitis of the acetabulum: case report and review of the literature," *Vector-Borne and Zoonotic Diseases*, vol. 15, no. 8, pp. 463–467, 2015.

[2] J. C. Garcia, M. J. Nunez, B. Castro, J. M. Fernandez, A. Portillo, and J. A. Oteo, "Hepatosplenic cat scratch disease in immunocompetent adults," *Medicine*, vol. 93, no. 17, pp. 267–279, 2014.

[3] S. Joychan, Y. Kuchipudi, P. J. Danielsky, K. M. Bovid, and G. Deepak, "Case of nonspinal osteomyelitis due to *Bartonella* and review of the literature," *Infectious Diseases in Clinical Practice*, vol. 25, no. 5, pp. 240–242, 2017.

[4] K. Mazur-Melewska, K. Jonczyk-Potoczna, A. Mania et al., "The significance of *Bartonella henselae* bacteria for oncological diagnosis in children," *Infectious Agents and Cancer*, vol. 10, no. 1, p. 30, 2015.

[5] P. Brouqui and D. Raoult, "Arthropod-borne diseases in homeless," *Annals of the New York Academy of Sciences*, vol. 1078, no. 1, pp. 223–235, 2006.

[6] S. A. Klotz, V. Ianas, and S. P. Elliot, "Cat-scratch disease," *American Family Physician*, vol. 83, no. 2, pp. 152–155, 2011.

[7] Cat-scratch disease, 2018, https://www.cdc.gov/healthypets/diseases/cat-scratch.html.

[8] E. Metzkor-Cotter, Y. Kletter, B. Avidor et al., "Long-term serological analysis and clinical follow-up of patients with cat scratch disease," *Clinical Infectious Diseases*, vol. 37, no. 9, pp. 1149-1150, 2018.

[9] Y. Kodama, N. Maeno, J. Nishi et al., "Multifocal osteomyelitis due to *Bartonella henselae* in a child without focal pain," *Journal of Infection and Chemotherapy*, vol. 13, no. 5, pp. 350–352, 2007.

[10] N. Hajjaji, L. Hocqueloux, R. Kerdraon, and L. Bret, "Bone infection in cat-scratch disease: a review of the literature," *Journal of Infection*, vol. 54, no. 5, pp. 417–421, 2007.

[11] I. Pons, I. Sanfeliu, N. Cardenosa, M. M. Nogueras, B. Font, and F. Segura, "Serological evidence of *Bartonella henselae* infection in healthy people in Catalonia, Spain," *Epidemiology and Infection*, vol. 136, no. 12, pp. 1712–1716, 2008.

[12] S. R. Boggs and R. G. Fisher, "Bone pain and fever in an adolescent and his sibling," *Pediatric Infectious Disease Journal*, vol. 30, no. 1, p. 89, 2011.

[13] V. Rozmanic, S. Banc, D. Miletic, K. Manestar, S. Kamber, and S. Paparic, "Role of magnetic imaging and scintigraphy in the diagnosis and follow-up of osteomyelitis in cat-scratch disease," *Journal of Paediatrics and Child Health*, vol. 43, no. 7-8, pp. 568–570, 2007.

[14] M. Al-Rahawan, B. Gray, C. Mitchell, and S. Smith, "Thoracic vertebral osteomyelitis with paraspinous mass and intraspinal extension: an atypical presentation of cat-scratch disease," *Pediatric Radiology*, vol. 42, no. 1, pp. 116–119, 2012.

[15] J. W. Bass, B. C. Freitas, A. D. Freitas et al., "Prospective randomized double blind placebo-controlled evaluation of azithromycin for treatment of cat-scratch disease," *Pediatric Infectious Disease Journal*, vol. 17, no. 6, pp. 447–452, 1998.

[16] D. Dornbos, J. Morin, J. R. Watson, and J. Pindrik, "Thoracic osteomyelitis and epidural abscess formation due to cat scratch disease: case report," *Journal of Neurosurgery: Pediatrics*, vol. 18, no. 6, pp. 713–716, 2016.

[17] D. L. Stevens, A. L. Bisno, H. F. Chambers et al., "Practice guidelines for the diagnosis and management of skin and soft tissue infections: 2014 update by the Infectious Diseases Society of America," *Clinical Infectious Diseases*, vol. 59, no. 2, pp. e10–e52, 2014.

A Pediatric Case of Cowden Syndrome with Graves' Disease

Cláudia Patraquim,[1] **Vera Fernandes,**[2,3,4] **Sofia Martins,**[5] **Ana Antunes,**[5] **Olinda Marques,**[2] **José Luís Carvalho,**[6] **Jorge Correia-Pinto,**[3,4,6] **Carla Meireles,**[7] **and Ana Margarida Ferreira**[8]

[1]*Pediatrics Department, Hospital de Braga, Sete Fontes, São Victor, 4710-243 Braga, Portugal*
[2]*Endocrinology Department, Hospital de Braga, Sete Fontes, São Victor, 4710-243 Braga, Portugal*
[3]*Life and Health Sciences Research Institute (ICVS), School of Health Sciences, University of Minho, Braga, Portugal*
[4]*ICVS/3B's-PT Government Associate Laboratory, Braga, Guimarães, Portugal*
[5]*Pediatric Endocrinology Department, Hospital de Braga, Sete Fontes, São Victor, 4710-243 Braga, Portugal*
[6]*Pediatric Surgical Department, Hospital de Braga, Sete Fontes, São Victor, 4710-243 Braga, Portugal*
[7]*Pediatrics Department, Hospital da Senhora da Oliveira, Creixomil, 4835-044 Guimarães, Portugal*
[8]*Anatomic Pathology Department, Hospital de Braga, Sete Fontes, São Victor, 4710-243 Braga, Portugal*

Correspondence should be addressed to Cláudia Patraquim; claudiapatraquim@gmail.com

Academic Editor: Yann-Jinn Lee

Cowden syndrome (CS) is a rare dominantly inherited multisystem disorder, characterized by an extraordinary malignant potential. In 80% of cases, the human tumor suppressor gene phosphatase and tensin homolog (PTEN) is mutated. We present a case of a 17-year-old boy with genetically confirmed CS and Graves' disease (GD). At the age of 15, he presented with intention tremor, palpitations, and marked anxiety. On examination, he had macrocephaly, coarse facies, slight prognathism, facial trichilemmomas, abdominal keratoses, leg hemangioma, and a diffusely enlarged thyroid gland. He started antithyroid drug (ATD) therapy with methimazole and, after a 2-year treatment period without achieving a remission status, a total thyroidectomy was performed. Diagnosis and management of CS should be multidisciplinary. Thyroid disease is frequent, but its management has yet to be fully defined. The authors present a case report of a pediatric patient with CS and GD and discuss treatment options.

1. Introduction

Cowden syndrome (CS) is a rare dominantly inherited multisystem complex disorder with high variability and susceptibility, incomplete penetrance, and an identifiable germline mutation [1–4]. The human tumor suppressor gene, phosphatase and tensin homolog (PTEN), is mutated in 80% cases; mutations in other genes such as KILLIN, SDH B/D, PIK3CA, and AKT1 are responsible for the rest of the cases [4]. After gene identification, the incidence of CS was calculated to be 1 in 200,000 [2, 5, 6], which is considered underestimated given the common manifestations and variable expression of the syndrome [5].

CS was first described in 1963 by Lloyd and Dennis referring to their 20-year-old patient who died of breast cancer, Rachel Cowden, after whom the syndrome was named [2–6].

A slight female predominance appears to be present [2, 7]. It usually occurs in the second or third decade of life and generally involves the skin, oral mucosa, thyroid, breast, gastrointestinal tract, genitourinary tract, central nervous system, and bone, being characterized by an extraordinary potential for malignant transformation [4–7].

Mucocutaneous manifestations, apparent in 99-100% of patients, are a pathognomonic feature and usually the first presenting lesions of the disease. These lesions include trichilemmomas (hamartomas of the infundibulum of the hair follicle), facial papules, acral keratoses, oral cavity verrucous or papillomatous papules, benign (e.g., angiomas, dermal fibromas, lipomas, and neurinomas) and malignant tumors (e.g., melanomas, basal cell carcinoma, and squamous cell carcinomas) [4–7]. Extracutaneous manifestations occur in about 90% of cases, most often involving the thyroid gland

(50–70%), with the majority of lesions being adenomatous goiters or multiple follicular adenomas [4, 5]. Thyroid carcinoma has been reported in 3–10%, mostly follicular or papillary carcinomas, but medullary carcinoma may also occur, even in children. Other frequent lesions related to CS are hamartomatous polyps of the digestive tract, fibrocystic disease of the breast, uterine leiomyoma, and macrocephaly [5, 8].

Graves' disease (GD) is an autoimmune disease that affects the thyroid gland and includes diffuse goiter, hyperthyroidism, and ophthalmopathy. Pathophysiology of GD involves a complex interplay between genetic and environmental influences, but the exact mechanisms are not yet known. GD is a rare condition in childhood, with an estimated incidence of 0,1–3 per 100,000. Antithyroid drugs (ATDs) are generally considered the first-line treatment. Nevertheless, long-term remission rates after 2 or more years of ATDs have been reported to be low and definitive treatment modalities with radioiodine (RAI) ablation or total thyroidectomy may be necessary [9].

There are no evidence-based guidelines for management of these conditions in childhood. Although patients with CS are known to have a predisposition for thyroid disease, the exact incidence and pathophysiology are still undefined, as is the best way to manage those children and adolescents [5].

To the best of our knowledge, reports of pediatric patients with CS and GD are exceedingly rare in literature. The authors present a case report of a pediatric patient with CS and GD and discuss treatment options.

2. Case Description

The patient is a 17-year-old Caucasian boy that presented with intention tremor, palpitations, and marked anxiety at age 15. He was medicated with propranolol and hydroxyzine with partial improvement of symptoms and was referred to a hospital pediatric appointment.

The adolescent and his father had genetically confirmed CS [heterozygous frameshift mutation in exon 5 of PTEN gene: c.405_406insA (C136Mfs∗44) NM_000314]. The patient's father was submitted to a total thyroidectomy for multinodular goiter at age 23 and died at 60 years old of brain tumor (anaplastic oligodendroglioma). His paternal grandfather had thyroid cancer.

Other notable features in our patient's previous medical history were macrocephaly, the presence of a hemangioma in his left lower limb, learning disabilities, and a cognitive evaluation that concluded that a global delay in cognitive development with an intelligence quotient (IQ) at the lower limit of the normal range was present. On physical examination, he had a coarse facies, slight prognathism, facial trichilemmomas, abdominal keratoses, and an irregular, elastic, and diffusely enlarged thyroid gland (Figures 1 and 2). Exophthalmia was not apparent.

Thyroid function tests were consistent with a hyperfunctioning thyroid state: thyrotropin (TSH) < 0,005 IU/mL (normal range 0,358–3,740 IU/mL), free thyroxine (fT4) 4,97 ng/dL (normal range 0,76–1,46 ng/dL), free triiodothyronine

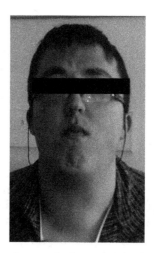

FIGURE 1: Patient photograph showing diffusely enlarged thyroid gland (frontal view).

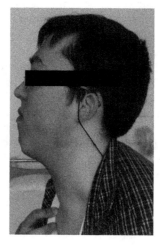

FIGURE 2: Patient photograph showing diffusely enlarged thyroid gland (left profile).

(fT3) 27,58 pg/mL (normal range 2,18–3,98 pg/mL), with positive anti-thyroid autoantibodies: thyroid peroxidase antibodies (anti-TPO) > 3340 IU/mL (normal range 0–100 IU/mL), thyroglobulin antibodies (anti-Tg) > 24400 IU/mL (normal range 0–344 IU/mL), and thyrotropin receptor antibodies (TRAbs) 14,3 IU/mL (normal range < 1,2 IU/mL). Thyroid ultrasonography at diagnosis showed a heterogeneous, hypoechoic, and high volume goiter (43 × 94 × 38 mm left lobe and 49 × 100 × 44 mm right lobe), with no visible nodules.

He was started on methimazole, maximum dose 20 mg/day, and propranolol treatment, lasting for a 2-year period, without achieving an euthyroid state.

Thyroid ultrasonography, 2 years after GD diagnosis, revealed dominant isoechoic solid nodules of 10 mm and 12 mm in the left and right lobes, respectively. Fine needle aspiration (FNA) cytology result was benign, consistent with hyperplastic/adenomatoid nodule (designed according to

The Bethesda System for Reporting Thyroid Cytopathology) (Figure 3).

A multidisciplinary team, including Pediatric Endocrinologist, Adult Endocrinologist, and Pediatric Surgeon, met in order to discuss the therapeutic options. Attending to the voluminous goiter and risks inherent to CS, a total thyroidectomy was the definite treatment consensus. That was also the patient's choice. Potassium iodide-iodine solution (Lugol) was used in preoperative preparation and surgery went uneventful. On gross examination, the surgical specimen weighed 218 g, with a larger left (95 mm) than right lobe (90 mm). The microscopic examination revealed lymphocytic thyroiditis (Figures 4–6). He was started on replacement therapy with oral levothyroxine 125 ug/day and he is currently compensated.

3. Discussion

Early recognition of individuals with CS is essential in order to start appropriate cancer screening and prevent potential complications associated with this disorder [1, 4].

Thyroid disease is an important concern among patients with CS [5]. Clinical guidelines from the National Comprehensive Cancer Network (NCCN) recommend that patients with CS should undergo an annual physical examination starting at the age of 18 years or 5 years before the youngest age of diagnosis of a component cancer in the family (whichever is earlier), with special care to thyroid examination. They also advocate an annual thyroid ultrasound since the age of 18 years or 5–10 years before the youngest age of diagnosis of a thyroid cancer in the family (whichever is younger) [10]. On the other hand, some authors recommend that all patients with CS should undergo baseline thyroid ultrasound at the age of diagnosis, with follow-up on a yearly basis, given that the risk of thyroid cancer begins early in childhood and that ultrasound is an innocuous screening procedure [3]. Other studies advocate that thyroid examinations and ultrasound should be performed from the age of 10 years [6]. Thyroid surgery, if needed, ought to be a total thyroidectomy, even if only one side of the thyroid seems to be affected, owing to the high probability for additional disease and need for future reoperation [1, 3]. Prophylactic thyroidectomy has been considered an option for selected patients in whom lifetime screening may be challenging (e.g., patients with autism or other developmental disorders) [1, 3]. It may also be reasonable for CS patients who have nodules and understand the risks associated with this surgical procedure [1].

For GD, definitive treatment options are RAI or total thyroidectomy. RAI has been increasingly used in children except for the very young (less than 5 years of age), although theoretical concerns of heightened cancer risk still persist. Surgical treatment is most commonly used in the following situations: very large goiters (more than 80 g), children younger than 5 years, planned pregnancy, or patient's choice [9]. Currently, the ideal therapeutic approach remains controversial.

Regarding our patient and the available therapeutic options, RAI could be related to an increased cancer risk,

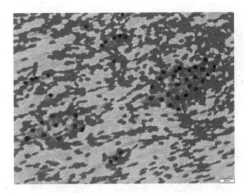

FIGURE 3: Fine needle aspiration (FNA) cytology: benign, consistent with hyperplastic/adenomatoid nodule (H&E, 400x).

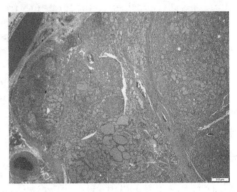

FIGURE 4: Thyroid gland presenting with lymphocytic thyroiditis and multinodular goiter (H&E, 20x).

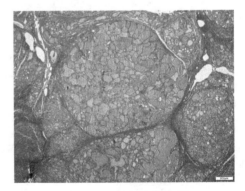

FIGURE 5: Multinodular goiter (H&E, 20x).

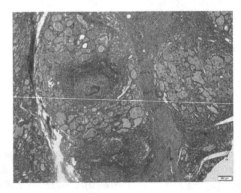

FIGURE 6: Lymphocytic thyroiditis (H&E, 40x).

which is of special concern in CS; possible surgical complications include anesthetic risk, recurrent laryngeal nerve injury, hypoparathyroidism, and wound infection [9]. The experience of treatment centers and specific characteristics of each patient are definitely decisive factors in the therapeutic choice.

In the present case, it was decided to perform a total thyroidectomy given the size of the goiter, increased risk of malignancy inherent to CS, and patient's will.

Lugol's solution was used in the preoperative preparation to reduce thyroid gland vascularity and potential surgical blood loss [11].

To the best of our knowledge, reports of pediatric patients with CS and GD are extremely uncommon. A meta-analysis from Hall and coworkers reported only 1 case of hyperthyroidism among 96 patients with CS and thyroid disease [5].

In conclusion, the diagnosis and the management of CS should be multidisciplinary. This syndrome has significant malignant associations, therefore requiring early clinical suspicion and aggressive screening. Thyroid disease occurs in about two-thirds of patients, being one of the most frequent extracutaneous manifestations, thus demanding special attention and careful monitoring. Despite that, the management of thyroid disease in CS has yet to be fully defined. Furthermore, meticulous evaluation of patient's family is essential, not only for identification of potential at risk relatives but also for genetic counseling.

Abbreviations

anti-Tg: Thyroglobulin antibodies
anti-TPO: Thyroid peroxidase antibodies
ATD: Antithyroid drug
CS: Cowden syndrome
FNA: Fine needle aspiration
fT3:   Free triiodothyronine
fT4:   Free thyroxine
GD: Graves' disease
IQ: Intelligence quotient
NCCN: National Comprehensive Cancer Network
PTEN: Phosphatase and tensin homolog
RAI: Radioiodine
TRAbs: Thyrotropin receptor antibodies
TSH: Thyrotropin.

Consent

Informed consent has been properly documented.

Authors' Contributions

All authors collected and analyzed the patient's clinical data and wrote the paper. All authors revised the final version of the manuscript. Dr. Ana Margarida Ferreira analyzed and provided the histological figures.

References

[1] M. Milas, J. Mester, R. Metzger et al., "Should patients with Cowden syndrome undergo prophylactic thyroidectomy?" *Surgery*, vol. 152, no. 6, pp. 1201–1210, 2012.

[2] P. Stathopoulos, A. Raymond, and M. Esson, "Cowden syndrome: mucocutaneous lesions as precursors of internal malignancy," *Oral and Maxillofacial Surgery*, vol. 18, no. 2, pp. 229–235, 2014.

[3] J. Mester and C. Eng, "Cowden syndrome: recognizing and managing a not-so-rare hereditary cancer syndrome," *Journal of Surgical Oncology*, vol. 111, no. 1, pp. 125–130, 2015.

[4] M. Molvi, Y. K. Sharma, and K. Dash, "Cowden syndrome: case report, update and proposed diagnostic and surveillance routines," *Indian Journal of Dermatology*, vol. 60, no. 3, pp. 255–259, 2015.

[5] J. E. Hall, D. J. Abdollahian, and R. J. Sinard, "Thyroid disease associated with cowden syndrome: a meta-analysis," *Head and Neck*, vol. 35, no. 8, pp. 1189–1194, 2013.

[6] S. Hammami, O. Berriche, H. B. Ali, O. Hellara, F. Ansar, and S. Mahjoub, "Managing the risk of cancer in Cowden syndrome: a case report," *Journal of Medical Case Reports*, vol. 6, article 225, 2012.

[7] A. Masmoudi, Z. M. Chermi, S. Marrekchi et al., "Cowden syndrome," *Journal of Dermatological Case Reports*, vol. 5, no. 1, pp. 8–13, 2011.

[8] Y. Koksal, M. Sahin, H. Koksal, D. Orhan, E. Unal, and E. Alagoz, "Thyroid medullary carcinoma in a teenager with Cowden syndrome," *The Laryngoscope*, vol. 117, no. 7, pp. 1180–1182, 2007.

[9] G. Jevalikar, J. Solis, and M. Zacharin, "Long-term outcomes of pediatric Graves' disease," *Journal of Pediatric Endocrinology and Metabolism*, vol. 27, no. 11-12, pp. 1131–1136, 2014.

[10] M. B. Daly, R. Pilarski, J. E. Axilbund et al., "Genetic/familial high-risk assessment: breast and ovarian, version 1.2014," *Journal of the National Comprehensive Cancer Network*, vol. 12, no. 9, pp. 1326–1338, 2014.

[11] Y. Erbil, Y. Ozluk, M. Giriş et al., "Effect of lugol solution on thyroid gland blood flow and microvessel density in the patients with Graves' disease," *Journal of Clinical Endocrinology and Metabolism*, vol. 92, no. 6, 2007.

5

Late Onset Cobalamin Disorder and Hemolytic Uremic Syndrome: A Rare Cause of Nephrotic Syndrome

Gianluigi Ardissino,[1] **Michela Perrone,**[1] **Francesca Tel,**[1] **Sara Testa,**[1] **Amelia Morrone,**[2,3] **Ilaria Possenti,**[4] **Francesco Tagliaferri,**[5] **Robertino Dilena,**[6] **and Francesca Menni**[5]

[1] *Center for HUS Prevention Control and Management, Fondazione IRCCS Ca' Granda Osp. Maggiore Policlinico, Milan, Italy*
[2] *Paediatric Neurology Unit and Laboratories, Neuroscience Department, Meyer Children's Hospital, Florence, Italy*
[3] *Neuroscience, Psychology, Pharmacology and Child Health Department, University of Florence, Florence, Italy*
[4] *Pediatric Unit, Pediatric Hospital C. Arrigo, Alessandria, Italy*
[5] *Pediatric Unit, Fondazione IRCCS Ca' Granda Osp. Maggiore Policlinico, Milan, Italy*
[6] *UOC Neurophysiology, Fondazione IRCCS Ca' Granda Osp. Maggiore Policlinico, Milan, Italy*

Correspondence should be addressed to Gianluigi Ardissino; ardissino@centroseu.org

Academic Editor: Anibh Martin Das

Hemolytic uremic syndrome (HUS) is an unrare and severe thrombotic microangiopathy (TMA) caused by several pathogenetic mechanisms among which Shiga toxin-producing *Escherichia coli* infections and complement dysregulation are the most common. However, very rarely and particularly in neonates and infants, disorders of cobalamin metabolism (CblC) can present with or be complicated by TMA. Herein we describe a case of atypical HUS (aHUS) related to CblC disease which first presented in a previously healthy boy at age of 13.6 years. The clinical picture was initially dominated by nephrotic range proteinuria and severe hypertension followed by renal failure. The specific treatment with high dose of hydroxycobalamin rapidly obtained the remission of TMA and the complete recovery of renal function. We conclude that plasma homocysteine and methionine determinations together with urine organic acid analysis should be included in the diagnostic work-up of any patient with TMA and/or nephrotic syndrome regardless of age.

1. Introduction

Atypical hemolytic uremic syndrome (aHUS) is a life-threatening disease characterised by thrombotic microangiopathy (TMA) that is mainly due to Shiga toxin-producing *Escherichia coli* infections and uncontrolled complement activation, although it may rarely be due to other causes, such as disorders of intracellular cobalamin (cbl) metabolism [1]. Methylmalonic aciduria and homocystinuria, cobalamin C type (cblC) (OMIM 277400) is likely the most common of such disorders and is caused by biallelic mutations in the *MMACHC* gene (Lerner-Ellis et al. 2006). cblC-related TMA has been almost mainly reported in neonates and infants [2–8], but we have recently encountered a case that developed it at the very unusual age of 13.6 years. Its clinical presentation was dominated by symptoms of nephrotic syndrome and hypertension that initially responded to eculizumab treatment.

2. Case Presentation

A Caucasian son of unrelated parents was referred to our centre because of severe hypertension, nephrotic range proteinuria, microhematuria, acute kidney injury, and signs of TMA. His family history was unremarkable for kidney diseases and his own previous medical history was uneventful until the age of 8 years, when he experienced an episode of generalised seizure in apyrexia that was not followed by any relevant event and did not require any specific treatment.

One month before the acute episode, the boy suffered from severe headache and recurrent emesis associated with a weight loss (from 47 to 43 kg) for which he was admitted to another hospital. Severe arterial hypertension was detected (150/110 mmHg) and laboratory tests revealed nephrotic range proteinuria (5 gr/day), associated with signs of kidney injury: serum creatinine 1.3 mg/dL, microscopic hematuria together with mild thrombocytopenia (121,000/mm^3) and hemolytic anemia (hemoglobin 10.2 g/dL, lactic dehydrogenase (LDH) 894 U/L, and undetectable haptoglobin). Renal ultrasonography revealed enlarged, hyperechogenic kidneys with reduced corticomedullary differentiation, and echocardiography showed left ventricular hypertrophy and a slightly enlarged aortic bulb. During the subsequent 3 weeks proteinuria increased further and renal function deteriorated until the patient was referred to our centre. Twenty-one days after the onset, laboratory tests at arrival were as follows: hemoglobin: 9.6 gr/dL; platelet count: 115.000/mm^3; plasma albumin: 3.2 gr/dL; serum creatinine: 2.7 gr/dL; LDH: 484 IU/L; haptoglobin: undetectable; cholesterol 234 mg/dL; urinary protein/urinary creatinine: 5.1 mg/mg.

Given the clinical picture of TMA, functional and genetic tests for complement dysregulation were requested, and eculizumab treatment was immediately started (900 mg followed by a second dose after seven days).

Despite efficient complement inhibition (AP$_{50}$: 1%) and a normalised platelet count (180,000/mm^3), the hemolysis persisted (haptoglobin < 20 mg/dL) and kidney function continued to decline reaching a peak serum creatinine level of 7.2 mg/dL. For these reasons and for the normal level of complement C3 (93 mg/dL), laboratory tests were extended to rule out less frequent inherited causes of TMA. Hyperhomocysteinemia (364 mMol/L, normal range < 15.4) and hypomethioninemia (8 uMol/L, normal range 15–20 uMol/L) and increased urinary excretion of methylmalonic acid (20 mMol/mol, normal range < 2 mMol/mol) were detected. Since these metabolic alterations strongly suggested a cblC disease, the specific treatment with intravenous hydroxycobalamin (5 mg/day), betaine (4 g/day), and folic acid (5 mg/day) was started on the fourteenth day. The first evidence of a response was observed as early as 4 days after starting the specific treatment with a clear-cut reduction in the urinary protein/urinary creatinine ratio from 6.4 to 2.6 mg/mg (Figure 1). In the meantime, complement dysregulation was ruled out by molecular analysis of the relevant genes (CFH, CFH-related, CFI, CFB, MCP, C3) and by the normal titre of anti-CFH antibodies. HIV, antinuclear, and anticardiolipin antibodies and ADAMTS13 were also normal. Molecular analysis of the MMACHC gene definitively confirmed the diagnosis of cblC by identifying the known causative c.271dupA (p.Arg91Lysfs*14) and c.388T>C (p.Tyr130His) mutations. The p.Tyr130His has been previously described in compound heterozygous state with

c.481C>T (p.Arg161*) mutation in a patient with onset of disease at 17 years. Since p.Tyr130 maps in the conserved cobalamin binding motif (122-HXXGX$_{126-154}$GG$_{156}$), the p.Tyr130His mutation may affect clb binding or protein structural integrity and it could be associated with a late onset phenotype.

Renal function gradually normalised during the following six weeks, as also the other TMA laboratory parameters, including proteinuria (Figure 1). Thirty-five days after admission, and while improving, the patient presented two episodes of generalised seizure, which were attributed to posterior reversible encephalopathy syndrome on the basis of magnetic resonance imaging.

The patient is currently well, and his hypertension only requires two drugs (atenolol and ramipril) and he is undergoing a maintenance treatment with oral hydroxycobalamin (1 mg once daily), betaine (4 g once daily), and folic acid (5 mg once daily).

3. Discussion

Both Shiga toxin-related and atypical HUS are unrare causes of acute kidney injury in children, but cblC disorder is responsible for fewer than 1% of TMA cases and is characterised by presentation very early in life (usually at an age of <1 year).

Our case underlines the importance of including homocysteine in the initial diagnostic work-up of all nephrotic patients beyond the typical age of idiopathic nephrotic syndrome of infancy (<6 years) as well as all cases of aHUS to screen for intracellular cobalamin metabolism disorders as these disorders are not limited to infancy.

Although most cases of aHUS are accompanied by various degrees of proteinuria due to endothelial damage at glomerular level, the development of overt nephrotic syndrome at the time of presentation is not common and may be misleading. However, it can be useful to mention that the loss of urinary proteins is not the only mechanism responsible for reduced albumin concentration in this setting: the disease is systemic (all of the microvasculature can be damaged); therefore widespread endothelial protein leakage takes place.

Although the pathogenetic mechanism of the endothelial damage in cblC-related TMA is very different from that of aHUS associated with complement dysregulation, a certain degree of complement involvement has been hypothesised also in other forms of TMA. In this regard, the partial but unequivocable response to eculizumab seems to provide indirect evidence that complement is involved in the mechanism of damage.

In conclusion, we strongly recommend including plasma homocysteine determination in the diagnostic work-up of any patient with nephrotic syndrome and/or with TMA in order to ensure timely diagnosis and effective treatment.

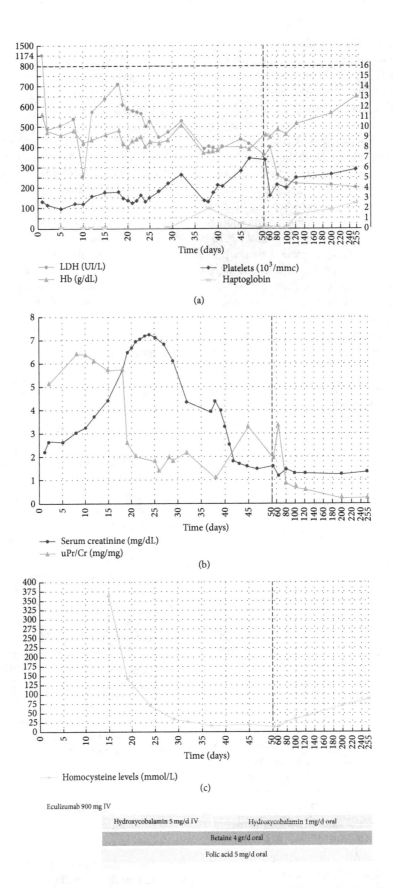

FIGURE 1: Laboratory relevant to TMA activity. (a) Hematological parameters: LDH (UI/L); Hb (g/dL); platelets (10^3/mmc); (b) renal parameters: serum creatinine (mg/dL); uPr/Cr (mg/mg); (c) homocysteine levels (mmol/L).

Acknowledgments

Due to limitation in the number of authors, the authors want to acknowledge the following physicians who collaborated in the management of the patient: Stefania Salardi, Martina Sgarbanti, Enrica Ciceri, and Catia Cavicchi. They are also thankful to Francesco Albano for the precious help in producing the presented graphs.

References

[1] B. B. Beck, F. van Spronsen, A. Diepstra, R. M. Berger, and M. Kömhoff, "Renal thrombotic microangiopathy in patients with cblC defect: review of an under-recognized entity," *Pediatric Nephrology*, vol. 32, no. 5, pp. 733–741, 2017.

[2] D. S. Froese, J. Zhang, S. Healy, and R. A. Gravel, "Mechanism of vitamin B12-responsiveness in cblC methylmalonic aciduria with homocystinuria," *Molecular Genetics and Metabolism*, vol. 98, no. 4, pp. 338–343, 2009.

[3] M. Koutmos, C. Gherasim, J. L. Smith, and R. Banerjee, "Structural basis of multifunctionality in a vitamin B 12-processing enzyme," *Journal of Biological Chemistry*, vol. 286, no. 34, pp. 29780–29787, 2011.

[4] J. P. Lerner-Ellis, J. C. Tirone, P. D. Pawelek et al., "Identification of the gene responsible for methylmalonic aciduria and homocystinuria, cblC type," *Nature Genetics*, vol. 38, no. 1, pp. 93–100, 2006.

[5] C. Nogueira, C. Aiello, R. Cerone et al., "Spectrum of MMACHC mutations in Italian and Portuguese patients with combined methylmalonic aciduria and homocystinuria, cblC type," *Molecular Genetics and Metabolism*, vol. 93, no. 4, pp. 475–480, 2008.

[6] Q.-L. Li, W.-Q. Song, X.-X. Peng, X.-R. Liu, L.-J. He, and L.-B. Fu, "Clinical characteristics of hemolytic uremic syndrome secondary to cobalamin C disorder in Chinese children," *World Journal of Pediatrics*, vol. 11, no. 3, pp. 276–280, 2015.

[7] M. H. Vaisbich, A. Braga, M. Gabrielle, C. Bueno, F. Piazzon, and F. Kok, "Thrombotic microangiopathy caused by methionine synthase deficiency: diagnosis and treatment pitfalls," *Pediatric Nephrology*, vol. 32, no. 6, pp. 1089–1092, 2017.

[8] F. Menni, S. Testa, S. Guez, G. Chiarelli, L. Alberti, and S. Esposito, "Neonatal atypical hemolytic uremic syndrome due to methylmalonic aciduria and homocystinuria," *Pediatric Nephrology*, vol. 27, no. 8, pp. 1401–1405, 2012.

6

Novel *HAX1* Gene Mutation in a Vietnamese Boy with Severe Congenital Neutropenia

Tham Thi Tran,[1] **Quang Van Vu** ⓘ**,**[1] **Taizo Wada,**[2] **Akihiro Yachie,**[2] **Huong Le Thi Minh,**[3] **and Sang Ngoc Nguyen**[1]

[1]*Department of Pediatrics, Haiphong University of Medicine and Pharmacy, Haiphong, Vietnam*
[2]*Department of Pediatrics, Institute of Medical, Pharmaceutical and Health Science, Kanazawa University, Kanazawa, Japan*
[3]*National Hospital of Pediatrics, Hanoi, Vietnam*

Correspondence should be addressed to Quang Van Vu; vvquang@hpmu.edu.vn

Academic Editor: Anselm Chi-wai Lee

Severe congenital neutropenia (SCN) is a rare disease that involves a heterogeneous group of hereditary diseases. Mutations in the *HAX1* gene can cause an autosomal recessive form of SCN-characterized low blood neutrophil count from birth, increased susceptibility to recurrent and life-threatening infections, and preleukemia predisposition. A 7-year-old boy was admitted due to life-threatening infections, mental retardation, and severe neutropenia. He had early-onset bacterial infections, and his serial complete blood count showed persistent severe neutropenia. One older sister and one older brother of the patient died at the age of 6 months and 5 months, respectively, because of severe infection. Bone marrow analysis revealed a maturation arrest at the promyelocyte/myelocyte stage with few mature neutrophils. In direct DNA sequencing analysis, we found a novel homozygous frameshift mutation (c.423_424insG, p.Gly143fs) in the *HAX1* gene, confirming the diagnosis of SCN. The patient was successfully treated with granulocyte colony-stimulating factor (G-CSF) and antibiotics. A child with early-onset recurrent infections and neutropenia should be considered to be affected with SCN. Genetic analysis is useful to confirm diagnosis. Timely diagnosis and suitable treatment with G-CSF and antibiotics are important to prevent further complication.

1. Introduction

Severe congenital neutropenia (SCN) is a rare disease that involves a heterogeneous group of inherited disorders. It is characterized by persistent severe neutropenia from birth, increased susceptibility to severe bacterial infections, and a preleukemic predisposition [1–3]. SCN presents several genetic inheritance states including autosomal dominant, autosomal recessive, and X-linked sporadic form, which could show association with several distinct genes [2, 4, 5]. Recent reports show that homozygous mutations in the *HAX1* gene are responsible for an autosomal recessive form of SCN, in about one-third of SCN patients [6]. *HAX1* is located mainly in the mitochondria and controls the integrity of the internal mitochondrial membrane potential and protects the myeloid cells from apoptosis [7]. Clinical signs of SCN are often overlapped with infectious diseases, sometimes causing delayed or missed diagnosis [3]. Herein, we report an SCN patient with a novel homozygous frameshift mutation in the *HAX1* gene in an attempt to improve the diagnosis and management of SCN.

2. Case Presentation

A 7-year-old boy was admitted to our hospital with a 4-day history of high fever and scalp swelling with ulcers. Physical examination revealed consciousness (Glasgow Coma Scale/core was 15), pus formation, and fistula with purulent discharge on the scalp, scalp peeling, face swelling, and poor eating (Figure 1). Laboratory findings exhibited severe neutropenia (white blood cells, 2.39×10^9/l; neutrophils, 0.25×10^9/l; and lymphocytes, 2.1×10^9/l) and increased acute-phase reactants (erythrocyte sedimentation rate 101 mm/hour and C-reactive protein 272 mg/dl). Pus culture exhibited *Enterococcus faecalis* and *Escherichia coli*. Blood culture and urine culture were negative. The chest X-ray and

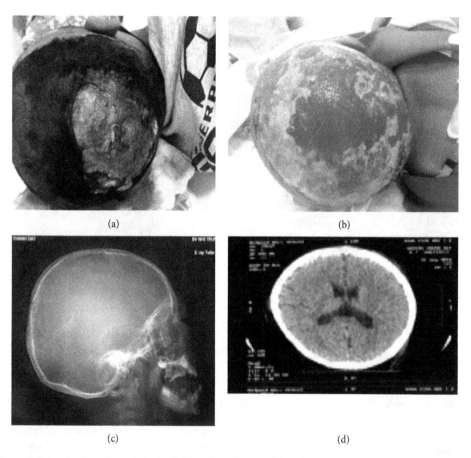

FIGURE 1: Some lesions of the patient's scalp and his skull. (a) Scalp infection. (b) Scalp peeling. (c, d) Subcutaneous emphysema of the scalp, neither brain injury nor skull fractures.

urinalysis results were normal. Cerebrospinal fluid (CSF) analysis was normal. Serum titers of IgG, IgM, IgA, and IgE and percentage of CD4$^+$ and CD8$^+$ T cells were normal. Tests of HIV, HBV, HCV, EBV, and CMV were negative. Bone marrow analysis revealed a maturation arrest at the promyelocyte/myelocyte stage with few mature neutrophils; there was no evidence of malignant involvement in the bone marrow. Computed tomography scan of the head and skull showed subcutaneous emphysema of the scalp, neither brain injury nor skull fractures (Figure 1). Necrotizing fasciitis of the scalp and septicaemia were diagnosed. The patient was treated with pentaglobin (0.5 g/kg) and the combination of three antibiotics: vancomycin, meropenem, and metronidazole, respectively. To maintain the neutrophil count, granulocyte colony-stimulating factor (G-CSF) was administered from 5 to 10 μg/kg/day and 15 μg/kg/day, respectively (Figure 2). The patient was discharged from our hospital after 46 days of treatment. Now, he is well under regular G-CSF therapy.

Due to severe neutropenia and infections, we analyzed the medical history, family history, and medical records of the patient carefully. The patient is the third child in his family. He has two healthy younger sisters, one older sister who died at the age of 6 months because of meningitis, and one older brother who died at the age of 5 months because of severe pneumonia. No consanguinity was reported among parents, but their origins are from the same commune. From 7 months

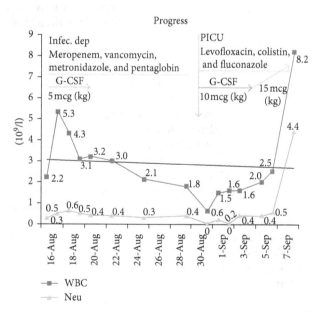

FIGURE 2: Absolute neutrophil count and total white blood cell count of the patient during treatment with G-CSF and antibiotics.

of age, the patient had recurrent severe infections such as cutaneous abscesses, otitis media, and respiratory infections, which were treated with appropriate antibiotics. In addition, he had neutropenia many times and mental retardation such as developmental delay, dysarthria, and linguistic immaturity.

Considering his past history, family history, and physical examination, SCN associated with *ELANE* or *HAX1* abnormality was suspected. The *ELANE* gene was analyzed by direct DNA sequencing analysis firstly but the mutation was not found. Due to mental retardation of the patient, the *HAX1* gene was analyzed next. In exon 3 of the *HAX1* gene, we found a homozygous frameshift mutation (c.423_424insG, p.Gly143fs). This is a novel mutation.

3. Discussion

SCN is a rare primary immunodeficiency syndrome [8] and is associated with multiple genes including the *ELANE*, *HAX1*, *WAS*, *GFI1*, and *G6PC3* genes [7]. There are two major subtypes of SCN: autosomal dominant subtypes such as neutrophil elastase mutations (about 60% of patients) and autosomal recessive subtypes such as *HAX1* mutation (about 30% of patients), both of which share the same clinical and morphological phenotype [9]. SCN is diagnosed when ANC is less than 0.5×10^9/l for at least 3 months; SCN patients suffer from recurrent life-threatening infections. The boy we report here showed typical SCN manifestations, including chronic severe neutropenia and recurrent bacterial infections. However, the diagnosis was missed and postponed to 7 years of age. This issue may be due to an inadequate knowledge about this very rare disease and because infectious diseases are popular in Vietnamese pediatric population [3, 10]. Therefore, it is important to stress this condition among health care professionals. After carefully analyzing clinical courses and bone marrow aspiration test of the patient, we excluded autoimmune neutropenia (AIN). In contrast to SCN patients, AIN patients often have mild phenotypes with minor intercurrent infections despite severe neutropenia. Because the patient had severe phenotypes with life-threatening infections, chronic severe neutropenia, and reduced granulocyte cell line on the bone marrow aspirate, SCN was diagnosed. After receiving G-CSF (from 5 to 15 μg/kg/24h), his neutrophil counts increased dramatically (Figure 2). To confirm SCN diagnosis, we analyzed the *ELANE* gene mutation firstly because it is the most common gene alteration in SCN; however, no mutation was found. Because the patient has had mental retardation, the *HAX1* gene was selected for analysis next. In exon 3, we found a novel homozygous frameshift mutation (c.423_424insG, p.Gly143fs), resulting in a completely different translation from the original. To our knowledge, this is the first *HAX1* mutation report from Vietnamese people. The *HAX1* gene provides instructions for producing a protein called HS-1, which is associated with the X-1 protein (HAX-1). This protein is involved in the modulation of apoptosis, in which cells destroy themselves when damaged or no longer necessary. HAX-1 protein is found mainly in the mitochondria, the centers of energy production in cells [11]. *HAX1* gene mutations that cause SCN lead to the production of nonfunctional HAX-1 protein. The lack of functional HAX-1 protein interrupts the regulation of apoptosis, leading to premature death of neutrophils. A lack of neutrophils causes recurrent infections, inflammatory episodes, and other immune problems in

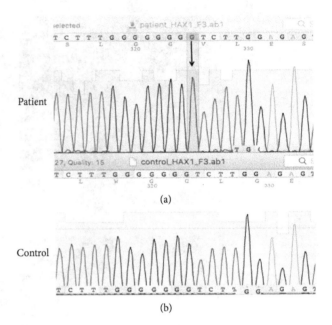

(a)

(b)

FIGURE 3: A novel homozygous frameshift mutation (c.423_424insG, p.Gly143fs) found in the *HAX1* gene (exon 3).

patients with SCN [11, 12]. Our patient had many superficial abscesses on his scalp, which caused scalp peeling (Figure 1). This rare condition in SCN can be explained by severe infections and sheath weakness, a connective tissue disorder caused by an HAX1 deficiency [1]. However, more studies are necessary to clarify the function of the HAX1 molecule in this regard [1]. Delayed mental development in this patient was a clue to help us decide on the *HAX1* gene analysis after excluding *ELANE* gene mutation. A novel homozygous frameshift mutation (c.423_424insG, p.Gly143fs) was found on exon 3 of the *HAX1* gene (Figure 3). To date, there are few reports about *HAX1* gene mutations in SCN patients, most of which are of Middle East descent [5, 7, 13]. The *HAX1* gene includes transcript variants 1 and 2. While neurological disorders are not present in mutations associated with transcript variant 1, mutations affecting both transcript variants 1 and 2 cause SCN and neurological abnormalities such as mental retardation, epilepsy, and developmental delay [4, 7, 13]. The *HAX1* mutation of our patient is found in exon 3 affecting transcript variants 1 and 2; the patient presents mental retardation.

In summary, we report a Vietnamese boy with SCN caused by a novel *HAX1* gene mutation. Every child with early-onset recurrent infections and neutropenia should be considered to have SCN. Genetic analysis is useful to confirm the diagnosis. Timely diagnosis and suitable treatment with G-CSF and antibiotics are important to prevent further complication.

Abbreviations

G-CSF: Granulocyte colony-stimulating factor
HAX1: HS1-associated protein X1
ELANE: ELA2 elastase, neutrophil expressed
SCN: Severe congenital neutropenia.

Consent

Written informed consent was obtained from the patient and his parents for publication of these data and for the accompanying images.

Authors' Contributions

QVV, TTT, SNN, and HTML participated in the study design, protocol development and performance, data analysis, interpretation of data, and writing of the manuscript and carried out the clinical data collection and data analysis. TW and AY reviewed and revised the manuscript, making important intellectual contributions. All authors read and approved the final manuscript.

Acknowledgments

The authors would like to thank the patient and his family in this study for their cooperation.

References

[1] A. Eghbali, P. Eshghi, F. Malek, H. Abdollahpour, and N. Rezaei, "HAX1 mutation in an infant with severe congenital neutropenia," *Turkish Journal of Pediatrics*, vol. 52, pp. 81–84, 2010.

[2] S.-L. Xue, J.-L. Li, J.-Y. Zou, J. Su, S.-N. Chen, and D.-P. Wu, "A novel compound heterozygous HAX1 mutation in a Chinese patient with severe congenital neutropenia and chronic myelomonocytic leukemia transformation but without neurodevelopmental abnormalities," *Haematologica*, vol. 97, no. 2, pp. 318–320, 2012.

[3] Q. V. Vu, T. Wada, T. T. Tran et al., "Severe congenital neutropenia caused by the ELANE gene mutation in a Vietnamese boy with misdiagnosis of tuberculosis and autoimmune neutropenia: a case report," *BMC Hematology*, vol. 15, no. 1, 2015.

[4] M. Faiyaz-Ul-Haque, A. Al-Jefri, F. Al-Dayel et al., "A novel HAX1 gene mutation in severe congenital neutropenia (SCN) associated with neurological manifestations," *European Journal of Pediatrics*, vol. 169, no. 6, pp. 661–666, 2010.

[5] B. N. Smith, P. J. Ancliff, A. Pizzey, A. Khwaja, D. C. Linch, and R. E. Gale, "Homozygous HAX1 mutations in severe congenital neutropenia patients with sporadic disease: a novel mutation in two unrelated British kindreds," *British Journal of Haematology*, vol. 144, no. 5, pp. 762–770.

[6] C. Klein, M. Grudzien, G. Appaswamy et al., "HAX1 deficiency causes autosomal recessive severe congenital neutropenia (Kostmann disease)," *Nature Genetics*, vol. 39, no. 1, pp. 86–92, 2007.

[7] C. Aydogmus, F. Cipe, and M. Tas, "HAX-1 deficiency: characteristics of five cases including an asymptomatic patient," *Asian Pacific Journal of Allergy and Immunology*, vol. 34, no. 1, pp. 73–76.

[8] M. Germeshausen, M. Grudzien, C. Zeidler et al., "Novel HAX1 mutations in patients with severe congenital neutropenia reveal isoform-dependent genotype-phenotype associations," *Blood*, vol. 111, pp. 4954–4957, 2008.

[9] C. Zeidler, M. Germeshausen, C. Klein, and K. Welte, "Clinical implications of ELA2-, HAX1-, and G-CSF-receptor (CSF3R) mutations in severe congenital neutropenia," *British Journal of Haematology*, vol. 144, no. 4, pp. 459–467, 2009.

[10] Q. V. Vu, T. Wada, H. T. M. Le et al., "Clinical and mutational features of Vietnamese children with X-linked agammaglobulinemia," *BMC Pediatrics*, vol. 14, no. 1, p. 129, 2014.

[11] HAX1 gene. Genetics Home Reference. https://ghr.nlm.nih.gov/gene/HAX1.

[12] C. Klein, "Kostmann's disease and HCLS1-associated protein X-1 (HAX1)," *Journal of Clinical Immunology*, vol. 37, no. 2, pp. 117–122, 2017.

[13] M. Lanciotti, S. Indaco, S. Bonanomi et al., "Novel HAX1 gene mutations associated to neurodevelopment abnormalities in two Italian patients with severe congenital neutropenia," *Haematologica*, vol. 95, no. 1, pp. 198–169, 2010.

7

Hemoglobin Sunshine Seth: A Case Report of Low-Oxygen-Affinity Hemoglobinopathy

Leah S. Heidenreich ⑩,[1] Jennifer L. Oliveira,[2] Peter J. Holmberg,[1,3] and Vilmarie Rodriguez ⑩[1,4]

[1]Mayo Clinic Children's Center, Mayo Clinic, Rochester, Minnesota, USA
[2]Division of Hematopathology, Mayo Clinic, Rochester, Minnesota, USA
[3]Division of General Pediatric and Adolescent Medicine, Mayo Clinic, Rochester, Minnesota, USA
[4]Division of Pediatric Hematology/Oncology, Mayo Clinic, Rochester, Minnesota, USA

Correspondence should be addressed to Vilmarie Rodriguez; rodriguez.vilmarie@mayo.edu

Academic Editor: Christophe Chantrain

Pulse oximetry is routinely used in the newborn nursery for clinical monitoring and to detect critical congenital heart disease. The differential diagnoses for reduced peripheral oxygen saturation in an infant include congenital heart disease, respiratory distress syndrome, transient tachypnea of the newborn, persistent pulmonary hypertension of the newborn, meconium aspiration syndrome, pneumonia, pneumothorax, and sepsis. The diagnostic evaluation for neonatal hypoxemia can be invasive and expensive. When this evaluation is unrevealing, other interventions may be tried without clear benefit to the patient, including, but not limited to, supplemental oxygen. Therefore, it is important to consider alternative, albeit rare, diagnoses, including hemoglobinopathies with abnormal oxygen binding properties. Mutations in the structure of alpha- and beta-globin chains can alter the affinity of hemoglobin for oxygen, and changes in oxygen affinity may result in changes in the oxygen saturation detected by pulse oximetry. These changes may or may not be of clinical significance. This case report describes Hemoglobin Sunshine Seth, a rare low-oxygen-affinity hemoglobin variant presenting as reduced peripheral oxygen saturation in an otherwise well-appearing infant male.

1. Introduction

Low peripheral oxygen saturation in newborns can be due to cardiac or pulmonary disease. In the absence of cardiopulmonary pathologic conditions, other causes, such as hemoglobinopathies associated with low oxygen affinity, should be considered. Normal adult hemoglobin (Hb) is composed of a tetramer of 2 α-globin and 2 β-globin chains. Genetic mutations in these chains can affect the affinity of Hb for oxygen. If Hb affinity for oxygen is increased, oxygen adheres tightly to Hb and oxygen delivery to peripheral tissues is impaired. More red blood cells are required to compensate for poor oxygen delivery, resulting in erythrocytosis. In contrast, if Hb affinity for oxygen is reduced, oxygen delivery to peripheral tissues increases [1]; this change may result in relative anemia, because fewer red blood cells are required for adequate oxygen delivery, and the patient may have cyanosis due to increased oxygen extraction by peripheral tissues [2].

Genetic mutations in Hb structure that alter its affinity for oxygen may or may not be clinically significant. Hb variants with high oxygen affinity, including Hb Chesapeake, Hb Montefiore, and Hb Crete, often result in erythrocytosis and no clinically significant downstream effects [3–8]. Variants with low oxygen affinity, including Hb Kansas, Hb Beth Israel, Hb Saint Mande, and Hb Sunshine Seth, may result in anemia, cyanosis, and low peripheral oxygen saturation [9–14]. Notably, although pulse oximetry shows low peripheral oxygen saturation, oxygen delivery to the peripheral tissues is actually increased; the oximeter is simply detecting the relatively low percentage of oxygenated Hb in the bloodstream in the setting of increased oxygen extraction by peripheral tissues. Often, no clinically significant downstream effects are present when Hb has low oxygen affinity, and no treatment of hypoxemia or mild anemia is required.

Diagnosis of oxygen affinity-altering genetic mutations in Hb first requires determination of the Hb-oxygen dissociation curve and P50 value, the oxygen tension at which Hb is 50% saturated [15]. If these appear abnormal, protein testing and globin DNA sequencing can help to establish the genetic mutation and diagnosis; these are necessary for future genetic counseling [15].

We present a case of persistently low peripheral oxygen saturation in a 17-month-old boy who underwent extensive evaluations for cardiopulmonary disease. The patient had been receiving supplemental oxygen therapy. We determined that the patient had a low-oxygen-affinity hemoglobinopathy (Hb Sunshine Seth), which explained his documented mild anemia and low peripheral oxygen saturation. Oxygen therapy was discontinued, and the patient continues to thrive. This case illustrates the need to consider evaluation for abnormal-oxygen-affinity hemoglobinopathy in children with hypoxemia but no cardiopulmonary pathologic conditions.

2. Case Presentation

2.1. History and Clinical Findings. A 17-month-old white boy was referred to our pediatric hematology clinic for evaluation of persistent low oxygen saturation without evidence of cardiac or pulmonary pathologic conditions. During pregnancy, the patient's mother had HELLP syndrome (hemolysis, elevated liver enzymes, and low platelet count), and she had an emergent late-preterm cesarean delivery. Newborn screening showed evidence of an abnormal Hb variant, which did not prompt immediate evaluation. After delivery, the patient required respiratory support with continuous positive airway pressure. Pulse oximetry showed that he had persistently low oxygen saturation (range, 80%–85%), and he was quickly transitioned to oxygen supplementation via low-flow nasal cannula (LFNC). He was discharged from the hospital and continued to receive 0.25 L/min oxygen via LFNC to maintain peripheral oxygen saturation greater than 93%. He required supplemental oxygen to maintain adequate peripheral saturation while awake and asleep.

Prior evaluation included computed tomography of the chest, flexible bronchoscopy, and multiple echocardiographic examinations, all of which showed normal findings. When the patient was nearly 1 year old, Hb electrophoresis showed an α-globin chain abnormality, 16.1% abnormal Hb (reference value, 0.0%), 2.0% HbA$_2$ (reference range, 2.0%–3.3%), and 0% fetal Hb (reference range, 0.0%–10.5%). The electrophoresis findings were thought to be unrelated to the patient's persistent hypoxemia. In addition, the patient had mild normocytic anemia. Laboratory evaluation demonstrated Hb 9.8 g/dL (mean (2 SD) reference value, 12 (10.5) g/dL) and mean corpuscular

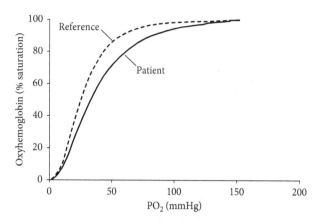

FIGURE 1: Hemoglobin-oxygen dissociation curve. The patient's curve is shifted to the right of the reference curve, consistent with reduced oxygen affinity. PO$_2$ indicates partial pressure of oxygen.

volume 86.1 fL (mean (2 SD) reference value, 78 (70) fL) [16, 17].

2.2. Clinical Course and Diagnosis. Because of the diagnostic uncertainty related to his care, the patient was referred to our institution for additional evaluation. The patient had no signs or symptoms suggestive of cardiopulmonary disease (e.g., cough, cyanosis, dyspnea, tachypnea, and wheezing), even when supplemental oxygen was suspended. His activity level was normal, and he had no history of recurrent respiratory infections. He was a well-appearing toddler. His body mass index was at the 36th percentile, and his weight was at the 23rd percentile. Physical examination showed no evidence of perioral or peripheral cyanosis, clubbing, or stigmata of chronic hypoxemia. We did not identify any heart murmurs, abnormal lung sounds, or other pertinent cardiopulmonary conditions. Evaluation of the family history did not identify individuals with a blood disorder, cyanosis, oxygen dependency, or other similar clinical presentations.

On the basis of these findings, further investigations were performed to identify possible abnormal-oxygen-affinity hemoglobinopathies. A P50 oxygen-Hb assay showed a right-shifted Hb-oxygen dissociation curve (P50, 33 mm Hg; reference range, 24–30 mm Hg) (Figure 1). Hb electrophoresis testing with cation-exchange high-performance liquid chromatography, capillary electrophoresis, and isoelectric focusing detected an abnormal variant peak (80.5% HbA, 2.2% HbA$_2$, 1.4% fetal Hb, and 15.9% Hb variant). DNA sequencing confirmed a heterozygous GAC > CAC, Asp > His missense mutation at codon 94 in the α-globin gene (Human Genome Variation Society nomenclature, *HBA2* c.283 G > C, p.D95H), resulting in Hb Sunshine Seth, an α-globin variant with low oxygen affinity. The Hb variant percentage was slightly lower than expected (15.9%; reference range, 26.3%–28.3%) [18]; however, the patient had concomitant iron deficiency (ferritin, 16 mcg/L; reference range, 24–336 mcg/L), which may have decreased the variant percentage. His parents were not tested for the genetic mutation.

2.3. Management and Outcome. The patient's diagnosis was Hb Sunshine Seth, an α-chain Hb variant with low oxygen affinity, resulting in reduced peripheral oxygen saturation without underlying cardiac or pulmonary pathologic conditions. For our patient, identification of this Hb variant with low oxygen affinity allowed for the cessation of diagnostic testing and discontinuation of unnecessary supplemental oxygen treatment. The patient is doing well without supplemental oxygen therapy.

3. Discussion

We described a case of low peripheral oxygen saturation in a child who received a diagnosis of oxygen dependency without a cardiopulmonary abnormality to explain his supplemental oxygen requirement. Our patient had a heterozygous genetic mutation for Hb Sunshine Seth, a Hb variant with low oxygen affinity that results from a mutation in the α-globin chain (histidine is substituted for an aspartic acid residue at position 94). This substitution is located in the α_1-β_2 contact site, which participates in the conversion of Hb from the oxygenated, relaxed state to the deoxygenated, taut state. Three of the 5 reported α-globin variants with amino acid substitutions at this position (Asp > Asn in Hb Titusville, Asp > Ala in Hb Bassett, and Asp > His in Hb Sunshine Seth) have decreased oxygen affinity and are associated with anemia, cyanosis, and decreased peripheral oxygen saturation [19].

Our patient did not have arterial blood gas studies performed. Therefore, the exact percentage of his Hb saturated by oxygen in the arterial blood (SaO$_2$) is not known. It is noted in the literature that some low-oxygen-affinity Hb variants will be characterized by concordant reduction in SaO$_2$ and SpO$_2$ (the oxygen saturation detected by pulse oximetry), while others will be characterized by discrepant values (reduced SpO$_2$ but normal SaO$_2$). There are no reported values of SaO$_2$ for patients with Hb Sunshine Seth in the literature, and it is challenging to predict if these values would be concordant or discrepant [20, 21]. In either case, there is no true tissue hypoxia. The pulse oximeter is simply detecting the relatively reduced ratio of oxygenated to deoxygenated Hb in the bloodstream, in the setting of increased oxygen extraction by peripheral tissues, resulting in a low peripheral SpO$_2$ measurement.

The sigmoidal Hb-oxygen dissociation curve emphasizes 2 characteristics of Hb-oxygen binding. The first is cooperativity, a phenomenon that improves oxygen affinity in high-oxygen environments (e.g., the lungs). When Hb is partially saturated by oxygen, the protein is in a relaxed state, and affinity for oxygen in the remaining binding sites is increased; therefore, Hb binds slowest to the first oxygen molecule, and the speed of binding increases for each subsequent oxygen molecule. This cooperativity accounts for variations in the slope and the sigmoidal shape of the dissociation curve. The second defining characteristic is the modifiable oxygen affinity, which can change in response to temperature, pH (acidosis vs. alkalosis), chemical binding of alternative compounds (e.g., carbon dioxide), and the presence of 2,3-bisphosphoglycerate (the major modulator of Hb-oxygen affinity in humans). These modifiers can increase or decrease affinity for oxygen and shift the dissociation curve along the x-axis [1].

Hb Sunshine Seth is a rare low-oxygen-affinity Hb variant. It has been sequenced only 11 times in more than 20 years at our institution, and an additional 10 to 15 cases have been reported in the literature [22–24]. All reported infants appeared normal or slightly cyanotic at birth, and pulse oximetry showed low peripheral oxygen saturation (range, 76%–84%) [18]. The genetic mutation has been detected with cord blood screening, maternal screening, or evaluation of known familial cases. The mutation has not been associated with obvious deleterious effects on the hematologic parameters or health of any described patient, and treatment, including oxygen supplementation, for anemia, and/or special precautions, has not been required [22–24]. Importantly, these points must be emphasized to patients, family members, and other health care providers, because unnecessary and costly evaluations and interventions for hypoxemia are common.

In summary, genetic mutations in Hb resulting in altered oxygen affinity are rare but important considerations for patients with unexplained erythrocytosis (associated with high-oxygen-affinity Hb variants) or unexplained anemia, cyanosis, and low peripheral oxygen saturation (associated with low-oxygen-affinity Hb variants). Early identification of these variants may prevent unnecessary and invasive diagnostic testing, such as cardiac and pulmonary studies, for patients with unexplained hypoxemia.

Abbreviations

Hb: Hemoglobin
LFNC: Low-flow nasal cannula.

References

[1] T. Somervaille, "Disorders of hemoglobin: genetics, pathophysiology, and clinical management," *Journal of the Royal Society of Medicine*, vol. 94, no. 11, pp. 602-603, 2001.

[2] A. Adeyinka and N. P. Kondamudi, "Cyanosis," *StatPearls*. Treasure Island (FL), 2019.

[3] S. Charache, D. J. Weatherall, and J. B. Clegg, "Polycythemia associated with a hemoglobinopathy," *Journal of Clinical Investigation*, vol. 45, no. 6, pp. 813–822, 1966.

[4] H. Wajcman, J. Kister, F. Galactéros et al., "Hb Montefiore (126(H9)Asp $\longrightarrow$ Tyr). High oxygen affinity and loss of cooperativity secondary to C-terminal disruption," *Journal of Biological Chemistry*, vol. 271, no. 38, pp. 22990–22998, 1996.

[5] A. Maniatis, T. Bousios, R. Nagel et al., "Hemoglobin Crete (beta 129 ala leads to pro): a new high-affinity variant interacting with beta o -and delta beta o -thalassemia," *Blood*, vol. 54, no. 1, pp. 54–63, 1979.

[6] J. L. Oliveira, L. M. Coon, L. A. Frederick et al., "Genotype-phenotype correlation of hereditary erythrocytosis mutations, A Single Center Experience," *American Journal of Hematology*, vol. 93, no. 8, pp. 1029–1041, 2018.

[7] J. L. Oliveira, K. Swanson, P. Wendt, T. D. Caughey, and J. D. Hoyer, "Hb cambridge-MA [β144(HC1)-β146(HC3)Lys-tyr-his $\longrightarrow$ 0 (HBB c.433 A>T)]: a new high oxygen affinity variant," *Hemoglobin*, vol. 34, no. 6, pp. 565–571, 2010.

[8] J. D. Hoyer, P. C. Wendt, W. J. Hogan, and J. L. Oliveira, "Hb Nebraska [β86(F2)Ala⟶Ile (HBB:c.259G>A;260C>T)]: a unique high oxygen affinity hemoglobin variant with a double nucleotide substitution within the same codon," *Hemoglobin*, vol. 35, no. 1, pp. 22–27, 2011.

[9] J. Bonaventura and A. Riggs, "Hemoglobin Kansas, a human hemoglobin with a neutral amino acid substitution and an abnormal oxygen equilibrium," *Journal of Biological Chemistry*, vol. 243, pp. 980–991, 1968.

[10] K. R. Reissmann, W. E. Ruth, and T. Nomura, "A human hemoglobin with lowered oxygen affinity and impaired heme-heme interactions," *Journal of Clinical Investigation*, vol. 40, no. 10, pp. 1826–1833, 1961.

[11] R. L. Nagel, J. Lynfield, J. Johnson, L. Landau, R. M. Bookchin, and M. B. Harris, "Hemoglobin Beth Israel. A mutant causing clinically apparent cyanosis," *New England Journal of Medicine*, vol. 295, no. 3, pp. 125–130, 1976.

[12] N. Arous, F. Braconnier, J. Thillet et al., "Hemoglobin Saint Mandé β102 (G4) Asn ⟶ Tyr: a new low oxygen affinity variant," *FEBS Letters*, vol. 126, no. 1, pp. 114–116, 1981.

[13] A. B. Collier 3rd, L. M. Coon, P. Monteleone et al., "A novel β-globin chain hemoglobin variant, Hb allentown [β137(H15) Val⟶Trp (GTG>TGG)HBB: c.412_413delinsTG, p.Val138Trp], associated with low oxygen saturation, intermittent aplastic crises and splenomegaly," *Hemoglobin*, vol. 40, no. 2, pp. 130–133, 2016.

[14] R. M. Taliercio, R. W. Ashton, L. Horwitz et al., "Hb grove city [β38(C4)Thr ⟶ Ser, ACC>AGC;HBB: c.116C>G]: a new low oxygen affinity β chain variant," *Hemoglobin*, vol. 37, no. 4, pp. 396–403, 2013.

[15] M. J. Percy, N. N. Butt, G. M. Crotty et al., "Identification of high oxygen affinity hemoglobin variants in the investigation of patients with erythrocytosis," *Haematologica*, vol. 94, no. 9, pp. 1321-1322, 2009.

[16] Harriet Lane Service (Johns Hopkins Hospital), H. Hughes, and L. Kahl, *The Harriet Lane Handbook: A Manual for Pediatric House Officers*, Elsevier, Philadelphia, PA, USA, 21st edition, 2018.

[17] D. G. Nathan, S. H. Orkin, and F. A. Oski, *Nathan and Oski's Hematology of Infancy and Childhood*, W.B. Saunders, Philadelphia, PA, USA, 5th edition, 1998.

[18] H. Bard, K. G. Peri, and C. Gagnon, "The biologic implications of a rare hemoglobin mutant that decreases oxygen affinity," *Pediatric Research*, vol. 49, no. 1, pp. 69–73, 2001.

[19] G. P. Patrinos, B. Giardine, C. Riemer et al., "Improvements in the HbVar database of human hemoglobin variants and thalassemia mutations for population and sequence variation studies," *Nucleic Acids Res*, vol. 32, pp. D537–D541, 2004.

[20] M. Verhovsek, M. P. A. Henderson, G. Cox, H.-y. Luo, M. H. Steinberg, and D. H. K. Chui, "Unexpectedly low pulse oximetry measurements associated with variant hemoglobins: a systematic review," *American Journal of Hematology*, vol. 85, no. 11, pp. 882–885, 2010.

[21] S. Wagner, S. Inbasi, S. Brunner-Agten, M. Gebauer, K. Hagemann, and J. McDougall, "Persistently low oxygen saturation in a neonate - there is more than meets the eye," *Swiss Society of Neonatology*, vol. 18, no. 2, pp. 1–18, 2018.

[22] W. A. Schroeder, J. B. Shelton, J. R. Shelton, and D. Powars, "Hemoglobin sunshine Seth-alpha 2 (94 (G1) Asp replaced by his) beta 2," *Hemoglobin*, vol. 3, no. 2, 3, pp. 145–159, 1979.

[23] H. Bard, A. Rosenberg, and T. Huisman, "Hemoglobinopathies affecting maternal-fetal oxygen gradient during pregnancy: molecular, biochemical and clinical studies," *American Journal of Perinatology*, vol. 15, no. 6, pp. 389–393, 1998.

[24] H. Bard, C. Gagnon, and K. G. Peri, "The biological implications of a rare hemoglobin mutant which decreases oxygen affinity discovered in newborns of several French Canadian families," *Pediatric Research*, vol. 45, no. 4, p. 143A, 1999.

8

A Case of Bilateral Spontaneous Chylothorax with Respiratory Syncytial Virus Bronchiolitis

Mario Briceno-Medina,[1] Michael Perez,[1,2] Jie Zhang,[3] Ronak Naik,[1] Samir Shah,[4] and Dai Kimura ⓘ[4]

[1]Division of Cardiology, Le Bonheur Children's Hospital, University of Tennessee Health Science Center, Memphis, TN, USA
[2]Division of Pediatric Cardiology, Ann & Robert H. Lurie Children's Hospital of Chicago, Northwestern University, Chicago, IL, USA
[3]Department of Pathology, Le Bonheur Children's Hospital, University of Tennessee Health Science Center, Memphis, TN, USA
[4]Division of Critical Care Medicine, Le Bonheur Children's Hospital, University of Tennessee Health Science Center, Memphis, TN, USA

Correspondence should be addressed to Dai Kimura; dkimura@uthsc.edu

Academic Editor: John W. Berkenbosch

A case of bilateral spontaneous chylothorax with respiratory syncytial virus (RSV) bronchiolitis has never been reported. We report the case of a 7-month-old boy born at 33 weeks gestation with a history of Down syndrome, atrial septal defect, pulmonary hypertension, and chronic lung disease, hospitalized due to RSV bronchiolitis who developed bilateral spontaneous chylothorax with exacerbation of pulmonary hypertension (PH). The patient died after 9 weeks of mechanical ventilation and treatment for PH. The autopsy showed acute infectious signs, a chronic interstitial lung disease with pulmonary hypertensive changes and subpleural cysts with no evidence of congenital lymphangiectasia. The cause of chylothorax in this child could be multifactorial. However, worsening pulmonary hypertension with RSV infection might have partially contributed to the development of chylothorax through elevated superior venous cava pressure. Thoracentesis should be considered for patients with Down syndrome and PH associated with congenital heart disease who develop persistent pleural effusion during RSV bronchiolitis to rule out chylothorax.

1. Introduction

Chylothorax, the accumulation of chylous pleural effusion, is very rare after neonatal period [1]. It can cause respiratory failure, malnutrition, and immunodeficiency if not treated. The cause of chylothorax includes lymphatic abnormality (pulmonary lymphangiomas and lymphangiectasia), trauma to the thoracic duct, venous thrombus in the superior vena cava (SVC) or subclavian vein, tumors such as lymphoma, and granulomatous infections such as tuberculosis, histoplasmosis, and sarcoidosis [1]. Chylothorax caused by other infectious diseases is extremely rare.

2. Case Description

The patient is a 7-month-old twin boy who presented to our institution's emergency department with increased work of breathing and desaturations (70 s). He was born at 33 weeks gestational age with Down syndrome, developed chronic lung disease (CLD) of prematurity, and was also found to have a moderate size secundum atrial septal defect (ASD) as a newborn. Prior to the current illness, he had been in the hospital multiple times for failure to thrive and respiratory distress, requiring mechanical ventilation with high amount of supplemental O_2 and inhaled nitric oxide (iNO) as he developed pulmonary hypertension (PH). Echocardiography showed progressive enlargement and hypertrophy of his right ventricle and at times bidirectional shunting across his ASD. A diagnostic cardiac catheterization as a preoperative evaluation was performed, which showed elevated pulmonary vascular resistance indexed (PVRi) at baseline (8.8 WU·m^2), which decreased with inhaled oxygen alone and iNO (3.8 WU·m^2). Additional catheterization data at baseline condition showed a right atrial mean pressure of

6 mmHg, right ventricular end diastolic pressure of 6 mmHg, and pulmonary artery pressure 51/19 mmHg with mean 32 mmHg. The patient was started on home O_2 therapy with nasal cannula. The current hospitalization occurred prior to a planned fenestrated patch repair of his ASD.

He was initially admitted to the general ward and soon transferred to the pediatric ICU for severe hypoxemic respiratory failure requiring mechanical ventilation. Respiratory syncytial virus (RSV) infection was diagnosed with the positive antigen test. He continued to have paroxysmal severe hypoxic events compatible with PH crisis. He was treated with sedation and neuromuscular paralysis, increased FiO_2, optimization of O_2 carrying capacity with packed red blood cells transfusions, and iNO. Milrinone infusion was added as the right ventricular function was depressed on echocardiogram (TAPSE 6 mm, Z-score −4), which demonstrated evidence of systemic to suprasystemic right ventricular pressure and bidirectional shunting across the ASD (Figures 1 and 2). No other cardiovascular intravenous drips were given during the ICU stay. Sildenafil was initiated enterally and escalated to maximal dose (2 mg/kg/day) without hemodynamic compromise. He was on diuretic therapy (bumetanide infusion up to 10 mcg/kg/hr) as chest X-ray demonstrated evidence of bilateral interstitial edema with bilateral pleural effusions on admission (Figure 3) and confirmed by chest ultrasound. Bilateral chest tubes were placed after failure of diuretic therapy to reduce effusions on hospital day #6. The drained fluid was milky in appearance bilaterally, with a white blood cell of 1,004/mm³ with lymphocyte predominance (88%) and elevated triglycerides (1008 mg/dl), and hence a diagnosis of chylothorax was made. Low IgG level (249 mg/dl) and hypoalbuminemia (2.5 g/dl) were noted at the time of pleural effusion drainage. Intravenous immunoglobulin and 25% albumin solution were administered. His feeding formula was changed to medium-chain triglyceride formula. The milky drainage became serous; however, the volume of chest tube drainage remained unchanged. Enteral feeding was discontinued and total parenteral nutrition was initiated, which decreased the volume of pleural effluent but small to moderate amount of pleural effusion was intermittently observed by chest X-ray for over sixty three days until the patient's death. Venous Doppler ultrasound of the upper extremities and the neck was performed on hospital day #7 and 4 weeks later, and compression, thrombosis or obstruction of the superior vena cava, and upper extremity were ruled out. A central venous catheter was placed in the right jugular vein soon after admission and was removed on hospital day #7 and replaced by a peripherally inserted central line. The patient required chest tubes for drainage until hospital day #22. Since then, intermittently small to moderate pleural effusion was observed by chest X-ray, but chest tubes were not placed.

He continued to be critically ill with persistent hypoxemic respiratory failure without improvement in PH with several PH crisis episodes. Therapy with an endothelin (ET) receptor antagonist (Bosentan) was added. The hospital course was complicated by bacterial tracheitis from

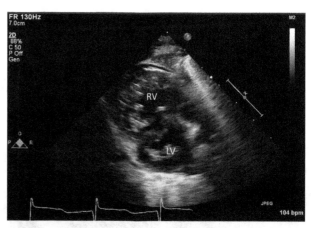

FIGURE 1: Parasternal short-axis view showing a flattening of the intraventricular septum during systole. Enlargement and hypertrophy of the right ventricle are also shown. RV, right ventricle; LV, left ventricle.

Pseudomonas and E. coli. The patient remained on mechanical ventilator support for 6 weeks due to failed weaning of ventilator support from hypoxemia despite high levels of supplementary FiO_2 and iNO. Cardiac catheterization performed 6 weeks after admission showed PVRi of 7 WU m² on 100% FiO_2 and 20 ppm of iNO under general anesthesia, pulmonary venous desaturation, and bidirectional shunting through ASD. Additionally, interval increases in right atrial pressure (mean 13 mmHg), right ventricular end diastolic pressure (12 mmHg), and pulmonary artery pressure (52/24 mean 36 mmHg) were noted. Given his severe and irreversible lung injury from mechanical ventilation in addition to baseline chronic lung disease, he was deemed not a candidate for lung transplant. Considering that the patient had Eisenmenger physiology due to severe PH and poor prognosis, the palliative care team was also consulted. Weaning from the mechanical ventilator was tried multiple times, but failed. At 9 weeks of his ICU hospitalization, he developed severe hypoxemia unresponsive to medical therapy that ultimately caused his death.

An autopsy showed bilateral small straw-colored pleural effusions (right 17 ml and left 10 ml), and the lung parenchyma was red-brown, poorly aerated, and diffusely congested with focal consolidation. The heart had an ASD (0.8 × 1.2 cm) with right ventricular hypertrophy secondary to PH. Microscopically, both lungs showed subpleural cysts lined by pneumocytes and containing macrophages, sloughed pneumocytes, and neutrophils. Acute multifocal bronchopneumonia was present with neutrophils in the bronchioles and alveoli. Chronic interstitial lung disease is diffusely present with alveolar septal thickening, capillary disorganization, and hemosiderosis. Small pulmonary arterial branches demonstrate moderate to marked medial smooth muscle hypertrophy with lumen narrowing, while large pulmonary arteries were normal with minimal changes. No lymphatic dilatation was observed on H&E or D2-40 immunostained slides; therefore, lymphangiectasia was ruled out (Figure 4). From the autopsy results, hypoxia due to progressive PH was considered as a cause of death.

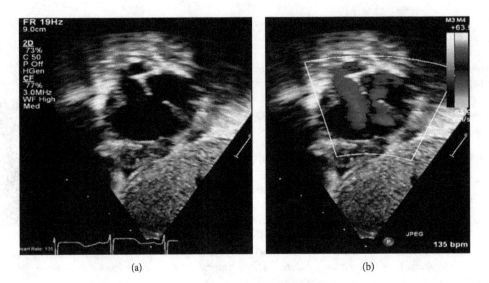

(a)   (b)

FIGURE 2: Color compared from the subcostal coronal view that shows moderate size secundum ASD with bidirectional shunting supporting findings of elevated RV pressure.

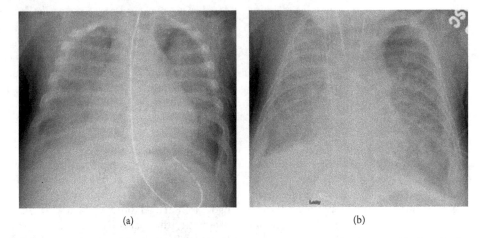

(a)   (b)

FIGURE 3: (a) Chest X-ray on admission showing bilateral pulmonary edema with pleural effusions. (b) Pleural effusion unresponsive to therapy with diuretics (hospital day #6).

3. Discussion

Chylothorax with granulomatous infection has been reported; however, there are no case reports of bilateral spontaneous chylothorax due to acute RSV bronchiolitis or bronchiolitis due to other viral infection [1]. The suspected mechanism of chylothorax in this child is multifactorial. However, worsening of PH with RSV bronchiolitis might have partially contributed to the development of chylothorax via elevated SVC pressure. PVRi measured by catheterization in this patient was not significantly different from the baseline, but the procedure was conducted at 6 weeks of admission after improvement in hypoxia. We suspect PVRi was even higher when the patient had severe respiratory failure with bilateral chylothorax soon after admission. Elevated SVC pressure is one of the etiologies of chylothorax resulting from the thoracic duct flow obstruction [2]. Another possible factor is an obstruction of SVC by a central venous catheter in the right jugular vein even though

Doppler ultrasound exams did not show signs of SVC thrombus and chest tube drainage continued until hospital day #22. We conducted Doppler ultrasound only twice and cannot completely rule out SVC thrombus before or between Doppler ultrasound exams. Many other factors possibly contributed to the development of chylothorax, including PH from congenital heart disease (CHD), chronic lung disease (CLD) of prematurity, and Down syndrome. Thoracentesis should be considered in patients with those risk factors for PH who develop persistent pleural effusion during RSV bronchiolitis to rule out chylothorax. Therapeutic drainage with chest tube placement may be necessary in patients with respiratory failure due to pleural effusions.

Transient or worsening PH in children with moderate to severe acute bronchiolitis has been reported and associated with a longer length of stay in the hospital [3–5]. The presence of PH in children with RSV infection was particularly associated with severity of the illness, with a mortality of 73% for children with CHD and PH [6]. Cardiac

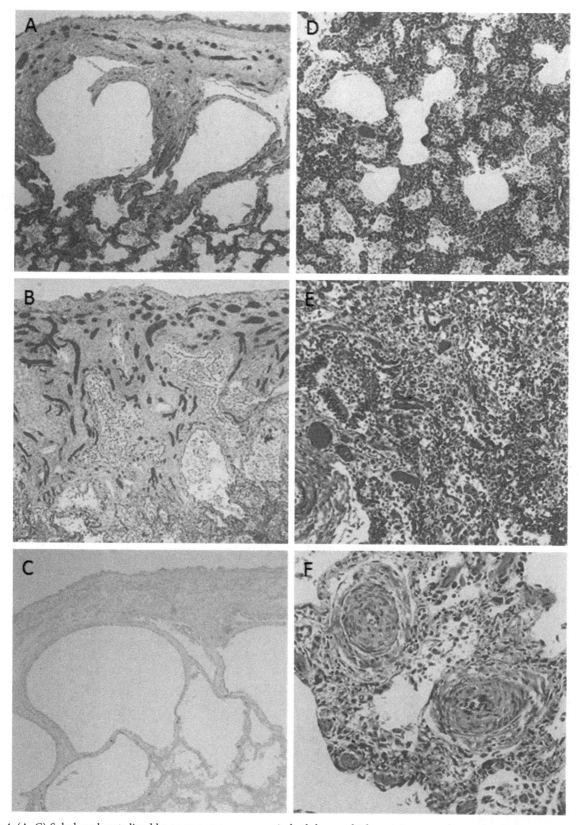

FIGURE 4: (A–C) Subpleural cysts lined by pneumocytes are seen in both lungs which contain macrophages, sloughed pneumocytes, and neutrophils ((A) H&E ×40 and (B) H&E ×20). (C) Immunohistochemistry with anti-D2-40 antibody, a marker for lymphatic endothelium, was negative. (D) Lung parenchyma demonstrates chronic interstitial lung disease with alveolar septal thickening, capillary disorganizing, and hemosiderosis (H&E ×40). (E) Acute bronchopneumonia is present (H&E ×40). (F) Pulmonary hypertensive changes are present with variable severities (H&E ×100).

surgery for children with CHD performed during the symptomatic period of RSV infection is associated with a high risk of postoperative complications, especially postoperative PH, and in a rare case, chylous effusion [7]. In the report, three patients with Down syndrome, CHD and PH died from RSV infection and could not receive cardiac surgery [7]. The pathophysiology of the development of PH during RSV bronchiolitis is unknown. In RSV bronchiolitis, hyperinflation and atelectasis secondary to lower airway obstruction and eventual hypoxia and hypercapnia can also cause increased pulmonary vascular resistance [8]. Therefore, multiple factors likely contribute to the development of PH in RSV bronchiolitis.

Patients with Down syndrome and CHD have a higher risk of developing PH quicker and with more damage to the pulmonary vascular bed than those without Down syndrome [9]. Persistently elevated serum ET-1 levels were observed in patients with Down syndrome after cardiopulmonary bypass for cardiac operations [10]. The imbalance between the prostacyclin and thromboxane and decreased arginine and NO production are other possible mechanisms of PH in Down syndrome [11]. Patients with Down syndrome also have a higher risk of developing chylothorax, most commonly congenitally [12, 13]. Furthermore, infants with Down syndrome were more likely to develop chylothorax after operation for CHD [14]. The etiology of chylothorax in patients with Down syndrome is not well understood, but it is likely associated with anomalous lymph drainage associated with aneuploidy syndromes (trisomy, Turner's syndrome, and Noonan's syndrome) [15]. In this patient, an autopsy showed subpleural cysts; however, there was no sign of congenital lymphangiectasis.

4. Conclusion

For patients with Down syndrome and PH associated with CHD who develop persistent pleural effusion during RSV bronchiolitis, thoracentesis should be considered to rule out chylothorax.

Consent

Informed consent was obtained from the patient's mother.

Acknowledgments

We thank Dr. Royce Joyner in the Department of Pathology, UTHSC, for kindly providing immunohistochemistry and comments and Dr. Amanda Preston in Le Bonheur Children's Hospital for scientific editing.

References

[1] J. D. Tutor, "Chylothorax in infants and children," *Pediatrics*, vol. 133, no. 4, pp. 722–733, 2014.

[2] M. Beghetti, G. La Scala, D. Belli, P. Bugmann, A. Kalangos, and C. Le Coultre, "Etiology and management of pediatric chylothorax," *Journal of Pediatrics*, vol. 136, no. 5, pp. 653–658, 2000.

[3] L. Bardi-Peti and E. P. Ciofu, "Pulmonary hypertension during acute respiratory diseases in infants," *Maedica (Buchar)*, vol. 5, no. 1, pp. 13–19, 2010.

[4] N. Sreeram, J. G. Watson, and S. Hunter, "Cardiovascular effects of acute bronchiolitis," *Acta Paediatrica*, vol. 80, no. 1, pp. 133–136, 1991.

[5] D. Fitzgerald, G. Davis, C. Rohlicek, and R. Gottesman, "Quantifying pulmonary hypertension in ventilated infants with bronchiolitis: a pilot study," *Journal of Paediatrics and Child Health*, vol. 37, no. 1, pp. 64–66, 2001.

[6] N. E. MacDonald, C. B. Hall, S. C. Suffin, C. Alexson, P. J. Harris, and J. A. Manning, "Respiratory syncytial viral infection in infants with congenital heart disease," *New England Journal of Medicine*, vol. 307, no. 7, pp. 397–400, 1982.

[7] A. Khongphatthanayothin, P. C. Wong, Y. Samara et al., "Impact of respiratory syncytial virus infection on surgery for congenital heart disease: postoperative course and outcome," *Critical Care Medicine*, vol. 27, no. 9, pp. 1974–1981, 1999.

[8] J. B. West and J. B. West, *Pulmonary Pathophysiology: The Essentials*, Wolters Kluwer/Lippincott Williams & Wilkins Health, Philadelphia, PA, USA, 2012.

[9] T. L. Chi and L. J. Krovetz, "The pulmonary vascular bed in children with Down syndrome," *Journal of Pediatrics*, vol. 86, no. 4, pp. 533–538, 1975.

[10] K. Kageyama, S. Hashimoto, Y. Nakajima, N. Shime, and S. Hashimoto, "The change of plasma endothelin-1 levels before and after surgery with or without Down syndrome," *Pediatric Anesthesia*, vol. 17, no. 11, pp. 1071–1077, 2007.

[11] H. Fukushima, K. Kosaki, R. Sato et al., "Mechanisms underlying early development of pulmonary vascular obstructive disease in Down syndrome: an imbalance in biosynthesis of thromboxane A2 and prostacyclin," *American Journal of Medical Genetics Part A*, vol. 152A, no. 8, pp. 1919–1924, 2010.

[12] B. S. Krovetz and P. J. Lipsitz, "Chylothorax in two mongoloid infants," *Clinical Genetics*, vol. 12, no. 6, pp. 357–360, 2008.

[13] J. Arena Ansotegui, A. Rey Otero, and J. Albisu Andrade, "Spontaneous neonatal chylothorax. Apropos of 5 cases," *Anales Españoles de Pediatría*, vol. 20, no. 1, pp. 49–54, 1984.

[14] C. Doell, V. Bernet, L. Molinari, I. Beck, C. Balmer, and B. Latal, "Children with genetic disorders undergoing open-heart surgery: are they at increased risk for postoperative complications?*," *Pediatric Critical Care Medicine*, vol. 12, no. 5, pp. 539–544, 2011.

[15] P. Moerman, K. Vandenberghe, H. Devlieger, C. Van Hole, J.-P. Fryns, and J. M. Lauweryns, "Congenital pulmonary lymphangiectasis with chylothorax: a heterogeneous lymphatic vessel abnormality," *American Journal of Medical Genetics*, vol. 47, no. 1, pp. 54–58, 1993.

9

Euglycemic Ketoacidosis in Spinal Muscular Atrophy

Dimitrios Stoimenis ⓘ,[1] **Christina Spyridonidou,**[2] **Sofia Theofanidou,**[3] **Nikolaos Petridis ⓘ,**[1] **Nikos Papaioannou,**[1] **Christina Iasonidou,**[4] **and Nikolaos Kapravelos**[4]

[1]*Department of Internal Medicine, General Hospital G. Papanikolaou, Thessaloniki, Greece*
[2]*Intensive Care Unit, General Hospital Papageorgiou, Thessaloniki, Greece*
[3]*Department of Internal Medicine, General Hospital G. Gennimatas, Athens, Greece*
[4]*Intensive Care Unit, General Hospital G. Papanikolaou, Thessaloniki, Greece*

Correspondence should be addressed to Dimitrios Stoimenis; dimitriosdoc@hotmail.com

Academic Editor: Stacey Tay

Euglycemic ketoacidosis is defined by the triad of high anion gap acidosis, increased plasma ketones, and the absence of hyperglycemia. Apart from diabetes mellitus, the disorder may occur in prolonged fasting, excessive alcohol consumption, pregnancy, and inborn errors of metabolism. Here, we highlight the diagnosis of euglycemic ketoacidosis in a pediatric nondiabetic patient with spinal muscular atrophy (SMA) type 1 (Werdnig–Hoffmann disease), who, subsequently to her postoperative admission to the intensive care unit following a spinal surgery, developed high anion gap metabolic acidosis. We discuss the pathophysiology of acid-base disorders in SMA, along with the glucose and fatty acids metabolism, the necessary knowledge for medical practitioners.

1. Introduction

Euglycemic ketoacidosis, albeit underrated, has been acknowledged since 1973, most commonly occurring in patients with diabetes mellitus (DM) [1]. The American Diabetes Association suggested the definition of euglycemic diabetic ketoacidosis as blood glucose <13.9 mmol/L combined with ketoacidosis [2]. This disorder, however, can develop in the absence of DM, under conditions characterized by severe ketosis, namely, starvation, alcohol intoxication, pregnancy, and inborn errors of metabolism [2]. Herein, we describe the diagnosis of euglycemic ketoacidosis in a pediatric nondiabetic patient with a known history of spinal muscular atrophy (SMA).

2. Case Presentation

A 13-year-old female patient was postoperatively admitted to the intensive care unit (ICU), following a spondylodesis procedure due to severe spinal malformation (Figure 1). The girl's medical history was remarkable for a genetically confirmed diagnosis of SMA type 1 (Werdnig–Hoffmann disease) within her first six months of age (homozygous deletion of the survival motor neuron 1 (SMN1) on exon 7, 5q chromosome, with two copies of the SMN2 gene).

On the third ICU day, the patient developed metabolic acidosis. Arterial blood gases revealed pH 7.17 (reference 7.35–7.45), partial pressure of oxygen (PaO_2) 12.40 kPa (reference 11–13 kPa), partial pressure of carbon dioxide ($PaCO_2$) 4 kPa (reference 4.7–6.0 kPa), bicarbonate (HCO_3^-) 10.7 mmol/L (reference 22–26 mmol/L), and base deficit −13 mmol/L. Lactate was normal with a value of 0.8 mmol/L (reference 0.56–2.0 mmol/L). The anion gap was 14 mmol/L, and the corrected value for the albumin anion gap was 26 mmol/L (reference 3–11 mmol/L).

Before admission, the patient's respiratory function was impaired. She had significant respiratory muscle weakness and poor cough ability, and she required at home the use of noninvasive ventilation (NIV) and mechanically assisted coughing (MAC). She was intubated prior to surgery and

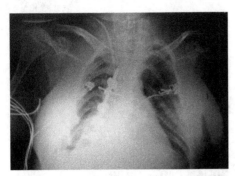

FIGURE 1: The spinal malformation and the spondylodesis materials of the pediatric patient.

extubated after a difficult and prolonged weaning following admission to the ICU. At the time of examination, she was breathing spontaneously and was supported intermittently with NIV. Despite her having had a gastrostomy tube at an earlier stage of life, during hospitalization, she was fasted for three consecutive days, the day of the surgery and the next two postoperative days, in light of the presumed risk of pulmonary aspiration. Furthermore, she was apyrexial, intravenously hydrated with 0.9% normal saline, and not on any inotropic or vasopressor support since her vital signs implied hemodynamic stability (systolic blood pressure > 110 mmHg and heart rate < 90 bpm). Common causes of metabolic acidosis with a high anion gap, namely, uremia, diabetic or alcoholic ketoacidosis, and lactic acidosis, were excluded. Renal and liver functions were normal, and no sign of infection was evident since inflammatory markers were negative and white blood cell account was normal. Total parenteral nutrition, and other agents, such as valproic acid and salicylates, which can potentially induce acidosis, had not been administered.

The pediatric patient had no history of DM, and she presented normal glycated hemoglobin (4.4%, reference 4.0–5.7%) and plasma glucose levels. However, her reduced body mass index-for-age (14.8 kg/m^2) and, accordingly, the extremely low levels of serum urea (1.78 mmol/L, reference 2.5–8.0 mmol/L) and serum creatinine (8.8 mmol/L, reference 52–96.8 mmol/L) prompted the ICU consultation team to investigate the likelihood of ketosis and ketoacidosis. Plasma β-hydroxybutyrate assay was unavailable on the premises; nevertheless, urine analysis revealed a severe degree of ketonuria (acetoacetate >7.84 mmol/L; urine value 4+).

Upon establishment of the diagnosis of euglycemic ketoacidosis, our patient was started on a fat-free enteral nutrition enriched with carbohydrates and proteins via her gastrostomy feeding tube. The acidosis resolved completely within 48 hours; urine ketones were negative at the time. No bicarbonate or insulin infusion was administered. The patient was discharged to the ward four days later.

3. Discussion

SMA comprises an autosomal recessive neuromuscular disorder and the most frequent inherited motor neuron disease, characterized by insufficient produced levels of the

survival motor neuron protein, which results in progressive neurodegeneration and atrophy of the skeletal muscles [3]. In patients with SMA, spinal deformity, respiratory complications, and orthopedic disorders constitute the major challenges of their clinical management. SMA is classified into four types, with type 1 representing the most severe form of the disease (Werdnig–Hoffmann disease) with infantile onset and multiorgan impairment [3]. Of note, due to the severity of the clinical course in SMA type 1, the majority of patients with this phenotype do not achieve the spinal developmental milestone that was described in our case, which was rather an atypically mild presentation. Suggestively, in a previous reported retrospect chart review and caregiver questionnaire for referred children with SMA type 1, only four patients with atypically mild SMA type 1 underwent a surgical correction of scoliosis, while none of the 74 typical SMA type 1 patients achieved this degree of spinal development in order to require such a surgical correction [4].

Additionally, SMA is associated with a complex disorder of fatty acids metabolism, which has raised controversy over the exact underlying pathogenesis. While it has been postulated that SMA patients are particularly susceptible to fasting hypoglycemia and ketosis mostly attributed to their reduced muscular mass [5, 6], several authors have indicated a mitochondrial β-oxidation abnormality in muscles as the primary pathogenic mechanism of fatty acids metabolism in SMA [3]. In fact, it has been reported that these patients may present increased levels of serum dicarboxylic acids, dicarboxylic aciduria, and potential metabolic acidosis during stress or fasting periods [7, 8].

In the case presented, over the first two postoperative days, the pediatric patient was fasted, given the high risk of pulmonary aspiration. In light of the absence of DM, typical predisposing factors of high anion gap acidosis [9], such as diabetic and alcoholic ketoacidosis, uremia, lactic acidosis, parenteral nutrition, and drug-induced acidosis, were ruled out from the differential diagnosis. Although no further anthropometric study, other than body mass index-for-age, was performed in order to assess the exact baseline nutritional status (e.g., skinfold thickness or dual energy X-ray absorptiometry), we considered that the patient had an element of chronic malnutrition. Hence, the reduced muscular mass combined with the fasting state, and the perioperative stress led the ICU consultation team to presume that the patient could have been subject to severe ketosis due to her proneness to rapid depletion of liver and muscle glycogen stores [10]. In fact, starvation and stress-induced acidosis perioperatively and in the ICU setting have previously been described in certain circumstances [11, 12], in which several factors in combination can result in moderate or severe ketoacidosis. Repeated episodes of stress-induced ketoacidosis were also reported in an adult patient with SMA type 2, and it was suggested that this metabolic disorder can be easily corrected within hours or few days, provided it is recognized early [13]. Of note, in our case, during the surgery and the first two postoperative days in the ICU, our patient was administered only normal saline solutions, and it is likely that should had we hydrated the patient more aggressively with crystalloids and dextrose solutions, she would rather not have developed the metabolic acidosis, at least to this degree.

Regarding our therapeutic approach, the applicable diet alone, a mixture of carbohydrates and proteins, resulted in the complete resolution of ketoacidosis, without applying any other treatment and thus confirmed the initial thought process of clinical diagnosis. The rationale for this fat-free dietary management was the reduction of the patient's further exposure to fatty acid substrates during the metabolic derangement in order to prevent additional accumulation of potentially toxic-free fatty acids [14] and the inhibition of ketosis by promoting glycolysis and glycogenesis, through appropriate enteral nutrition and adequate carbohydrate intake [10]. Certainly, apart from the need for sufficient continuous carbohydrate intake, we do not recommend or imply that a long-term fat-free diet could represent a suitable nutrition in patients with SMA, given that the deprivation of lipids or vital fat-soluble vitamins in the diet would have unknown implications and risks. Furthermore, it is worth noting that we did not assess the patient with tandem mass spectrometry analyses of the acylcarnitine profile and free fatty acids or with urine organic acid investigations for known inborn errors of metabolism, such as organic acidemias and ketolytic defects [2, 8]. Therefore, post hoc, we cannot definitely exclude the presence of other acids, including dicarboxylic acids, which could have contributed in the metabolic acidosis and neither can we determine the exact pathogenic mechanisms of abnormal fatty acids metabolism in our patient.

In conclusion, this case emphasizes the metabolic derangement in a patient with SMA type 1 after short-term fasting in the ICU setting and in a state of perioperative stress. Moreover, our report points out that clinicians and pediatric physicians should not forget the entity of non-diabetic euglycemic ketoacidosis when deciphering high anion gap acidosis. In conjunction with a pertinent medical history and clinical indication, urine ketones testing, a rapid and low-cost assay, can have particular diagnostic value with regard to abnormal glucose and fatty acids metabolism, and therefore, should not be neglected in the absence of DM.

References

[1] J. F. Munro, I. W. Campbell, A. C. McCuish, and L. J. P. Duncan, "Euglycaemic diabetic ketoacidosis," BMJ, vol. 2, no. 5866, pp. 578–580, 1973.

[2] F. Le Neveu, B. Hywel, and J. N. Harvey, "Euglycaemic ketoacidosis in patients with and without diabetes," Practical Diabetes, vol. 30, no. 4, pp. 167–171, 2013.

[3] M. Shababi, C. L. Lorson, and S. S. Rudnik-Schöneborn, "Spinal muscular atrophy: a motor neuron disorder or a multi-organ disease?," Journal of Anatomy, vol. 224, no. 1, pp. 15–28, 2013.

[4] J. R. Bach, "Medical considerations of long-term survival of Werdnig–Hoffmann disease," American Journal of Physical Medicine & Rehabilitation, vol. 86, no. 5, pp. 349–355, 2007.

[5] A. K. Bruce, E. Jacobsen, H. Dossing, and J. Kondrup, "Hypoglycemia in spinal muscular atrophy," The Lancet, vol. 346, no. 8975, pp. 609-610, 1995.

[6] B. Lakkis, A. El Chediak, J. G. Hashash, and S. H. Koubar, "Severe ketoacidosis in a patient with spinal muscular atrophy," CEN Case Reports, vol. 7, no. 2, pp. 292–295, 2018.

[7] R. I. Kelley and J. T. Sladky, "Dicarboxylic aciduria in an infant with spinal muscular atrophy," Annals of Neurology, vol. 20, no. 6, pp. 734–736, 1986.

[8] T. O. Crawford, J. T. Sladky, O. Hurko, A. Besner-Johnston, and R. I. Kelley, "Abnormal fatty acid metabolism in childhood spinal muscular atrophy," Annals of Neurology, vol. 45, no. 3, pp. 337–343, 1999.

[9] P. Reddy and A. D. Mooradian, "Clinical utility of anion gap in deciphering acid-base disorders," International Journal of Clinical Practice, vol. 63, no. 10, pp. 1516–1525, 2009.

[10] L. Laffel, "Ketone bodies: a review of physiology, pathophysiology and application of monitoring to diabetes," Diabetes/Metabolism Research and Reviews, vol. 15, no. 6, pp. 412–426, 1999.

[11] H. L. Toth and L. A. Greenbaum, "Severe acidosis caused by starvation and stress," American Journal of Kidney Diseases, vol. 42, no. 5, pp. e22.1–e22.4, 2003.

[12] M. Mostert and A. Bonavia, "Starvation ketoacidosis as a cause of unexplained metabolic acidosis in the perioperative period," American Journal of Case Reports, vol. 17, pp. 755–758, 2016.

[13] E. Mulroy, S. Gleeson, and M. J. Furlong, "Stress-induced ketoacidosis in spinal muscular atrophy: an under-recognized complication," Journal of Neuromuscular Diseases, vol. 3, no. 3, pp. 419–423, 2016.

[14] I. Tein, A. E. Sloane, E. J. Donner, D. C. Lehotay, D. S. Millington, and R. I. Kelley, "Fatty acid oxidation abnormalities in childhood-onset spinal muscular atrophy: primary or secondary defect(s)?," Pediatric Neurology, vol. 12, no. 1, pp. 21–30, 1995.

10

A Case of Kikuchi's Disease Without Cervical Lymphadenopathy

Shinya Tomori [ID],[1] **Seigo Korematsu,**[1] **Taichi Momose,**[1] **Yasuko Urushihara,**[1] **Shuji Momose,**[2] **and Koichi Moriwaki**[1]

[1]*Department of Pediatrics, Saitama Medical Center Saitama Medical University, Kamoda, Kawagoe Saitama 350-8550, Japan*
[2]*Department of Pathology, Saitama Medical Center, Saitama Medical University, Kamoda, Kawagoe Saitama 350-8550, Japan*

Correspondence should be addressed to Shinya Tomori; stomori-teikyo@med.teikyo-u.ac.jp

Academic Editor: Nur Arslan

Background. Kikuchi's disease with only extracervical lymphadenopathy is rare. *Case Presentation.* A 15-year-old male has presented with a fever lasting more than 1 week and right axillary lymphadenopathy. An axillary lymph node biopsy revealed coagulation necrosis, nuclear decay products, infiltration of histiocytes, and enlarged lymphocytes; he was diagnosed with Kikuchi's disease. The only four adult patients with Kikuchi's disease presenting without cervical lesions have been previously reported. *Conclusion.* This is the only pediatric case of Kikuchi's disease presenting without cervical lymphadenopathy. Kikuchi's disease should be included in the differential diagnosis even in cases of extracervical lymphadenopathy alone.

1. Introduction

Kikuchi's disease, also called Kikuchi-Fujimoto disease or histiocytic necrotizing lymphadenitis, is a benign condition of unknown cause characterized by a fever and cervical lymphadenopathy [1]. It was first reported from Japan by Kikuchi and Fujimoto in [2, 3]. The disease is thought to involve a viral immune response, and many triggers have been proposed, including Epstein-Barr virus, human herpesvirus 6, human herpesvirus 8, human immunodeficiency virus, parvovirus B19, paramyxovirus, parainfluenza virus, Yersinia enterocolitica, and toxoplasma [4]. Fever combined with cervical lymphadenopathy is the most typical clinical feature of Kikuchi's disease [5]. Other sites of lymphadenopathy other than the cervical lymph nodes include the axilla, mediastinum, groin, abdomen, and pelvis [5]. Kikuchi's disease without cervical lymphadenopathy is rare [6, 7].

We herein report a case of Kikuchi's disease presenting only with axillary lymphadenopathy, along with a review of previous reports.

2. Case Presentation

A 15-year-old boy born to healthy Japanese parents developed a fever, headache, and malaise 13 days before admission. He visited his local doctor one week prior to admission due to his persistent fever, and a blood test was performed but revealed no abnormalities. He was prescribed acetaminophen, but as the fever did not resolve, he visited our hospital three days prior to admission and was prescribed ampicillin/clavulanic acid. However, he was admitted due to his continued fever. He had never been scratched by a cat or other animals.

On admission, his consciousness was clear. His temperature was 39.0°C, and he had no respiratory disturbance or tachycardia. There was a 3-cm smooth, mobile, and tender lymphadenopathy in the right axilla. There were no scratches or injuries on his right arm. Other physical examination findings were normal. Laboratory results are shown in Table 1. Contrast-enhanced computed tomography (CT) showed multiple lymphadenopathies in the right axilla but no solid tumor.

TABLE 1: Laboratory data on admission.

Parameter	Recorded value	Standard value
White blood cell count (/μL)	4,400	4,500–13,000
Neutrophils (%)	65.8	
Hemoglobin (g/dL)	15.4	12.0–14.5
Hematocrit (%)	45.8	44–50
Platelet count (×10^4/μl)	29.5	15–40
ESR (mm/h)	33	1–10
Total protein (g/dL)	8.1	6.5–8.1
Albumin (g/dL)	4.4	3.8–4.8
Aspartate aminotransferase (U/L)	33	13–30
Alanine aminotransferase (U/L)	26	9–35
γ-glutamyl transpeptidase (U/L)	22	0–50
Creatinine (mg/dL)	0.75	0.48–0.93
Urea nitrogen (mg/dL)	11	6–20
Na (mEq/L)	137	138–145
K (mEq/L)	4.3	3.4–4.7
Cl (mEq/L)	98	98–106
C-reactive protein (mg/dL)	1.19	<0.2
CH50 (U/mL)	>60	25–48
C3 (mg/dL)	149	86–160
C4 (mg/dL)	56	17–45
β2-microglobulin (mg/L)	2.9	0.9–2.0
Serum amyloid A (μg/mL)	236.3	<8.0
IgG (mg/dL)	1374	770–1690
IgM (mg/dL)	103	67–291
IgA (mg/dL)	211	78–376
T-spot *tuberculosis*	Negative	
Antinuclear antibody	Negative	
CMV-IgM	Negative	
VCA-IgM	Negative	
Serum IL-2 receptor (U/mL)	847	145–519
CD4/CD8 ratio	0.64	0.4–2.3

Initially, we suspected pyogenic lymphadenitis and started treatment with cefepime and vancomycin. However, since the fever did not resolve and there was a discrepancy between inflammatory findings on blood tests and clinical findings, an axillary lymph node biopsy was performed on the fourth day of admission in order to differentiate malignant lymphoma. The pathology showed indistinct lymph node structure and an infiltrate of large lymphocytes and histiocytes from cortical to paracortical areas. In addition, the central part of the lymph node was necrotic, and macrophages with numerous nuclear karyorrhectic debris were observed in the necrotic tissue. The biopsied lymph node showed no neutrophilic infiltration (Figure 1(a) and 1(b)). Based on these pathological findings, a diagnosis of Kikuchi's disease was made.

Antimicrobial therapy was discontinued on day 9 of hospitalization. On the same day, small erythematous plaques without fusion appeared on the extremities and trunk. The patient was diagnosed with a skin rash associated with Kikuchi's disease. Olopatadine was administered because itching also appeared. On the 13th day of hospitalization, the patient's symptoms improved, and the inflammatory findings became negative, so he was discharged. Since then, the patient's symptoms have not flared up.

3. Discussion

Differential diagnoses of regional lymphadenopathy include hematologic malignancies, cancer metastases, hypersensitivity syndromes, infections, connective tissue disorders, atypical lymphoproliferative disorders, granulomatous disease, and Kikuchi disease. Among these, axillary lymphadenopathy is generally differentiated from infections (staphylococcal and streptococcal skin infections, cat scratch disease), sarcoidosis, and malignancies (breast cancer, lymphomas, and leukemia) [8].

In this case, a lymph node biopsy was performed because it was difficult to exclude malignant lymphoma, although Kikuchi's disease was suspected in addition to pyogenic lymphadenitis based on the clinical course, blood tests, and imaging studies. Although Kikuchi disease was diagnosed by lymph node biopsy, the histological differential diagnosis of Kikuchi disease is mainly reactive lesions such as lymphadenitis associated with systemic lupus erythematosus, lymphadenitis caused by microorganisms such as herpes simplex, nonHodgkin's lymphoma, plasmacytic T-cell leukemia, Kawasaki disease, metastatic adenocarcinoma, or acute myeloid leukemia [9]. The characteristic pathology of Kikuchi's disease is the absence of neutrophilic infiltration in the necrotic areas [10]. The outcome is usually good, with spontaneous resolution of symptoms in most cases and recurrence in 3%–4% of cases. If no complications arise, the disease resolves within a few months. Symptomatic treatment is the mainstay of therapy, and there is no specific treatment. Corticosteroids are used only in severe cases or in cases of recurrence [10, 11].

In Kikuchi's disease, lymphadenopathy is most commonly located in the neck. Almost all patients with pathologically diagnosed Kikuchi disease had cervical lymphadenopathy [6, 7].

In order to search case reports of Kikuchi's disease with axillary lesions, we checked the academic article database PubMed and the Japanese article database Ichushi with the key words "Kikuchi's disease and/or axillary lymphadenopathy" and "histiocytic necrotizing lymphadenitis and/or axillary lymphadenopathy." Mannu et al. reported a 19-year-old girl with no underlying disease who visited the hospital because of a mass in the right axilla that had been noted 2 months earlier [12]. There were no lesions in the breast. After an excisional biopsy of the axillary lesion, she was diagnosed with Kikuchi's disease. In the case of Verroiotou et al., a 56-year-old man with no underlying disease presented with left axillary lymphadenopathy [13]. Norris et al. reported a 63-year-old man with diabetes mellitus who was admitted to the hospital with fatigue, myalgia, a fever, and weight loss that persisted for 4 weeks [14]. Facial flushing and bilateral axillary lymphadenopathy were noted, as well as a decreased white blood cell count, elevated LDH, and elevated erythrocyte sedimentation. An axillary lymph node biopsy revealed a diagnosis of Kikuchi's disease.

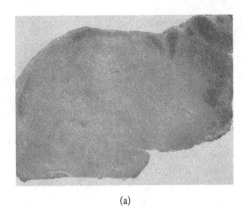
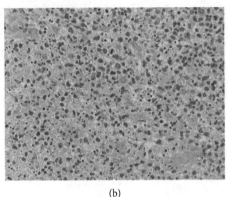

(a)   (b)

FIGURE 1: A histopathological image of axillary lymph node biopsy performed on the fourth day of admission. (a) Low power field, the central part of the lymph node was necrotic. (b) Hyper power field, macrophages with numerous nuclear karyorrhectic debris were observed in the necrotic tissue. The biopsied lymph node showed no neutrophilic infiltration.

4. Conclusion

To our knowledge, this is the only pediatric case of Kikuchi's disease presenting exclusively with axillary lymph node involvement. Why lymphadenopathy in Kikuchi's disease is often located in the neck is unclear, but it should be noted that lymphadenopathy outside the neck may also be present in Kikuchi's disease.

References

[1] S. Ifeacho, T. Aung, and M. Akinsola, "Kikuchi-Fujimoto Disease: a case report and review of the literature," *Cases Journal*, vol. 1, no. 1, p. 187, 2008.

[2] M. Kikuchi, "Lymphadenitis showing focal reticulum cell hyperplasia with nuclear debris and phagocytosis," *Nippon Ketsueki Gakkai Zasshi*, vol. 35, pp. 379-380, 1972.

[3] Y. Fujimoto, Y. Kojima, and K. Yamaguchi, "Cervical subacute necrotizing lymphadenitis," *New Clin Ent*, vol. 20, pp. 920-927, 1972.

[4] Y. Kucukardali, E. Solmazgul, E. Kunter, O. Oncul, S. Yildirim, and M. Kaplan, "Kikuchi-Fujimoto Disease: analysis of 244 cases," *Clinical Rheumatology*, vol. 26, no. 1, pp. 50-54, 2007.

[5] F. Jun-Fen, W. Chun-Lin, L. Li, C. Dayan, D. Guan-Ping, and H. Fang, "Kikuchi-Fujimoto disease manifesting as recurrent thrombocytopenia and Mobitz type II atrioventricular block in a 7-year-old girl: a case report and analysis of 138 Chinese childhood Kikuchi-Fujimoto cases with 10 years of follow-up in 97 patients," *Acta Paediatrica*, vol. 96, no. 12, pp. 1844-1847, 2007.

[6] L. C. Chen, C. J. Wang, Y. C. Chang et al., "Distribution of lymphadenopathy in patients with Kikuchi disease," *Journal of Microbiology, Immunology, and Infection*, vol. 54, no. 2, pp. 299-304, 2021.

[7] C. H. Chuang, D. C. Yan, C. H. Chiu et al., "Clinical and laboratory manifestations of Kikuchi's disease in children and differences between patients with and without prolonged fever," *The Pediatric Infectious Disease Journal*, vol. 24, no. 6, pp. 551-554, 2005.

[8] S. Mohseni, A. Shojaiefard, Z. Khorgami, S. Alinejad, A. Ghorbani, and A. Ghafouri, "Peripheral lymphadenopathy: approach and diagnostic tools," *Iranian Journal of Medical Sciences*, vol. 39, no. 2, pp. 158-170, 2014.

[9] X. Bosch, A. Guilabert, R. Miquel, and E. Campo, "Enigmatic Kikuchi-Fujimoto disease: a comprehensive review," *American Journal of Clinical Pathology*, vol. 122, no. 1, pp. 141-152, 2004.

[10] A. M. Perry and S. M. Choi, "Kikuchi-Fujimoto disease: a review," *Archives of Pathology & Laboratory Medicine*, vol. 142, no. 11, pp. 1341-1346, 2018.

[11] C. B. Hutchinson and E. Wang, "Kikuchi-Fujimoto disease," *Archives of Pathology & Laboratory Medicine*, vol. 134, no. 2, pp. 289-293, 2010.

[12] G. S. Mannu, F. Ahmed, G. Cunnick, and K. Sheppard, "A rare cause of axillary lymphadenopathy: Kikuchi's disease," *BMJ Case Reports*, vol. 2014, 2014.

[13] M. Verroiotou, S. A. Mogrampi, I. Polytidis, and I. Fardellas, "Kikuchi-fujimoto disease: a rare case of axillary lymphadenopathy," *Lymphatic Research and Biology*, vol. 9, no. 2, pp. 115-116, 2011.

[14] A. H. Norris, A. M. Krasinskas, K. E. Salhany, and S. J. Gluckman, "Kikuchi-Fujimoto disease: a benign cause of fever and lymphadenopathy," *The American Journal of Medicine*, vol. 101, no. 4, pp. 401-405, 1996.

11

Apnea in a Two-Week-Old Infant Infected with SARS-CoV-2 and Influenza B

Radhika Maddali ⑩,[1] Kelly L. Cervellione,[2] and Lily Q. Lew ⑩[1]

[1]*Department of Pediatrics, Flushing Hospital Medical Center, Flushing, NY 11355, USA*
[2]*Department of Clinical Research, Medisys Health Network, Jamaica, NY 11418, USA*

Correspondence should be addressed to Radhika Maddali; rmaddali.flushing@jhmc.org and Lily Q. Lew; llew2.flushing@jhmc.org

Academic Editor: Mohammad M. A. Faridi

Paucity of data exists on presenting symptoms and outcomes in infants with COVID-19. Reports of coinfection with COVID-19 and influenza B are sparse in the literature. Coinfection was uncovered during evaluation of neonatal apnea. Apnea has been reported in infants with SARS-CoV-2 infection, though it is rare. We describe a 2-week-old healthy term infant presenting with apnea and coinfection. The infant had a mild clinical course and complete recovery.

1. Introduction

Severe acute respiratory syndrome coronavirus 2 also known as SARS-CoV-2 causes coronavirus disease 2019 or COVID-19 [1]. Infected infants and children have a lower risk for symptomatic and severe infection than adults. Commonly reported clinical signs and symptoms of COVID-19 in infants include respiratory distress, cough, fever, nasal congestion, and poor feeding [2]. Since symptomatic COVID-19 in infants is not as common as in adults, presenting symptoms and disease course remain poorly characterized. Apnea has not been included as a symptom of COVID-19.

Infants who contract influenza are known to have a higher risk for severe illness than adults due to their immature immune system and smaller airway [3]. Infants combating coinfection may be at a risk for poorer outcomes than those with COVID-19 alone. Adults coinfected with COVID-19 and influenza [4–7] encountered higher morbidity and mortality than having COVID-19 alone [6–8]. We describe a 2-week-old healthy term infant presenting with apnea who was coinfected with SARS-CoV-2 and influenza B. The infant had a mild clinical course and complete recovery.

2. Case

A 2-week-old previously healthy girl presented with an apneic episode lasting three minutes while lying supine after a feed. The apneic episode was associated with stiffening of the body and turning red in color. There was no history of rhythmic or unusual facial movements. She experienced nasal congestion in the preceding two days that was not associated with fever, cough, or vomiting. She was born at term having a birth weight of 3365 grams (75th percentile), length of 48.9 centimeters (50th percentile), and head circumference of 33.5 centimeters (25th–50th percentile). The mother tested COVID-19 negative at delivery. The patient's household consisted of two school-age siblings in addition to the parents. At admission, the infant's weight was 4082 grams (75th percentile), temperature was 37.2°Celsius, pulse was 154 beats per minute, respiratory rate was 33 breaths per minute, and O_2 saturation was 100% in room air. The heart and lung examinations were normal. There were no neurological deficits. Laboratory findings *included* a white blood cell count of 16.9×10^9/L (16.9 K/uL), serum glucose of 6.27 mmol/L (113 mg/dL), calcium of 2.82 mmol/L (11.3 mg/dL), total carbon dioxide of 18 mmol/L, and C-reactive protein (CRP) of 0.00 nmol/L (<0.05 mg/dL). Urinalysis was *normal*. Chest radiograph revealed hyperinflated lungs with prominent central markings, no focal consolidation, no pleural abnormality, and unremarkable cardiothymic silhouette. SARS-CoV-2 PCR-NP (BioGX SARS-CoV-2 Reagents for BD MAX™ System) and influenza B viral antigens tested positive. A second SARS-CoV-2 PCR-NP was not obtained. Tests for influenza A virus, respiratory syncytial virus, and human metapneumovirus were negative. Electrocardiogram traced normal sinus rhythm without abnormal QT interval. Cranial imaging and cerebral spinal fluid analysis were not performed. She had an uneventful clinical course and was discharged after two days of observation.

3. Discussion

Children have fewer symptoms compared to adults [9] when coinfected with SARS-CoV-2 and influenza. Our patient experienced only nasal congestion in the two days preceding the apneic episode. She was feeding well and gaining weight. Domestic exposure to school-age siblings or by community spread was likely the mode of transmission. The siblings were asymptomatic and not tested. The mother tested COVID-19 negative at delivery, making vertical transmission unlikely. Our patient also did not have leukopenia or elevated CRP as previously reported in children infected with SARS-CoV-2 [10]. SARS-CoV-2 coinfection occurs at a higher rate with other respiratory pathogens [6]. Coinfection of SARS-CoV-2 with influenza A or B remains rare [8] and has been reported mainly in adults [11]. Influenza A is three times more common than influenza B and has been associated with apnea. Influenza B does not usually present with apnea. Coinfection with a second virus does not increase the frequency of apnea [12]. Similar to all respiratory viral illnesses, the most common symptoms of influenza B in children include fever, cough, and rhinorrhea. Those infected with influenza B tend to have milder symptoms and are symptomatic late into influenza season. Our patient presented at the beginning of influenza season and was too young to be protected by influenza vaccine. Whether one virus predisposed the infant to a second virus remains to be determined. The long-term effects of SARS-CoV-2 on young infants also remain to be determined. Our patient demonstrated full recovery without medical intervention.

Apnea occurs rarely in healthy full-term infants compared to preterm infants [13] with an incidence rate of one in 1000 [14]. Apnea presenting during the first weeks of life hints of "brief resolved unexplained event" (BRUE). In 2016, the American Academy of Pediatrics defined BRUE as an "acute event described by an observer with change in breathing, appearance, muscle tone and altered level of responsiveness lasting less than one minute in an infant younger than 12 months of age." The term BRUE replaced "apparent life-threatening event" (ALTE) and "near-miss sudden infant death syndrome" (SIDS), terms previously used to designate apnea [15]. The history and physical examination of our patient met criteria for high-risk BRUE for age (<60 days) and duration of event (>one minute). Apnea

associated with SARS-CoV-2 infection has been reported [13, 16, 17] and may be the presenting symptom [16, 17]. The COVID-19 pandemic and season for epidemic respiratory illnesses resulted in screening for viral respiratory illnesses. Tests for influenza A virus, respiratory syncytial virus, and human metapneumovirus, all known to be associated with apnea, were negative. BRUE was excluded when our patient tested positive for SARS-CoV-2 and influenza B.

4. Conclusion

We report the first case of apnea as the presenting symptom of SARS-CoV-2 and influenza B coinfection in a term infant. Apnea may be a symptom of COVID-19, of influenza B, or of coinfection. Healthcare providers should have a high index of suspicion for SARS-CoV-2 infection when infants have apnea and subtle respiratory symptoms. Based on our single case, coinfection does not necessarily predispose the infant to poor outcomes. Much larger studies are needed to characterize more accurately presenting symptoms and disease course in infants. It remains unclear from whom the infant contracted SARS-CoV-2 and influenza B.

References

[1] World Health Organization, "Novel coronavirus (2019-nCoV)," Report, World Health Organization, Geneva, Switzerland, 2020.

[2] P. Zimmermann and N. Curtis, "COVID-19 in children, pregnancy and neonates: a review of epidemiologic and clinical features," *Pediatric Infectious Disease Journal*, vol. 39, no. 6, pp. 469–477, 2020.

[3] M. A. Alexander-Miller, "Challenges for the newborn following influenza virus infection and prospects for an effective vaccine," *Frontiers in Immunology*, vol. 11, 2020.

[4] J. L. Miatech, N. N. Tarte, S. Katragadda, J. Polman, and S. B. Robichaux, "A case series of coinfection with SARS-CoV-2 and influenza virus in Louisiana," *Respiratory Medicine Case Reports*, vol. 31, Article ID 101214, 2020.

[5] B. Singh, P. Kaur, R.-J. Reid, F. Shamoon, and M. Bikkina, "COVID-19 and influenza co-infection: report of three cases," *Cureus*, vol. 12, no. 8, Article ID :e9852, 2020.

[6] J. S. Musuuza, L. Watson, V. Parmasad, N. Putman-Buehler, L. Christensen, and N. Safdar, "Prevalence and outcomes of co-infection and superinfection with SARS-CoV-2 and other pathogens: a systematic review and meta-analysis," *PLoS One*, vol. 16, no. 5, Article ID e0251170, 2021.

[7] J. Stowe, E. Tessier, H. Zhao et al., "Interactions between SARS-CoV-2 and influenza, and the impact of coinfection on disease severity: a test-negative design," *International Journal of Epidemiology*, vol. 50, no. 4, pp. 1124–1133, 2021.

[8] R. Ozaras, R. Cirpin, A. Duran et al., "Influenza and COVID-19 coinfection: report of six cases and review of the literature," *Journal of Medical Virology*, vol. 92, no. 11, pp. 2657–2665, 2020.

[9] G. Wehl, M. Laible, and M. Rauchenzauner, "Co-infection of SARS CoV-2 and influenza A in a pediatric patient in Germany," *Klinische Pädiatrie*, vol. 232, no. 04, pp. 217-218, 2020.

[10] A. Hoang, K. Chorath, A. Moreira et al., "COVID-19 in 7780 pediatric patients: a systematic review," *EClinicalMedicine*, vol. 24, Article ID 100433, 2020.

[11] D. Kim, J. Quinn, B. Pinsky, N. H. Shah, and I. Brown, "Rates

of Co-infection between SARS-CoV-2 and other respiratory pathogens," *JAMA*, vol. 323, no. 20, pp. 2085-2086, 2020.

[12] S. Ricart, N. Rovira, J. J. Garcia-Garcia et al., "Frequency of apnea and respiratory viruses in infants with bronchiolitis," *Pediatric Infectious Disease Journal*, vol. 33, no. 9, pp. 988–990, 2014.

[13] G. Loron, T. Tromeur, P. Venot et al., "COVID-19 associated with life-threatening apnea in an infant born preterm: a case report," *Frontiers in Pediatrics*, vol. 8, p. 568, 2020.

[14] J. C. Levin, J. Jang, and L. M. Rhein, "Apnea in the otherwise healthy, term newborn: national prevalence and utilization during the birth hospitalization," *The Journal of Pediatrics*, vol. 181, pp. 67–73, 2017.

[15] J. S. Tieder, J. L. Bonkowsky, R. A. Etzel et al., "Brief resolved unexplained events (formerly apparent life-threatening events) and evaluation of lower-risk infants," *Pediatrics*, vol. 137, no. 5, Article ID e20160590, 2016.

[16] J. S. Needleman and A. E. Hanson, "COVID-19-associated apnea and circumoral cyanosis in a 3-week-old," *BMC Pediatrics*, vol. 20, no. 1, p. 382, 2020.

[17] A. González Brabin, M. I. Iglesias-Bouzas, M. Nieto-Moro, A. Martínez de Azagra-Garde, and A. García-Salido, "Apnea neonatal como manifestación inicial de infección por SARS-CoV-2 [Neonatal apnea as initial manifestation of SARS-CoV-2 infection]," *Anales de Pediatría*, vol. 93, no. 3, pp. 215-216, 2020.

12

Thanatophoric Dysplasia: A Report of 2 Cases with Antenatal Misdiagnosis

Lamidi Audu ⓘD,[1] Amina Gambo,[1] Tokan Silas Baduku,[1] Bilkisu Farouk,[1] Anisa Yahaya,[2] and Kefas Jacob[2]

[1]Department of Paediatrics and Child Health, Barau Dikko Teaching Hospital, Kaduna State University, Kaduna, Nigeria
[2]Department of Radiology, Barau Dikko Teaching Hospital, Kaduna State University, Kaduna, Nigeria

Correspondence should be addressed to Lamidi Audu; lamidi.audu@npmcn.edu.ng

Academic Editor: Maria Moschovi

Thanatophoric dysplasia (TD) is a rare but uniformly lethal inherited disorder of the skeletal system resulting from defects in the fibroblast growth factor receptor-3 gene on the short arm of chromosome ##4. It is characterised by pronounced shortening of the tubular bones resulting in significant short stature, macrocephaly, a funnel-shaped chest, protuberant abdomen, redundant skin in the limbs, and typical facies among others. The two clinical types of TD are differentiated by typical cranial and tubular bone configurations. Antenatal diagnosis is usually made in the last trimester and corroborated at birth. We present 2 cases of TD seen at Barau Dikko Teaching Hospital (BDTH) between January and August 2021 to highlight the potential difficulty with antenatal diagnosis, its diagnostic features, and associated early postnatal fatality. The antenatal diagnosis was missed in both cases in spite of repeated 2nd and 3rd-trimester sonographic examinations. Both babies presented with remarkable micromelic short stature with the telephone-handle appearance of the femoral bones characteristic of type 1 TD, developed progressive respiratory distress at birth, and died within 36 hours of life despite respiratory support with Bubble CPAP. These cases are discussed along with a review of existing relevant literature.

1. Introduction

Thanatophoric dysplasia, (TD) was reportedly used for the first time in 1967 by Marateaux, Lamy, and Roberts who differentiated this condition from classical achondroplasia. [1] It is a rare autosomal dominant disease resulting from genetic mutations affecting the fibroblast growth factor receptor-3 (FGFR3) gene located on the short arm of chromosome number 4. [2]. While there are 3 known mutations responsible for type 1 TD (R248C, Y373C, and S249C), type 2 is associated with only 1 mutation (K650E, also known as p.Lys650Glu). This mutation has 100% penetrance [3]. Despite its rarity, TD is the most common lethal chondrodysplasia with population-based incidence ranging from 1.1/100000 in Japan [4] to 2.1–3.0/100000 in the US [5].

Babies with thanatophoric dysplasia characteristically present with macrocephaly, depressed nasal bridge, extreme shortening of tubular bones and ribs, narrow bell-shaped thorax, redundant skin folds in the extremities, vertebral body thinning, malformed temporal lobe, as well as hypoplastic lungs. Two clinical subtypes are differentiated by the presence of curved long bones shaped like table telephone handle seen in type 1 TD and cloverleaf-shaped head with straight long bones and less severe flatness of the vertebral bodies in type 2 TD [6].

Affected babies develop severe respiratory distress as a result of pulmonary hypoplasia, rapidly progressing to death within 24 hours. [6, 7]. Death may also be due to asphyxiating thoracic constriction or compression of the spinal cord and brainstem from a narrow foramen magnum [8].

In Nigeria, obstetric care is characterised by low antenatal-care attendance [9] and a high rate of out-of-hospital delivery. [10] In this setting, uncommon and lethal congenital abnormalities such as TD would rarely be seen by health workers and the resultant clinical knowledge gap

TABLE 1: Physical examination and radiographical features of babies 1 and 2.

Physical and radiological findings	Baby 1	Baby 2
Short stature	+	+
Macrocephaly	+	+
Cloverleaf head	−	−
Wide suture	+	+
Low-set ears	+	+
Depressed nasal bridge	+	+
Multiple skin folds	+	+
Narrow bell-shaped chest	+	+
Protuberant abdomen	+	+
Respiratory distress	+	+
Hypoplastic lung	+	+
Curved, telephone-handle femur	+	+
Curved telephone-handle humerus	+	−
Brachydactyly	+	+
Cyanosis	+	+

TABLE 2: Anthropometry of babies 1 and 2.

Measurements	Baby 1	Baby 2	Normal values
Birth weight	2.5 kg	2.2 kg	3.1 ± 0.5 kg[xx]
Length	38 cm	38 cm	49.9 ± 2.9 cm
Occipitofrontal circumference (OFC)	40 cm	43 cm	34.4 ± 1.7 cm
Chest circumference (CC)	27 cm	25 cm	33 ± 2.8 cm
Upper: Lower segment	2.45	2.54	1.41[y]
OFC: CC	1.5	1.72	1.04

[xx] Reference 15. [y] Reference 16

creates room for antenatal and postnatal misdiagnosis. This publication is informed by our conviction that individual case reports of such patients are important to create awareness to bridge the existing clinical knowledge gap.

2. Case Report (Baby 1)

Baby 1 was a term female neonate delivered spontaneously per vagina with "multiple malformations" at BDTH Kaduna, to a 25-year-old para 2 + 0 (all alive and normal) mother. The APGAR scores were 6 and 7 at the 1st and 5th minute, respectively. Before the plan for NICU admission was concluded, the parents left the hospital with the baby of their volition but returned 14 hours later to the hospital because of inability to suck and progressive breathing difficulty.

The mother received antenatal care and took both orthodox and herbal medications but was not exposed to any known teratogens. She was neither hypertensive nor diabetic pre- or postconception and there was no family history of congenital abnormalities. A 3rd-trimester ultrasound reported the "presence of polyhydramnios but no evidence of fetal abnormalities." The father was a 40-year-old businessman who had no consanguineous relationship with the mother.

On examination, she was severely dyspneic with chest wall recessions, nasal flaring, tachypnea, and central cyanosis. She was visibly dysmorphic with macrocephaly,

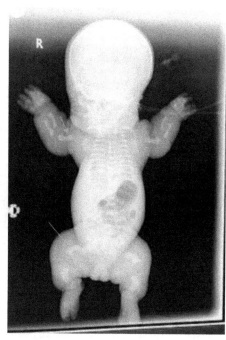

FIGURE 1: Plain radiograph of baby 1 with features of TD type 1. Arrows show telephone-handle shaped humerus and femur.

frontal bossing, sutural diastasis, depressed nasal bridge, and low-set ears. Other notable abnormalities included very short upper and lower limbs, with multiple excessive skin folds, short and stubby digits (brachydactyly), a narrow chest, and a protuberant abdomen. The head was not tri-lobed. Anthropometry revealed a weight of 2.5 kg, length of 38 cm (upper segment = 27 cm, lower segment = 11 cm, US : LS ratio = 2.45), occipitofrontal circumference (OFC) = 40 cm, and chest circumference (CC) = 27 cm, OFC : CC = 1.5 cm. The clinical examination findings are summarized in Tables 1 and 2.

A clinical diagnosis of congenital dwarfism most likely thanatophoric dysplasia was made with differential diagnoses of achondroplasia and achondrogenesis. The radiological findings (Figure 1 and Table 1) included macrocephaly with craniofacial disproportion, narrow chest with flattened ribs, poorly aerated lung fields, shortening of the long bones with telephone-handle appearance of the humerus and femur bilaterally, and widening of vertebral bodies with reduced heights. These along with the clinical features were in keeping with a diagnosis of thanatophoric dysplasia type 1. She was nursed on bubble CPAP and glucose infusion in spite of which respiratory distress deteriorated rapidly, and she died at a postnatal age of 20 hours.

3. Case Report (Baby 2)

Baby 2 (male) was brought into SCBU 2 hours postdelivery. He was delivered to a 35-year-old gravida 10 Para 9 + 2 (9 alive) mother by elective caesarean section at term. The APGAR scores were 6 and 8 in the 1st and 5th minute, respectively, and the birth weight was 2.2 kg.

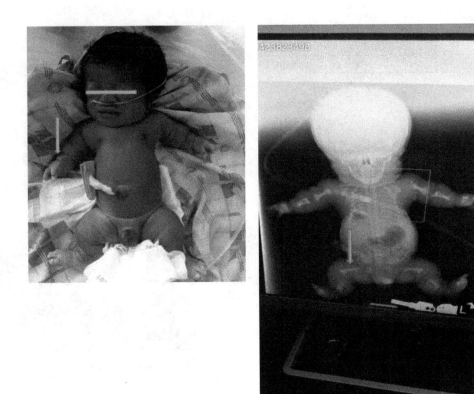

(a)

(b)

FIGURE 2: (a) A clinical photograph of baby 2 with thanatophoric dysplasia: large head prominent skin folds (arrow), narrow chest, and short limbs. (b) A plain radiograph of baby 2 with features of TD type 1. The arrow shows a curved telephone-handle femur.

The pregnancy was booked for antenatal care at about 32 weeks gestation at a private health facility from where the mother was referred to BDTH on account of an abdominal ultrasound examination which revealed "fetal abnormalities," but the details were not specified. A repeat USS at our facility at 35 weeks showed polyhydramnios and shortening of fetal long bones and a diagnosis of achondrogenesis was made.

There was no maternal history of hypertension, diabetes mellitus, or sickle cell disease. The mother received routine antenatal medications and was not exposed to any known teratogens. The father was a 45 years old self-employed businessman. The family was monogamous, non-consanguineous, and had no history of congenital malformations. However, 2nd and 4th pregnancies ended as 1st-trimester spontaneous abortions.

Examination revealed a term baby with obvious abnormalities characterised by short stature, macrocephaly, depressed nasal bridge, narrow chest, and distended abdomen, but no palpably enlarged organs. Other prominent features included micromelia and multiple segmented circumferential skin folds on all the limbs. He was in severe respiratory distress with central cyanosis and poor, barely audible breath sounds. Respiratory rate was 65/min, heart rate = 134 beats/min, heart sounds were 1 and 2 only, no murmur. He was conscious with patent fontanels and widened sutures while muscle tone and primitive reflexes were slightly depressed. Anthropometry: weight = 2.2 kg, length = 38 cm, occipitofrontal circumference (OFC) = 43 cm, chest circumference (CC) = 25 cm, OFC : CC = 1.72, arm span = 28 cm, upper segment (crown-rump length) = 28 cm, lower segment (rump-heel length) = 11 cm, upper: and lower segment ratio = 2.54. The clinical and radiographical features are summarized in Tables 1 and 2 and shown in Figures 2(a) and 2(b). A diagnosis of TD type 1 was made, and he received intranasal oxygen and intravenous glucose infusion, and the parents were counseled. There was a transient noticeable improvement in oxygenation but the baby subsequently developed progressive dyspnea and poor saturation despite continuous positive airway pressure (CPAP) support and died at the age of 32 hours.

4. Discussion

We have presented the first 2 cases of "neonatal dwarfs" with clinical and radiological features of thanatophoric dysplasia type 1, a rare form of congenital chondrodysplasias, from our center. In spite of 2nd and 3rd-trimester sonography, prenatal diagnosis was not made. This highlights the difficulty that may be associated with antenatal diagnosis. Several authors have, on the contrary, reported cases of TD correctly diagnosed in-utero with sonographic examination [11, 12]. Skeletal dysplasias can be diagnosed in-utero with increasing accuracy as the pregnancy advances. Increased nuchal translucency and shortened limbs are seen in the first trimester while polyhydramnios, narrow chest cavity and ribs, bowed femur, and macrocephaly become prominent in later trimesters [11]. Therefore, timely, meticulous, and skillful application of abdominal sonographic examination should accurately diagnose TD in-utero (polyhydramnios, macrocephaly, micromelic short stature, and straight or curved femur/humerus) and clearly differentiate this from other micromelic dwarfs [1]. Genetic counseling can then be initiated promptly.

There was no family history of the disease in both patients. TD is an autosomal dominant (AD) disease with remarkably high perinatal fatality and each case invariably results from a "de novo" genetic mutation. The parents are phenotypically normal, recurrence risk in subsequent offspring is nonexistent, and positive family history is unlikely. This was alluded to by Waller et al. [5] who reported that none of the 48 cases of TD seen in a population-based study in Texas US was inherited. An interesting observation in their study was the increased prevalence of TD with higher paternal age giving rise to the postulation of a possible paternal origin for the mutated gene. Although the genetic basis for the speculated paternal origin of this mutation is yet unproven, it is noteworthy that the paternal ages of our patients were high; 40 years and 45 years for babies 1 and 2, respectively and this information may contribute to the buildup of epidemiologic evidence for this observation.

Thanatophoric dysplasia is defined by unique anthropometry and skeletal morphology. In the babies here presented, we demonstrated extreme short stature with crown-heel length greater than 3SD below the mean length of Nigerian newborn babies (49.2 ± 2.4 M, 48.8 ± 2.5 F) [13], as well as remarkable micromelia and disproportionate short stature; (upper segment: lower segment = 2.45, normal = 1.41) [14]. They both coincidentally had a length of 38 cm which is similar to the documented average length of thanatophoric dwarfs [3, 8] in addition to other features detailed in the table. The presence of curved telephone handle-shaped femora confirmed type 1 TD while the absence of cloverleaf head excluded type 2 TD in both cases. Very rarely, however, clinical overlaps have been reported. For example, Salinas–Torres [15] described a female dichorionic twin with thanatophoric dysplasia phenotype who presented with both curved femur and cloverleaf head but classified this as type 1 TD. Corsello et al. [16] reported a set of monozygotic twins who were concordant for short and curved femur but discordant for cloverleaf head and both were designated type 1 TD. This suggests that the telephone-handle appearance of the femur is a more specific feature of TD than the cloverleaf head, the presence of the cloverleaf head defines type 2 TD only when the long bones are straight; the cloverleaf head can also be seen in type I TD.

We did not conduct genetic analysis on our patients for lack of appropriate facilities. However, in spite of being a genetic disorder with clearly defined molecular abnormality, clinical and radiological features are sufficiently characteristic and therefore often suffice in its diagnosis [5, 17]. Therefore, a combination of postnatal clinical and radiological examination clinches the diagnosis even without molecular testing.

Extrauterine survival is usually severely impaired, resulting in early postneonatal death if respiratory support is not provided [4]. Aggressive respiratory support and surgical decompression of the foramen magnum followed by comprehensive physical rehabilitation may result in prolonged survival [18]. Death is attributed to a number of factors and particularly, asphyxiating thoracic constriction and pulmonary hypoplasia [6, 8]. In the absence of postmortem examination, the exact immediate cause of death in our cases can only be speculative.

The differential diagnoses of thanatophoric dysplasia include achondrogenesis and achondroplasia among others. Achondrogenesis is associated with extreme dwarfism and postnatal fatality but lacks the classical multiple skin folds of the extremities [19], while achondroplasia is compatible with long-term survival [20]. The typical configuration of the femur and humerus in TD is absent in both conditions.

5. Conclusion

Thanatophoric dysplasia, a rare genetic skeletal dysplasia, is a distinct clinical and radiological entity that requires a thorough and skillful antenatal sonographic fetal diagnosis for early family counseling. Antenatal misdiagnosis can be avoided by creating awareness to bridge the existing knowledge gap.

Additional Points

(i) In spite of the unique prenatal sonographic and postnatal clinical and radiological features of TD, antenatal misdiagnosis can occur presumably because of its rarity and similarity to other micromelic dwarfs. (ii) Anthropometric computations may provide more specific information to define the phenotypic characteristics of thanatophoric dysplasia. (iii) There is a need to further explore the speculated association of TD with high paternal age.

Acknowledgments

The authors acknowledge the contribution of the entire staff of the Neonatal Unit for their contribution to the care of the babies before their demise.

References

[1] K. Shah, R. Astley, and A. H. Cameron, "Thanatophoric dwarfism," *Journal of Medical Genetics*, vol. 10, no. 3, pp. 243–252, 1973.

[2] "What is the gene that causes thanatophoric dysplasia? ThinkGenetic," 2022, http://www.thinkgenetic.com/diseases/thanatophoric-dysplasia/causes/56759.

[3] G. L. Defendi, "Thanatophoric dysplasia," 2022, http://www.emedicine.medscape.com.

[4] H. Sawai, K. Oka, M. Ushioda et al., "National survey of prevalence and prognosis of Thanatophoric dysplasia in Japan," *Pediatrics International*, vol. 61, no. 8, pp. 748–753, 2019.

[5] D. Waller, A. Correa, T. M. Vo et al., "The population-based prevalence of Achondroplasia and thanatophoric dysplasia in selected regions of the US," *American Journal of Medical Genetics, Part A*, vol. 146A, no. 18, pp. 2385–2389, 2008.

[6] U. Jahan, A. Sharma, N. Gupta, S. Gupta, F. Usmani, and A. Rajput, "Thanatophoric dysplasia: a case report," *International Journal of Reproduction, Contraception, Obstetrics and Gynecology*, vol. 8, no. 2, pp. 758–761, 2019.

[7] B. Dereje, Y. Gebrehiwot, and J. Schenider, "A case Of thanatophoric dysplasia type I: The first clinicopathologic report from Ethiopia Ethiopian," *Journal of Reproductive Health (EJRH)*, vol. 10, no. 3, pp. 65–70, 2018.

[8] T. French and R. Savarirayan, *Thanatophoric Dysplasia*, University of Washington, Seattle, WA, USA, 2004.

[9] A. F. Fagbamigbe, O. Olaseinde, and V. Setlhare, "Sub-national analysis and determinants of numbers of antenatal care contacts in Nigeria: assessing the compliance with the WHO recommended standard guidelines," *BMC Pregnancy and Childbirth*, vol. 21, no. 1, p. 402, 2021.

[10] S. T. Adedokun and O. A. Uthman, "Women who have not utilized health facility for delivery in Nigeria: who are they and where do they live?" *BMC Pregnancy and Childbirth*, vol. 19, 2019.

[11] B. B. Jimah, T. A. Mensah, K. Ulzen-Apiah et al., "Prenatal diagnosis of skeletal dysplasia and review of the literature," *Case Reports in Obstetrics and Gynaecology*, vol. 2021, Article ID 9940063, 5 pages, 2021.

[12] O. W. Daniyan, O. Ezeanosike, C. Ogbonna-Nwosiu, and U. C. Ulodiba, "Thanatophoric Dysplasia type 1as seen in a tertiary institution in South-East Nigeria," *Nigerian Journal of Paediatrics*, vol. 47, no. 3, pp. 277–279, 2020.

[13] O. Oluwafemi, F. Njokanma, E. Disu, and T. Ogunlesi, "The current pattern of gestational age-related anthropometric parameters of term Nigerian Neonates," *South African Journal of Child Health*, vol. 7, no. 3, pp. 100–104, 2013.

[14] S. Kondpalle, R. Lote-Oke, P. Patel, V. Khadilkar, and A. V. Khadilkar, "Upper and lower body segment ratios from birth to 18 years in children from western Maharashtra," *Indian Journal of Pediatrics*, vol. 86, no. 6, pp. 503–507, 2019.

[15] V. M. Salinas-Torres, "Thanatophoric dysplasia type 1 with cloverleaf skull in a dichorionic twin," *Genetic Counseling*, vol. 26, no. 1, pp. 61–65, 2015.

[16] G. Corsello, E. Maresi, C. Rossi, L. Giuffrè, and E. Cittadini, "Thanatophoric dysplasia in monozygotic twins discordant for cloverleaf skull: prenatal diagnosis, clinical and pathological findings," *American Journal of Medical Genetics, Part A*, vol. 42, no. 1, pp. 122–126, 1992.

[17] D. E. Donnelly, V. McConnell, A. Paterson, and P. J. Morrison, "The prevalence of thanatophoric dysplasia and lethal osteogenesis imperfecta type II in Northern Ireland—a complete population study," *Ulster Medical Journal*, vol. 79, no. 3, pp. 114–118, 2010.

[18] R. S. Carolle, A. L. Duker, A. J. Schelhaas, M. E. Little, E. J. Miller, and M. B. Bober, "Should we stop calling thanatophoric dysplasia a lethal condition? A case report of a long term survivor," *Palliative Medicine Reports*, vol. 1, 2020.

[19] Z. Villines, "Achondrogenesis: definition, causes, diagnosis, and more (medicalnewstoday.Com)," 2022, https://www.medicalnewstoday.com/article/Achondrogenesis.

[20] W. A. Horton, J. G. Hall, and J. T. Hecht, "Achondroplasia," *The Lancet*, vol. 370, no. 9582, pp. 162–172, 2007.

13

Persistent Atraumatic Knee Pain in a Teenage Female with Bony Protuberance Secondary to Hook-Shaped Osteochrondroma

Adityanarayan Rao ⓘ,[1] Joshua Pryor,[1] Jaclyn Otero,[2] and Molly Posa ⓘ[2]

[1]University of Florida College of Medicine, Gainesville, FL 32610, USA
[2]University of Florida-Pediatrics Department, Gainesville, FL 32610, USA

Correspondence should be addressed to Molly Posa; mollyposa@ufl.edu

Academic Editor: Juan Mejía-Aranguré

A 13-year-old female presented at her pediatrician's office with a complaint of sharp, intermittent, right-sided knee pain that had been present for the previous three days without any known trauma and no association with activity. Her medical history was significant for fractures, and on physical exam, there was a hard mass palpated on the medial aspect of her distal thigh that was nontender, nonmobile, and without overlying skin changes. The plain radiograph findings were consistent with a hook-shaped osteochondroma of the right medial distal metaphysis. Orthopedics recommended conservative management with continued ibuprofen for pain and six-week follow-up with repeat Deletedradiograph to evaluate for progression. The follow-up Deletedradiograph showed no interval growth. However, due to continued pain, the patient had surgical excision of the osteochondroma six months after initial presentation, allowing her to finish her current soccer season. The surgery was successful, and the patient did well after operation with no residual pain.

1. Background

Osteochondromas are the most common type of benign bone lesions accounting for nearly 30% of benign bone tumors. This condition is more common in males than in females at an approximate ratio of 2 : 1 and most frequently presents in children under 21 years of age [1]. This case highlights the need for holistic evaluation of each patient and under what circumstances to proceed with surgical intervention for this condition.

2. Case Presentation

A 13-year-old female presents at her pediatrician's office with a complaint of sharp, intermittent, right-sided knee pain that has been present for the previous three days. The patient first noticed the pain when she awoke three days ago. She denies any recent physical activity or known trauma. The pain occurs 2-3 times a day and is rapid in onset, lasting anywhere from 30 minutes to 3 hours. There is no association with time of day, activity, or rest. She states it feels like "someone hit her with a hammer," and she has not found any aggravating factors. ibuprofen provides only minimal relief. The adolescent reports that she has recently had a growth spurt. The pain has not hindered her daily activities, and she has not noticed knee swelling, redness, or decreased range of motion. On pertinent review of systems, she denies fevers, chills, night sweats, weight loss, rash, palpitations, abdominal pain, vomiting, diarrhea, constipation, back pain, or pain in any additional joints.

Her medical history is significant for right radial and ulnar fractures requiring short arm casting after closed reduction, as well as a 5th metatarsal fracture (Jones fracture) on her right foot. All of these occurred due to sports-related injuries and falls. She is not currently taking any medication other than ibuprofen as needed for knee pain. Her family history is negative for autoimmune disorders and childhood cancer.

On physical exam, there is a hard mass palpable on the medial aspect of her distal thigh that is nontender, nonmobile, and without overlying skin changes. She has full painless range of motion of her right knee on both extension and flexion, with negative anterior and posterior drawer, Lachman's, valgus and varus manipulation, and Thessaly's tests. There is no joint line, tibial plateau, patellar, or quadriceps tendon tenderness. There is no motor deficit, and there is normal sensation in the right lower extremity. The patient has normal gait. Due to a visual and palpable mass being present on physical examination, a radiograph Deleted of the right knee and femur is obtained with concerns for osteochondroma versus malignancy. The plain radiograph findings are consistent with a hook-shaped osteochondroma of the right medial distal metaphysis (Figures 1 and 2), and the patient was referred to orthopedics due to the significant pain.

3. Outcome

Orthopedics recommended conservative management with continued ibuprofen for pain and six-week follow-up with repeat Deletedradiograph to evaluate for progression. Physical therapy was not recommended during the six-week observation period. The patient continued to have pain consistent with initial presentation throughout the interceding six weeks. The follow-up radiograph Deleted showed no interval growth. Due to continued pain, the patient had surgical excision of the osteochondroma six months after initial presentation, allowing her to finish her current soccer season. The surgery was successful, and the patient did well after operation with no residual pain (Figure 3).

4. Discussion

Classic presentation of osteochondroma includes a single painless palpable mass located at the ends of the long bones or along the axial skeleton found incidentally on imaging after a trauma. The most common sites of growth are the ends of the long bones with special affinity for the distal and proximal femur as well as the proximal humerus [2]. While these lesions are usually painless, their frequency in the pediatric population and the possibility for pain and restriction of movement emphasize the importance of further clinical evaluation.

The lesion itself consists of a bony spur (sessile or pedunculated shape) with a cartilaginous cap, usually located at the epiphysis or metadiaphysis of the bone. The exact cause of formation is unknown, but osteochondroma pathophysiology manifests as a peripheral chondroblast growing outward from a metaphysis forming a cap over the bone [3]. The cartilaginous cap serves as the source of growth which typically continues until skeletal maturity occurs. Malignant changes are rare and occur in about 1% of the patient population: if this does occur, it typically occurs at 20–30 years of age with transformation of the lesion to chondrosarcoma [3, 4]. However, an autosomal dominant condition Multiple Hereditary Osteochondromatosis (germline mutations in EXT1

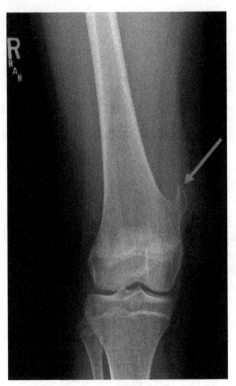

FIGURE 1: An anterior posterior radiograph of the patient's right knee with limited view of the femur showing the hook-shaped osteochondroma (red arrow).

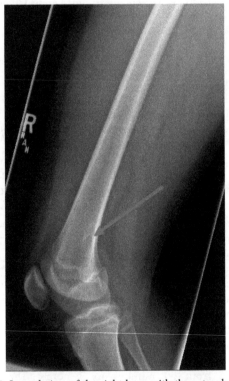

FIGURE 2: Lateral view of the right knee with the osteochondroma (red arrow).

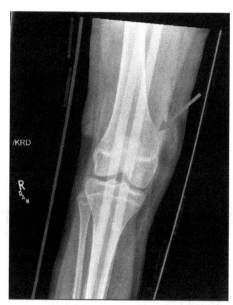

FIGURE 3: Plain radiograph of the right knee status after surgical excision of the osteochondroma with an immobilizer in place.

or EXT2 tumor suppressor genes) manifests as multiple lesions with a significantly higher probability of progression to malignancy (1% to 20%) [2, 5].

For a child presenting with a palpable bony mass, further investigation is recommended to rule out malignancy. The most common methodology of imaging is conventional radiology with specific attention to the anatomic location and the presence of transition zones [1]. A key radiological finding in osteochondroma is mineralization of the matrix, without which diagnosis is more difficult. In these cases, a computer tomography (CT) or magnetic resonance imaging (MRI) to identify additional features of osteochondromas, including endosteal scalloping, thick periosteal reaction, and cortical hook, is recommended [1].

Most cases of osteochondromas do not require surgical treatment, as osteochondromas will cease to grow after the patient reaches skeletal maturity. As such, first-line treatment involves conservative observation with imaging to monitor growth [6]. Surgical excisions are primarily reserved for patients with pain and/or reduced range of motion: persistent, significant pain was present in our patient, which is why surgical resection was recommended. In addition, cases of deformity and potential malignant transformation should be treated surgically [6].

Prognosis for osteochondromas, in both surgical resection as well as conservative management, is excellent. If surgical resection is considered, it is recommended after skeletal maturity occurs to decrease the risk of recurrence [4]. If surgery is necessary prior to skeletal maturity, due to pain or restriction of movement, a partial excision is recommended to preserve the physis, so as not to affect growth potential [7].

Our patient is an excellent reflection of the above findings. After diagnosis with an osteochondroma, the patient was managed conservatively for six months with the use of non-steroidal anti-inflammatory drugs before finally opting for surgical excision due to pain. Further follow-up

demonstrated no residual pain and full range of motion reflecting the curative ability of surgical intervention for osteochondroma treatment.

References

[1] G. R. Gaumer, D. S. Weinberg, C. D. Collier, P. J. Getty, and R. W. Liu, "An osteological study on the prevalence of osteochondromas," *The Iowa Orthopaedic Journal*, vol. 37, pp. 147–150, 2017.

[2] D. N. Hakim, T. Pelly, M. Kulendran, and J. A. Caris, "Benign tumours of the bone: a review," *Journal of Bone Oncology*, vol. 4, no. 2, pp. 37–41, 2015.

[3] L. Copley and J. P. Dormans, "Benign pediatric bone tumors," *Pediatric Clinics of North America*, vol. 43, no. 4, pp. 949–966, 1996.

[4] L. Hameetman, J. V. Bovée, A. H. Taminiau, H. M. Kroon, and P. C. Hogendoorn, "Multiple osteochondromas: clinicopathological and genetic spectrum and suggestions for clinical management," *Hereditary Cancer in Clinical Practice*, vol. 2, no. 4, p. 161, 2004.

[5] M. N. Baig, S. O'Malley, C. Fenelon, and K. Kaar, "Osteochondroma of acromioclavicular joint," *BMJ Case Reports*, vol. 12, no. 8, Article ID e230246, 2019.

[6] J. V. Bovée, "Multiple osteochondromas," *Orphanet Journal of Rare Diseases*, vol. 3, p. 3, 2008.

[7] K. R. Chin, F. D. Kharrazi, B. S. Miller, H. J. Mankin, and M. C. Gebhardt, "Osteochondromas of the distal aspect of the tibia or fibula," *Journal of Bone and Joint Surgery American Volume*, vol. 82, no. 9, pp. 1269–1278, 2000.

14

Successful Treatment with Antibiotics Alone for Infant Rib Osteomyelitis

Yasuaki Matsumoto ⓘ,[1] Katsuyoshi Shimozawa ⓘ,[1,2] Junko Yamanaka ⓘ,[1] Yukari Atsumi ⓘ,[1] Tomomi Ota ⓘ,[1,3] Shinji Mochizuki ⓘ,[1] and Hiroyuki Shichino ⓘ[1]

[1]*Department of Pediatrics, National Center for Global Health and Medicine Hospital, 1-21-1 Toyama, Shinjuku-ku, Tokyo 162-8655, Japan*
[2]*Department of Pediatrics and Child Health, Nihon University School of Medicine, 30-1 Oyaguchikami-cho, Itabashi-ku, Tokyo 173-8610, Japan*
[3]*Division of Neonatology, Nagano Children's Hospital, 3100 Toyoshina, Azumino-shi, Nagano 399-8288, Japan*

Correspondence should be addressed to Yasuaki Matsumoto; ymatsumoto@hosp.ncgm.go.jp and Junko Yamanaka; jyamanak@hosp.ncgm.go.jp

Academic Editor: Vjekoslav Krzelj

Pediatric rib osteomyelitis is a rare disease occurring predominantly in the neonatal period and early childhood and accounting for about 1% of all pediatric osteomyelitis. Compared to osteomyelitis in other parts of the body, pediatric rib osteomyelitis shows few localized findings (such as redness and swelling) and often an indolent lesion as well either of which may delay diagnosis and thus make treatment more difficult. A previously healthy one-year-old girl came to our department with a chief complaint of fever lasting for three days. She was admitted to our department to investigate her fever. At the time of admission, radiographs showed decreased permeability in the left lung field; so, we started antimicrobial therapy on the assumption of pneumonia. On the second day of admission, methicillin-susceptible *Staphylococcus aureus* was detected in the blood culture. A further, more detailed physical examination revealed some slight left anterior chest swelling. We performed a contrast-enhanced CT scan and an MRI and diagnosed her with rib osteomyelitis complicated with a chest wall abscess. She was given intravenous cefazolin for two weeks, switched to oral cephalexin for four weeks, and then recovered completely. She was treated without surgical intervention, having showed a good response to antimicrobial therapy. Osteomyelitis of the ribs in children is reported to be more common in the lower ribs and to occur more frequently in infants. In many cases, the earliest symptoms are nonspecific, so careful examination to detect any subtle abnormalities—such as swelling or mass—is of key importance for early diagnosis in infants. Regarding treatment, most cases of hematogenous osteomyelitis resolve with antimicrobial therapy alone—although surgical intervention may be required in cases of poor response to antimicrobial therapy. Therefore, early diagnosis of rib osteomyelitis through careful physical examination may reduce the chances of requiring surgical intervention.

1. Introduction

Pediatric rib osteomyelitis is a rare disease accounting for approximately 1% of all pediatric osteomyelitis cases [1, 2]. It occurs predominantly in the neonatal period and early childhood, making it difficult for patients to articulate their symptoms [2]. Pediatric rib osteomyelitis is more difficult to diagnose than osteomyelitis of other sites because often the earliest symptoms are nonspecific and lack local findings (such as redness and swelling) and may also present indolent lesions [3] that can further impede diagnosis. We present a case of an infant with rib osteomyelitis complicated with chest wall abscess. The patient was treated successfully with antimicrobial therapy alone and avoided surgical intervention due to early, careful physical examination.

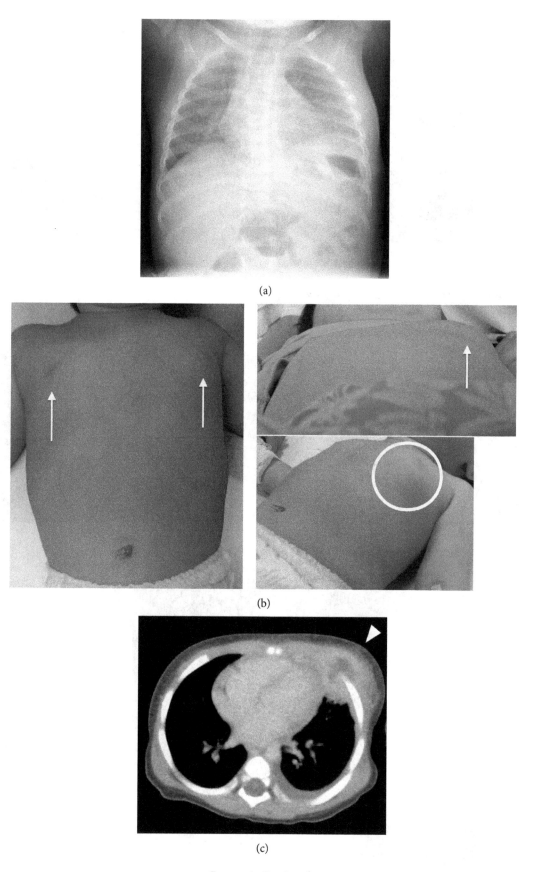

Figure 1: Continued.

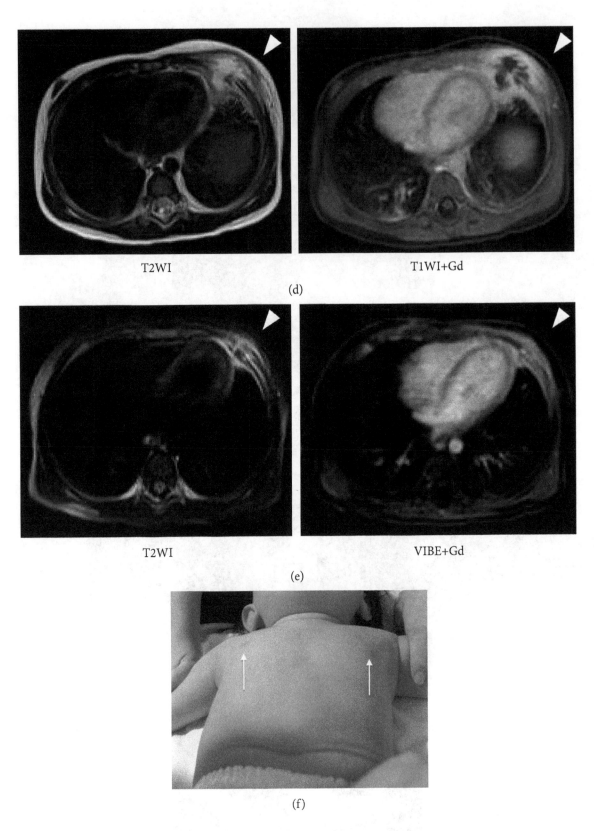

T2WI T1WI+Gd

(d)

T2WI VIBE+Gd

(e)

(f)

FIGURE 1: Continued.

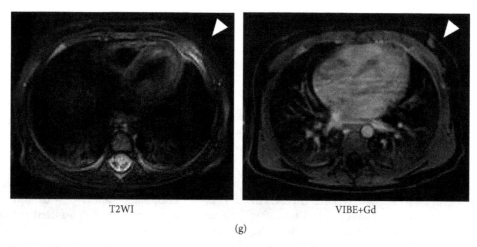

T2WI   VIBE+Gd

(g)

FIGURE 1: (a) Chest X-ray at admission. The permeability in the left middle and lower lung fields is decreased. The left diaphragm is elevated and the left costophrenic angle is dull. (b) Physical findings of the left anterior chest at the time of diagnosis. The left anterior chest is swollen without redness, and the nipple on the affected side is displaced to the upper left. (c) Initial enhanced chest computed tomography (CT) scan on the second day of admission. A low absorption lesion with a contrast effect is detected around the fifth rib, which suggested a chest wall abscess. Left pleural effusion with low volume is detected. (d) T2-weighted and T1-weighted + gadolinium (Gd) chest magnetic resonance imaging (MRI) on the 3rd day of admission. A high signal on T2-weighted images was observed from the anterior part of the left fifth rib to the transitional part of the costal cartilage. (e) T2-weighted and gadolinium-enhanced chest MRI on the 15th day of admission. The size of the abscess around the left fifth rib is greatly reduced. A contrast-enhanced area can be seen from the anterior part of the left fifth rib to the transitional part of the costal cartilage, resulting in the diagnosis of left fifth rib osteomyelitis. (f) Physical findings of the left anterior chest at the time of after 38 days of treatment. Swelling around the left fifth rib and papillary deviation are improving. (g) T2-weighted and gadolinium-enhanced chest MRI on after 38 days of treatment. The contrast area of the anterior portion of the fifth rib to the costochondral transition of the ribs is also reduced.

2. Case Presentation

A previously healthy one-year-old girl was admitted to our hospital with a fever lasting for three days. She had no medical history, and her vaccination status was satisfactory for her age. There were no apparent epidemics nor any known contact with infected people at her nursery schools. At the time of admission, her body temperature was 39.2°C, heart rate was 169 beats/min, respiratory rate was 28 breaths/min, blood pressure was 102/68 mmHg, and oxygen saturation was 98% in room air. Her chest sounds were clear, and there was pharyngeal redness. A laboratory test showed a white blood cell count of 21,290/μL with 66% neutrophils and a C-reactive protein concentration of 9.9 mg/dL. Urinalysis result showed no urinary tract infection. Chest X-ray on the day of admission showed a cardiothoracic ratio of 55%; the left costophrenic angle was dull, and permeability of the left middle and lower lung fields was decreased (Figure 1(a)). Therefore, she was diagnosed with pneumonia and antibiotic therapy was started with cefotaxime.

On the second day of admission, methicillin-sensitive *Staphylococcus aureus* was detected in blood culture, and the antibiotic was changed to cefazolin (150 mg/kg/day). A physical examination revealed slight swelling on the left anterior chest; her mother had been unaware of the swelling before admission (Figure 1(b)). We suspected that her swollen chest was the cause of the fever, and thus an enhanced chest computed tomography (CT) scan was performed. This scan showed a low absorption lesion centered on the left fifth costal cartilage junction, with adjacent soft tissue swelling and ring enhancement. Additionally, mild left

pleural effusion was detected (Figure 1(c)). These findings led to the diagnosis of left anterior chest wall abscess and suspected rib osteomyelitis. On the third day of admission, a contrast-enhanced magnetic resonance imaging (MRI) was performed in order to diagnose rib osteomyelitis. MRI findings showed a 30-mm-large mass in the costochondral transition of the left fifth rib, extending across the ribs to the chest wall and thoracic cavity (Figure 1(d)). In the center of the mass, there was an irregular contrast-enhancing area that extended into the left thoracic cavity and was accompanied by pleural thickening. These results supported the presence of a left anterior chest wall abscess which might have developed from osteomyelitis at the costochondral transition but we were not able to identify osteomyelitis at this time because of the strong signal from the abscess. No methicillin-sensitive *Staphylococcus aureus* was detected in a repeated blood culture after starting cefazolin. On the ninth day of admission, CT scan showed that the abscess had greatly improved. Thus, no surgical treatment was required. On the 15th day of hospitalization, contrast MRI was performed to evaluate for osteomyelitis (Figure 1(e)). The MRI showed that the abscess around the left fifth rib had markedly shrunk, and the swelling in the same area had decreased. At the same time, a contrast area was observed in the anterior part of the left fifth rib to the costochondral transition, leading to the diagnosis of osteomyelitis of the left fifth rib and abscess of the left anterior chest wall. She was treated with cefazolin intravenously for two weeks, and then, this was switched to oral cephalexin (120 mg/kg/day). Subsequently, she was discharged on the 24th day of admission and continued to take cephalexin. Antibiotic therapy was administered for six weeks. Follow-up MRI at 38 days after starting treatment showed that the inflammation around the left fifth rib had improved, and no recurrence was detected (Figures 1(f) and 1(g)).

We evaluated her immune function during her hospitalization which showed no immunological abnormality.

3. Discussion

Rib osteomyelitis in children is an extremely rare disease, accounting for approximately 1% of childhood osteomyelitis [1, 2]. While pediatric osteomyelitis in other areas of the body typically occurs during puberty, osteomyelitis of the ribs typically occurs during infancy [2]. Thus, it is difficult for patients to explain their symptoms. In this case, the patient's mother did not notice chest swelling initially, and neither did the attending physicians. The general presentation of rib osteomyelitis has been reported as fever, chest or back pain, and an abscess [1]; however, other articles have reported that such findings are not always presented—instead, patients may display nonspecific clinical features [3, 4]. Because of these nonspecific symptoms, the lack of local findings (such as redness and swelling), and the indolent lesion that often occurs in cases of rib osteomyelitis [3], it is difficult to diagnose this disease early. This may lead to delays in treatment initiation compared with osteomyelitis affecting other parts, such as the long bones [2–4].

Regarding pathogenesis of osteomyelitis, once the bacterial foci are established, phagocytes travel to the site, producing inflammatory exudate [5], forming abscesses, and impacting multiple regions including the bone marrow, cortex, periosteum, and surrounding soft tissues [6]. Our case is also assumed to have developed a chest wall abscess after the onset of osteomyelitis of the ribs because of the complication of bacteremia which established bacterial foci and produced inflammation to spread out to the surrounding tissues, although from the initial MRI image findings, we were not able to diagnose rib osteomyelitis due to the strong signal from the abscess. However, we followed up on the image after the improvement of the abscess; thus, we were able to diagnose the rib osteomyelitis and administer the appropriate term of antibiotics.

In the case of hematogenous osteomyelitis, the most common causative organism is *Staphylococcus aureus*, for which antibiotic therapy alone is sufficient [2]. Although surgical drainage is required when pus revel from the subperiosteal space or metaphysis [5], this procedure is highly invasive for infants. Existing data show no clear evidence of the efficacy of surgical intervention for osteomyelitis [1]. If acute osteomyelitis is diagnosed at a sufficiently early stage, antibiotic treatment alone is sufficient in most cases [1]. A previous case report and literature review found that many cases of rib osteomyelitis required surgical drainage [4] and surgical debridement was required as the optimal treatment for cases of osteomyelitis associated with contiguous infections, or chronic osteomyelitis [4, 5, 7]. Our case was diagnosed early and treatment response was good; thus, surgical drainage was avoided.

This case was typical of rib osteomyelitis in terms of age and site of onset, but the diagnosis was difficult at the time of admission because of the lack of specific symptoms. The clinical symptoms of rib osteomyelitis are less severe than those of typical osteomyelitis in other parts of the body; as such, for early diagnosis in infants, it is important to examine the patient carefully for any subtle abnormalities such as swelling or masses. In our case, it was initially difficult to evaluate the presence of osteomyelitis due to the presence of an abscess, but after the abscess shrank in response to treatment, we were able to diagnose osteomyelitis via MRI. Owing to this early diagnosis, our patient's clinical and imaging symptoms improved with antimicrobial therapy alone, and treatment was completed without the need for surgical intervention.

Acknowledgments

The authors thank Scott McCleary for editing a draft of this manuscript.

References

[1] H. Peltola and M. Pääkkönen, "Acute osteomyelitis in children," *New England Journal of Medicine*, vol. 370, no. 4, pp. 352–360, 2014.

[2] J. Dartnell, M. Ramachandran, and M. Katchburian, "Haematogenous acute and subacute paediatric osteomyelitis," *Journal of Bone and Joint Surgery British Volume*, vol. 94-B, no. 5, pp. 584–595, 2012.

[3] A. M. Crone, M. R. Wanner, M. L. Cooper, T. G. Fox, S. G. Jennings, and B. Karmazyn, "Osteomyelitis of the ribs in children: a rare and potentially challenging diagnosis," *Pediatric Radiology*, vol. 50, no. 1, pp. 68–74, 2020.

[4] M. Nascimento, E. Oliveira, S. Soares, R. Almeida, and F. Espada, "Rib osteomyelitis in a pediatric patient case report and literature review," *The Pediatric Infectious Disease Journal*, vol. 31, no. 11, pp. 1190–1194, 2012.

[5] S. L. Kaplan, "Osteomyelitis," in *Nelson Textbook of Pediatrics*, R. M. Kligman, B. F. Stanton, and J. W. Geme III, Eds., pp. 2394–2398, WB. Saunders, Philadelphia, PA, USA, 19th edition, 2011.

[6] N. Kavanagh, E. J. Ryan, A. Widaa et al., "Staphylococcal osteomyelitis: disease progression, treatment challenges, and future directions," *Clinical Microbiology Reviews*, vol. 31, no. 2, p. 17, Article ID e00084, 2018.

[7] D. P. Lew and F. A. Waldvogel, "Osteomyelitis," *The Lancet*, vol. 364, no. 9431, pp. 369–379, 2004.

15

A Case of Suspected Adverse Reactions to Sirolimus in the Treatment of Generalized Lymphatic Anomaly

Takayuki Fujii ⓘ, Ryuichi Shimono ⓘ, Aya Tanaka, and Hiroto Katami

Department of Pediatric Surgery, Faculty of Medicine, Kagawa University, 1750-1 Ikenobe, Mikicho, Kitagun, Kagawa 761-0793, Japan

Correspondence should be addressed to Ryuichi Shimono; shi-mono@med.kagawa-u.ac.jp

Academic Editor: Carmelo Romeo

Generalized lymphatic anomaly (GLA) is characterized by diffuse or multicentric proliferation of dilated lymphatic vessels resembling common lymphatic malformation, and thoracic lesions can be related to a poor prognosis. Sirolimus, an inhibitor of the mammalian target of rapamycin, is effective against vascular anomalies with few severe adverse drug reactions. Here, we report the case of a patient with intractable hemothorax pleural effusion due to GLA who was treated with sirolimus and experienced disseminated intravascular coagulation. Although a standard treatment for GLA has not been established, pleural fluid might be reduced using the Kampo medicine Eppikajyutsuto.

1. Introduction

Generalized lymphatic anomaly (GLA) is characterized by diffuse or multicentric proliferation of dilated lymphatic vessels resembling common lymphatic malformation, and thoracic lesions can be related to a poor prognosis [1].

In recent years, several studies have reported that sirolimus, an inhibitor of the mammalian target of rapamycin (mTOR), is effective and well tolerated in the treatment of vascular anomalies [2–4]. Adverse drug reactions to sirolimus include leukopenia, mucositis, gastrointestinal manifestations, and hyperlipidemia; however, severe adverse drug reactions are rare [2–4].

Here, we report the case of a patient with intractable hemothorax pleural effusion due to GLA who was treated with sirolimus and developed disseminated intravascular coagulation (DIC). Although a standard treatment for GLA has not been established, pleural fluid might be reduced using a Kampo medicine called Eppikajyutsuto (TJ-28; Tsumura & Co., Tokyo, Japan), which is reportedly effective against lymphatic malformations (LMs) [5–7].

2. Case Presentation

A 13-year-old boy underwent pericardial fenestration and thoracic duct ligation for pericardial and pleural effusion at 3 years of age and was diagnosed with GLA after a pleural biopsy. The patient experienced no pleural effusion before his 11th birthday. The patient had a history of cerebrospinal fluid leakage due to a skull fracture at 7 years of age. The patient was referred to our department immediately following pleural effusion when he was 11 years old. A hematological examination showed high values for D-dimer (22.2 μg/mL) and P-FDP (50.9 μg/mL). A radiograph showed pleural effusion in the right lung (Figure 1). Thoracentesis revealed chylothorax mixed with blood components. Magnetic resonance imaging showed additional lesions on the lymph ducts on both sides of the inner auditory channels; computed tomography (CT) showed diffuse osteolytic changes on both sides of the femoral neck and thoracic vertebra. Figure 2 shows the patient's clinical course. Although the patient abstained from eating and parenteral nutrition was provided in addition to octreotide testing and pulse steroid therapy, pleural effusion worsened and became bilateral. Two or more liters were drained on

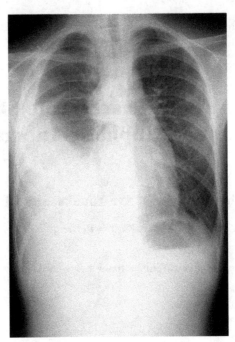

FIGURE 1: A radiograph showing massive pleural effusion in the right lung.

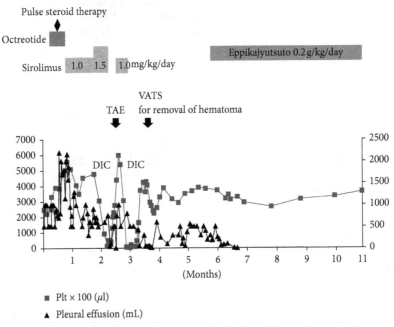

FIGURE 2: Clinical course of treatment in a 13-year-old male patient. (■) platelets (Plt); (▲) pleural effusion. TAE, transcatheter arterial embolization; VATS, video-assisted thoracic surgery; DIC, disseminated intravascular coagulation.

days when there was a large amount of pleural effusion. We were unable to locate the site of the leakage even though we conducted a lymphogram to treat the pleural effusion and identify the leakage site. Sirolimus administration was initiated at 0.88 mg/m^2/day, which proved to be an insufficient dosage. However, when the dosage was increased to 1.3 mg/m^2/day after 1 month, the patient experienced an onset of disseminated intravascular coagulation (DIC) after 1 week. At that time, a blood examination showed platelet (1.4×10^4/

μL), P-FDP (590 μg/mL), fibrinogen (114 mg/dL), prothrombin time rate (1.35), antithrombin (129%), and no liver dysfunction. The urine and blood cultures were negative. Viral serology was negative for cytomegalovirus, and aspergillus antigen was negative. Rheumatoid factor and antinuclear antibody were normal levels. The CT scan showed no sign of pneumonia or pyothorax. We diagnosed him with DIC using DIC score [8]. Although we temporarily paused the administration of sirolimus, the patient experienced an

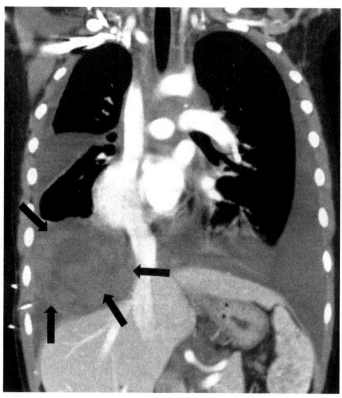

FIGURE 3: A chest contrast-enhanced computed tomography scan showing massive pleural effusion in both lungs. The black arrow shows a high-density hematoma in the right lung.

additional onset of DIC 10 days after we resumed administration. Thus, he underwent thoracoscopic removal of the hematoma (Figure 3). The trough level of sirolimus during administration was 3.4–8.9 ng/mL, which does not represent abnormal elevation. Although an additional pause in the administration of sirolimus did not reduce the amount of pleural fluid, there were no additional onsets of DIC. Subsequently, there was a significant decrease in pleural fluid once Eppikajyutsuto was administered at 0.2 g/kg/day. We were able to proceed with tube thoracostomy removal 40 days after the initiation of oral administration. There was no re-accumulation of pleural fluids in the 18 months following the initiation of oral administration.

3. Discussion

In total, 89.2% of GLA cases involve chest lesions. Many cases are intractable despite drainage of the thoracic cavity, pleurodesis, and steroid treatment [1].

In recent years, sirolimus has been considered as a new therapeutic option for vascular anomalies [2–4]. mTOR is a serine threonine kinase regulated by phosphoinositide 3 kinase (PI3K) and protein kinase B (Akt). The PI3K/Akt/mTOR pathway is the basis for cell growth and proliferation and also increases the expression of vascular endothelial growth factor, regulating angiogenesis as well and lymphangiogenesis. mTOR inhibitors directly inhibit mTOR, blocking downstream protein synthesis and eliciting antitumoral and antiangiogenic effects [2, 9].

Adverse drug reactions to sirolimus include leukopenia, mucositis, gastrointestinal manifestations, and hyperlipidemia; however, severe adverse drug reactions that threaten life are rare [2–4]. The range of sirolimus concentration appropriate for the treatment of vascular anomalies was reported as 5–15 ng/mL [2]. Our patient had no abnormal high blood levels of sirolimus. GLA including kaposiform lymphangiomatosis may cause the severe thrombocytopenia and coagulopathy. Therefore, it might be associated with the patient's diseases. However, our patient experienced DIC consistent with the timing of sirolimus administration. Although DIC has not been reported as a side effect of sirolimus, we believe that it is important to note the onset of DIC when using sirolimus. On the other hand, Hammer et al. reported that sirolimus decreased coagulation abnormalities [4]. Further studies are needed to elucidate the mechanism of the effect of sirolimus on the blood coagulation system.

The Kampo medicine Eppikajyutsuto was created to conform to other Kampo formulations such as Mao, Sekko, and so on. It has an irrigation effect that normalizes the disequilibrium of fluids in the body. It is also reported to have an anti-inflammatory effect and is effective against lymphatic malformations [5–7]. Mao (ephedra herb) is a main component of Eppikajyutsuto. The herb ephedra is suggested to suppress of vascular endothelial growth factor activity by inhibiting prostaglandin E2 synthesis and cyclooxygenase protein synthesis, which might contribute to the shrinkage of LMs [7, 10–12]. Hashizume et al. reported the mean LM volume shrinkage rate of 54.5 ± 38.3% in eight patients who received the medicine [6].

In the present case, because we performed various treatments, it was difficult to determine which treatment was effective in reducing pleural effusion. However, because pleural effusion decisively decreased after the administration of Eppikajyutsuto and we were able to proceed with tube thoracostomy removal, we assume that Eppikajyutsuto influenced the disequilibrium of fluids in the body (pleural effusion) in this patient. Further research based on this finding is necessary.

Consent

Written informed consent was obtained from the patient's family.

References

[1] M. Ozeki, A. Fujino, K. Matsuoka, S. Nosaka, T. Kuroda, and T. Fukao, "Clinical features and prognosis of generalized lymphatic anomaly, kaposiform lymphangiomatosis, and Gorham-Stout disease," *Pediatric Blood & Cancer*, vol. 63, no. 5, pp. 832–838, 2016.

[2] P. Triana, M. Dore, V. N. Cerezo et al., "Sirolimus in the treatment of vascular anomalies," *European Journal of Pediatric Surgery*, vol. 27, no. 1, pp. 86–90, 2017.

[3] D. M. Adams, C. C. Trenor III, A. M. Hammill et al., "Efficacy and safety of sirolimus in the treatment of complicated vascular anomalies," *Pediatrics*, vol. 137, no. 2, article e20153257, 2016.

[4] J. Hammer, E. Seront, S. Duez et al., "Sirolimus is efficacious in treatment for extensive and/or complex slow-flow vascular malformations: a monocentric prospective phase II study," *Orphanet Journal of Rare Diseases*, vol. 13, no. 1, p. 191, 2018.

[5] K. Ogawa-Ochiai, N. Sekiya, Y. Kasahara et al., "A case of mediastinal lymphangioma successfully treated with Kampo medicine," *Journal of Alternative and Complementary Medicine*, vol. 17, no. 6, pp. 563–565, 2011.

[6] N. Hashizume, M. Yagi, H. Egami et al., "Clinical efficacy of herbal medicine for pediatric lymphatic malformations: a pilot study," *Pediatric Dermatology*, vol. 33, no. 2, pp. 191–195, 2016.

[7] T. Shinkai, K. Masumoto, F. Chiba, and N. Tanaka, "A large retroperitoneal lymphatic malformation successfully treated with traditional Japanese Kampo medicine in combination with surgery," *Surgical Case Reports*, vol. 3, no. 1, p. 80, 2017.

[8] H. Asakura, H. Takahashi, T. Uchiyama et al., "Proposal for new diagnostic criteria for DIC from the Japanese Society on Thrombosis and Hemostasis," *Thrombosis Journal*, vol. 14, no. 42, 2016.

[9] C. M. Hartford and M. J. Ratain, "Rapamycin: something old, something new, sometimes borrowed and now renewed," *Clinical Pharmacology & Therapeutics*, vol. 82, no. 4, pp. 381–388, 2007.

[10] Y. Kasahara, H. Hikino, S. Tsurufuji, M. Watanabe, and K. Ohuchi, "Antiinflammatory actions of ephedrines in acute inflammations," *Planta Medica*, vol. 51, no. 4, pp. 325–331, 1985.

[11] K. Matsuo, K. Koizumi, M. Fujita et al., "Efficient use of a crude drug/herb library reveals ephedra herb as a specific antagonist for T_H2-specific chemokine receptors CCR3, CCR4 and CCR8," *Frontiers in Cell and Developmental Biology*, vol. 4, no. 54, 2016.

[12] K. Aoki, T. Yamakuni, M. Yoshida, and Y. Ohizumi, "Ephedorae herba decreases lipopolysaccharide-induced cyclooxgenase-2 protein expression and NF-κB-dependent transcription in C6 rat glioma cells," *Journal of Pharmacological Sciences*, vol. 98, no. 3, pp. 327–330, 2005.

16

Onychomadesis in a 20-Month-Old Child with Kawasaki Disease

Alexander K. C. Leung[1,2], **Kin Fon Leong**,[3] and **Joseph M. Lam**[4]

[1]Clinical Professor of Pediatrics at The University of Calgary, Calgary, Alberta, Canada T2M 0H5
[2]Pediatric Consultant at The Alberta Children's Hospital, Calgary, Alberta, Canada T2M 0H5
[3]Consultant Pediatric Dermatologist at the Pediatric Institute, Kuala Lumpur General Hospital, Kuala Lumpur, Malaysia
[4]Clinical Associate Professor of Pediatrics and Associate Member at the Department of Dermatology and Skin Sciences, University of British Columbia, Vancouver, Canada

Correspondence should be addressed to Alexander K. C. Leung; aleung@ucalgary.ca

Academic Editor: Piero Pavone

Kawasaki disease is characterized by fever for ≥ five days, bilateral bulbar conjunctival injection without exudate, polymorphous rash changes in the extremities, oral mucosal changes, and cervical lymphadenopathy. We report a 20-month-old boy with Kawasaki disease who had onychomadesis affecting the fingernails and toenails bilaterally. To our knowledge, there were three reported cases of onychomadesis associated with Kawasaki disease, to which we add another one. We suggest keeping in mind the possibility of onychomadesis as a nail sequela of Kawasaki disease.

1. Introduction

Kawasaki disease, also known as Kawasaki syndrome, is one of the most common acute systemic vasculitides that predominantly affects medium-sized arteries, with a predilection for coronary arteries [1]. The condition occurs mostly in children younger than five years of age [1]. The disease is characterized by fever of at least five days and a constellation of clinical features that are used as diagnostic criteria [2]. Onychomadesis has rarely been reported following Kawasaki disease [3–5]. A perusal of the literature revealed three cases, to which we are going to add another one.

2. Case Report

A 20-month-old Chinese boy was seen with a 7-day history of high-spiking fevers. The child broke out with a non-pruritic widespread reddish rash 1 day after the onset of fever. On the third day of the fever, he developed nonpurulent conjunctival injection. The child was irritable and had decreased oral intake. His mother brought him to see a family physician who treated the child with azithromycin and acetaminophen. The fever persisted in spite of the treatment. The child had not been exposed to anyone with a known infectious disease. His past medical history was unremarkable. The family history was noncontributory.

On examination, the child was irritable and lethargic. His weight was 10.4 kg, height 82 cm, and head circumference 48.5 cm. His temperature was 39°C, heart rate 115 beats per minute, blood pressure 84/40 mm·Hg, and respiratory rate 33 breaths per minute. The child was noted to have bilateral nonpurulent bulbar conjunctival injection; fissured red lips (Figure 1); strawberry tongue diffuse erythema of the oropharyngeal mucosa; a generalized blanching polymorphous maculopapular rash over his face, trunk (Figure 1), and groin; erythema and firm edema of the dorsa of the hands and feet with sharp demarcation at the ankles and wrists and two enlarged firm tender lymph nodes each measuring 2 × 3 cm in the right cervical area. The rest of the physical examination was normal. In particular, there was no hepatosplenomegaly or a heart murmur.

The child was admitted to the hospital for investigations and management. Laboratory tests on admission revealed the following results: hemoglobin 12.6 g/dL (126 g/L), white blood cell count 21.3/μL (×10⁹/L) with 88% neutrophils, platelet count 277 × 10³/μL (×10⁹/L), and C-reactive protein

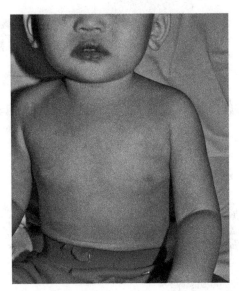

FIGURE 1: A 20-month-old boy with Kawasaki disease presenting with red cracked lips and an erythematous maculopapular rash on the anterior chest and upper arms.

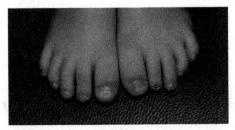

FIGURE 2: Onychomadesis noted at 2-month follow-up. The toenails on both feet were partially shed.

21.2 mg/L (201.7 nmol/L). Urinalysis showed 15 white blood cells per high-power field with no bacteria. Serum electrolytes, albumin, liver enzymes, and renal function were normal. Urine culture and throat swab culture were negative. The baseline chest radiograph, electrocardiograph, and echocardiograph were normal.

A diagnosis of Kawasaki disease was made based on the findings of fever for seven days, conjunctival injection, polymorphous rash, oral mucosal changes, changes in extremities, and cervical lymphadenopathy. The child was treated with intravenous immunoglobulin (2 g/kg) infused over 12 hours and high-dose aspirin (80 mg/kg/day divided into 4 doses) given orally. Over the next 36 hours, the child became afebrile, and the maculopapular rash resolved completely. He was discharged after 4 days of hospitalization on high-dose aspirin (80 mg/kg/day divided into 4 doses) for a total of 14 days followed by low-dose aspirin (4 mg/kg/day) in once-daily dosing for 8 weeks. At 2-month follow-up, the child's fingernails and toenails were found to be partially shed on both hands and feet, with the proximal nail beds covered by new nail (Figure 2). At 4-month follow-up, the old fingernails and toenails were fully shed, and the new fingernails and toenails were normal. Follow-up echocardiogram at 4 weeks and 3 months was normal.

3. Discussion

The diagnosis of classic or typical Kawasaki disease is based on clinical criteria established by the American Heart Association [2]. These criteria include fever for ≥ five days (first calendar day of temperature is illness day 1) plus ≥ four of the five primary or principal clinical features without plausible alternative explanations for the clinical findings. The five principal clinical features are bilateral bulbar conjunctival injection without exudate, polymorphous rash (diffuse maculopapular, erythroderma, urticarial, erythema

multiforme-like, but not bullous or vesicular), changes in the extremities (periungual desquamation, indurated edema and erythema of the feet and hands, and sharp demarcation at the ankles and wrists), oral mucosal changes (erythematous, fissured cracked lips, diffuse erythema of the oral pharynx, and strawberry tongue), and cervical lymphadenopathy (unilateral, nonfluctuant, >1.5 cm in diameter) [2]. According to the 2017 scientific statement for health professions from the American Heart Association, in the presence of ≥4 major features, mainly when swelling and redness of the feet and hands are present, the diagnosis can also be made even if the fever has only been present for four days [2]. In this regard, the Japanese criteria include those cases in whom the fever has subsided before the fifth day in response to treatment [6]. Patients who have a fever for five or more days and only three major clinical features can also be diagnosed as having classic Kawasaki disease when coronary artery disease is detected by two-dimensional (2D) echocardiography or coronary angiography [2].

Periungual desquamation of the fingers and toes is a characteristic feature of Kawasaki disease and usually occurs 2 to 3 weeks after the onset of fever [1]. Nail changes in Kawasaki disease include Beau lines (linear nail creases), transverse orange-brown or red chromonychia, transverse leukonychia (leukonychia striata), pincer nails, and onychomadesis, usually occurring four to six weeks after onset of fever [7–11].

Onychomadesis refers to the separation of the nail plate from the matrix starting at the proximal edge and is the result of temporary arrest of growth of the nail bed matrix [12]. The mechanism of nail matrix arrest is unknown but may be secondary to inhibition of cellular proliferation [13]. It is also possible that the quality of the newly formed nail may be temporarily altered, leading to separating of the nail plate [13]. As the new nail begins its growth proximally, it extends underneath the previous nail, pushing the previous nail forward, resulting in shedding of the previous nail [13, 14]. Typically, the condition is painless and self-limited [14]. New nail growth will be normal [14]. Onychomadesis may occur in fingernails and/or toenails. Although onychomadesis is usually easily recognizable, it can be mistaken for onychomycosis, trachyonychia, or psoriatic nails. Onychomadesis has been shown to be associated with infections (notably hand-foot-mouth disease, varicella, scarlet fever, onychomycosis, and paronychia), systemic medical illnesses (Kawasaki disease, Steven-Johnson syndrome, toxic epidermal necrolysis, lichen planus, Cronkhite–Canada syndrome, Guillain-Barré syndrome, myocardial infarction, renal failure, and immunodeficiency), direct trauma to the nail matrix, medications (chemotherapeutic agents [doxorubicin, capecitabine, etoposide, and cytosine arabinoside], antibiotics [penicillin, cloxacillin, azithromycin, and cephalosporin], antiepileptics [valproic acid and carbamazepine], retinoids, lithium, and lead), and autoimmune diseases (alopecia areata and pemphigus vulgaris) [5,12–14]. Onychomadesis can also be familial or idiopathic [13].

Onychomadesis associated with Kawasaki disease is very rare. To our knowledge, only three cases have been reported in the literature [3–5]. In 1990, Pilapil and Quizon reported a 4-year-old Caucasian boy with features of Kawasaki disease for 7 days before he was hospitalized and treated as such for 20 days [5]. The patient was noted to have onychomadesis affecting his fingernails and toenails when he was examined 36 days after discharge from the hospital. In 2002, Ciastko described an 8-year-old boy with Kawasaki disease who was noted to have onychomadesis of the fingernails and toenails 6 weeks from the onset of the illness [3]. In 2015, Kalasekhar and Venkatesh reported a 2-year-old boy with Kawasaki disease [4]. On the 10th day of the illness, the child was noted to have orange-brown discoloration on the right ring fingernail, transverse nail crease on his right middle fingernail, and onychomadesis of the right index fingernail [4]. We report a 20-month-old child with Kawasaki disease who had onychomadesis on the fingernails and toenails bilaterally two months from the onset of the disease.

Our impression is that onychomadesis associated with Kawasaki disease may be more common than is generally appreciated. We suggest keeping in mind the possibility of onychomadesis as a nail sequela of Kawasaki disease.

References

[1] A. K. Leung, "Kawasaki disease," in *Common Problems in Ambulatory Pediatrics*, A. K. Leung, Ed., vol. 1, pp. 385–390, Nova Science Publishers, Inc., Hauppauge, NY, USA, 2011.

[2] B. W. McCrindle, A. H. Rowley, J. W. Newburger et al., "Diagnosis, treatment, and long-term management of Kawasaki disease: a scientific statement for health professionals from the American Heart Association," *Circulation*, vol. 135, no. 17, pp. e927–e999, 2017.

[3] A. R. Ciastko, "Onychomadesis and Kawasaki disease," *Canadian Medical Association Journal*, vol. 166, no. 8, p. 1069, 2002.

[4] V. Kalasekhar and C. Venkatesh, "A constellation of nail changes in a child with Kawasaki disease," *Journal of Clinical and Diagnostic Research*, vol. 9, no. 7, p. SJ01, 2015.

[5] V. R. Pilapil and D. F. Quizon, "Nail shedding in Kawasaki syndrome," *American Journal of Diseases of Children*, vol. 144, no. 2, pp. 142-143, 1990.

[6] JCS Joint Working Group, "Guidelines for diagnosis and management of cardiovascular sequelae in Kawasaki disease (JCS 2013)," *Circulation Journal*, vol. 78, no. 10, pp. 2521–2562, 2014.

[7] R. Berard, R. Scuccimarri, and G. Chédeville, "Leukonychia striata in Kawasaki disease," *Journal of Pediatrics*, vol. 152, no. 6, p. 889, 2008.

[8] A. P. George, C. E. Gaby, and R. A. Broughton, "Red chromonychia in Kawasaki disease," *Pediatric Infectious Disease Journal*, vol. 34, no. 6, pp. 675-676, 2015.

[9] P. Pal and P. P. Giri, "Orange-brown chromonychia, a novel finding in Kawasaki disease," *Rheumatology International*, vol. 33, no. 5, pp. 1207–1209, 2012.

[10] L. Tessarotto, G. Rubin, L. Bonadies, E. Valerio, and M. Cutrone, "Orange-brown chromonychia and Kawasaki disease: a possible novel association?," *Pediatric Dermatology*, vol. 32, no. 3, pp. e104–e105, 2015.

[11] S. L. Vanderhooft and J. E. Vanderhooft, "Pincer nail deformity after Kawasaki's disease," *Journal of the American Academy of Dermatology*, vol. 41, no. 2, pp. 341-342, 1999.

[12] N. Y. Hoy, A. K. Leung, A. I. Metelitsa, and S. Adams, "New concepts in median nail dystrophy, onychomycosis, and hand, foot, and mouth disease nail pathology," *ISRN Dermatology*, vol. 2012, Article ID 680163, 5 pages, 2012.

[13] J. Hardin and R. M. Haber, "Onychomadesis: literature review," *British Journal of Dermatology*, vol. 172, no. 3, pp. 592–596, 2015.

[14] N. A. Kuehnel, S. Thach, and D. G. Thomas, "Onychomadesis as a late complication of hand-foot-mouth disease: a case series shedding light on nail shedding," *Pediatric Emergency Care*, vol. 33, no. 11, pp. e122–e123, 2017.

17

A Case of Descending Necrotizing Mediastinitis in a Previously Healthy Child

Toshihiko Okumura,[1] **Nobuyuki Tetsuka,**[2] **Makoto Yamaguchi,**[1] **Takako Suzuki,**[1] **Yuka Torii,**[1] **Jun-ichi Kawada,**[1] **and Yoshinori Ito** (iD)[1]

[1]*Department of Pediatrics, Nagoya University Graduate School of Medicine, 65 Tsurumai-cho, Showa-ku, Nagoya 466-8550, Japan*
[2]*Department of Infectious Disease, Nagoya University Hospital, 65 Tsurumai-cho, Showa-ku, Nagoya 466-8550, Japan*

Correspondence should be addressed to Yoshinori Ito; yoshi-i@med.nagoya-u.ac.jp

Academic Editor: Nan Chang Chiu

Descending necrotizing mediastinitis (DNM) is a rare complication of oropharyngeal and cervical infection, especially in children. We report a case of DNM secondary to a cervical abscess in a previously healthy 1-year-old boy. The patient presented with redness and swelling of the neck and fever. He was treated with an antimicrobial agent for the diagnosis of cervical lymphadenitis. On the sixth day, a huge mediastinal abscess was found, and he was admitted to the intensive care unit. He was successfully treated with surgical drainage and appropriate antimicrobial therapy. The pus culture isolated multiple bacteria, including methicillin-resistant *Staphylococcus aureus* (MRSA). Although we did not use an antimicrobial agent covering MRSA, the symptoms and test results improved. Washing with drainage was effective. The patient required multidisciplinary treatment, and we collaborated with specialists in other departments. DNM is a severe disease in which team medical care is needed to provide appropriate treatment.

1. Introduction

Descending necrotizing mediastinitis (DNM) is a rare complication of oropharyngeal and cervical infection, especially in children. We report a case of DNM secondary to a cervical abscess in a previously healthy 1-year-old boy. The patient presented with redness and swelling of the neck and fever. He was treated with an antimicrobial agent for the diagnosis of cervical lymphadenitis. On the sixth day, a huge mediastinal abscess was found, and he was admitted to the intensive care unit. He was successfully treated with surgical drainage and appropriate antimicrobial therapy. The pus culture isolated multiple bacteria, including methicillin-resistant *Staphylococcus aureus* (MRSA). Although we did not use an antimicrobial agent covering MRSA, the symptoms and test results improved. Washing with drainage was effective. The patient required multidisciplinary treatment, and we collaborated with specialists in other departments.

DNM is a severe disease in which team medical care is needed to provide appropriate treatment.

2. Case Presentation

Descending necrotizing mediastinitis (DNM) is a severe acute inflammation of the mediastinum secondary to oropharyngeal and cervical infection spreading rapidly through the space between cervical fasciae. Common primary origins include tonsillar and pharyngeal infection and odontogenic infection [1, 2]. DNM is a rare complication and has a high mortality rate of 6–15% as reported in recent studies [1–3]. Although the mortality rate in children may be lower than that in adults [4–7], DNM is a clinically important disease that requires early diagnosis and appropriate treatment because it can cause septic shock and airway emergency. We report the case of a child with DNM who was successfully treated without permanent damage despite the presence of a huge mediastinal abscess. Written informed consent was obtained from the patient's guardians for publication of this case report and the accompanying images.

A 1-year-and-5-month-old previously healthy boy presented with redness and swelling of the neck and fever. He was admitted to a general hospital for the diagnosis of cervical lymphadenitis. Although ceftriaxone was administered at 60 mg/kg per day, the fever persisted, the right side of the neck became red, and swelling of the region worsened. On the sixth day, a contrast-enhanced computed tomography (CT) scan of the head revealed a right cervical abscess spreading to the mediastinum. He was admitted to our hospital for intensive care, including surgical management. On admission, his vital signs were as follows: temperature, 39.1°C; pulse rate, 112 beats/min; blood pressure, 77/42 mmHg; respiration rate, 34 times/min; and 90% oxygen saturation in ambient air. The results of the laboratory examinations were as follows: white blood cell count, 22,300/μL; aspartate aminotransferase, 80 U/L; alanine aminotransferase, 60 U/L; C-reactive protein, 24.72 mg/dL; and procalcitonin, 2.1 ng/mL. A contrast-enhanced CT scan of the head and chest revealed an abscess in the right submandibular region and a sequential abscess of the anterior mediastinum (Figure 1) that touched the posterior surface of the sternum. The patient was therefore diagnosed with DNM associated with a cervical abscess.

After admission to the intensive care unit, anesthesiologists anesthetized him and performed intratracheal intubation considering the possibility of tracheal obstruction. Pediatric surgeons performed percutaneous drainage from the neck and placed two drainage tubes (Figure 2). Foul-smelling cream-colored pus was drained. Pediatricians began intravenous administration of piperacillin/tazobactam (PIPC/TAZ) at 330 mg/kg per day for the purpose of broadening the antibacterial spectrum to include *Pseudomonas aeruginosa* and obligate anaerobes. On hospital day 2, PIPC/TAZ was changed to ampicillin/sulbactam at 300 mg/kg per day because the results of the pus culture ruled out *Pseudomonas aeruginosa*. On hospital day 4, several bacteria were identified, including a large amount of *Prevotella oris* and *Fusobacterium nucleatum* and a small amount of *Streptococcus constellatus*, *Eikenella corrodens*, and methicillin-resistant *Staphylococcus aureus* (MRSA). We did not add an antimicrobial agent to target MRSA because the high fever dropped, the results of blood examinations improved, and the abscess was reduced in size on the CT scan. The blood culture for only aerobes was negative. On hospital day 6, as the fluid from the drainage tubes gradually decreased and the tubes seemed to be clogged; pediatric surgeons replaced the drainage tubes with thicker tubes and washed out the cavity. On hospital day 11, the patient was extubated after an otolaryngologist assessed the edema of the respiratory tract. On hospital days 18 and 19, the drainage tubes were removed one by one. Antibiotic therapy in our hospital was continued for a total of 23 days after confirming that the patient did not develop osteomyelitis as a complication on magnetic resonance imaging. He was discharged on hospital day 26 without any complications.

3. Discussion

DNM is caused by the downward spread of oropharyngeal and cervical infections. Pharyngeal infection is the most frequent causative infection for DNM in adults [1, 2], and DNM is a rare complication that develops in 9% of deep neck infections [8, 9]. Meanwhile, in children, retropharyngeal abscess is the most frequent cause of DNM. DNM is a critical illness that requires appropriate treatment because pharyngeal and mediastinal abscesses can cause airway emergencies [10, 11]. Airway management is the most important treatment for deep neck abscesses and mediastinal abscesses. In this case, as the abscess reached the anterior aspect of the trachea and the oxygen saturation decreased, we emergently conducted intratracheal intubation. When the patient was extubated, an otolaryngologist evaluated the condition of the larynx so that airway obstruction due to edema after extubation would not occur.

The main symptoms of DNM are fever, odynophagia, cervical swelling, cervical pain, and dyspnea [1]. Infrequent symptoms include thoracic pain and back pain. It is difficult to diagnose DNM only based on clinical symptoms and physical examination because these symptoms are not specific to DNM. If a patient has cervical and chest symptoms, we must consider the possibility of DNM developing. It is very important to perform a CT scan when we suspect DNM to make an early diagnosis.

Prior studies reported that the most commonly isolated pathogen in pus cultures in children was *S. aureus*, most of which were MRSA [4, 5, 7]. Over 50% of adult patients with DNM were reported to have a polymicrobial infection with aerobic and anaerobic organisms [1, 3]. In this case, the pus culture isolated two anaerobes, *P. oris* and *F. nucleatum*, in addition to MRSA. Although we did not use an antimicrobial agent covering MRSA when MRSA was discovered, the symptoms and the test results tended to improve. We would have added an antimicrobial agent if the patient had become ill. Since the number of anaerobes was large, these bacteria were identified as the main pathogen, and antibiotic therapy and washing with drainage were considered sufficiently effective. It was suggested that MRSA detected in the culture does not necessarily have to be covered.

Drainage is very important for the treatment of DNM, and surgical management was performed in all cases in several studies [1, 3, 5]. As surgical management is required two times on average [2, 5], it should be remembered that the initial drainage is not always sufficient. It is necessary to always consider the possibility of relapse of the abscess and evaluate treatment efficacy using imaging tests, such as contrast-enhanced CT, as appropriate. In this case, the amount of pus from drainage tubes was decreased due to clogging; therefore, we placed thicker tubes again 5 days after the first drainage, and the clinical course of the patient was subsequently good.

In conclusion, this case report confirms that early diagnosis by a CT scan and early treatment with drainage, which is often needed multiple times, are important for the medical care of DNM. MRSA detected in pus culture may not always be covered. We should continue to accumulate case reports to further improve the treatment of DNM in children.

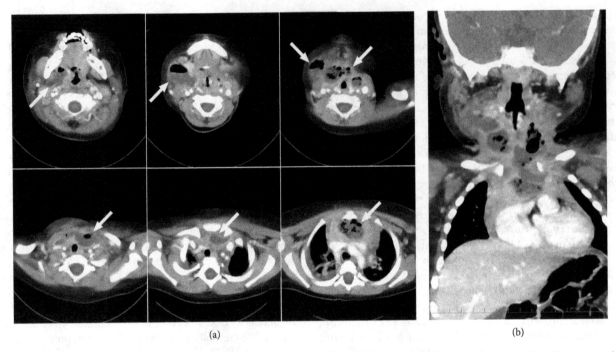

(a)   (b)

FIGURE 1: Axial (a) and coronal (b) images from the contrast-enhanced CT scan of the head and chest on admission. The white arrows show an abscess ranging from the neck to the anterior mediastinum.

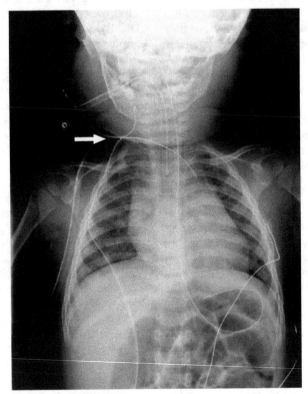

FIGURE 2: Chest radiograph after percutaneous drainage tubes were placed. The white arrow shows the insertion site. One was placed in the right neck, and the other was placed in the anterior mediastinum.

References

[1] G. J. Ridder, W. Maier, S. Kinzer, C. B. Teszler, C. C. Boedeker, and J. Pfeiffer, "Descending necrotizing mediastinitis," *Annals of Surgery*, vol. 251, no. 3, pp. 528–534, 2010.

[2] Y. Sumi, "Descending necrotizing mediastinitis: 5 years of published data in Japan," *Acute Medicine & Surgery*, vol. 2, no. 1, pp. 1–12, 2015.

[3] D. M. Palma, S. Giuliano, A. N. Cracchiolo et al., "Clinical features and outcome of patients with descending necrotizing mediastinitis: prospective analysis of 34 cases," *Infection*, vol. 44, no. 1, pp. 77–84, 2016.

[4] C. T. Wright, R. M. S. Stocks, D. L. Armstrong, S. R. Arnold, and H. J. Gould, "Pediatric mediastinitis as a complication of methicillin-resistant *Staphylococcus aureus* retropharyngeal abscess," *Archives of Otolaryngology - Head and Neck Surgery*, vol. 134, no. 4, pp. 408–413, 2008.

[5] C. D. Wilson, K. Kennedy, J. W. Wood et al., "Retrospective review of management and outcomes of pediatric descending mediastinitis," *Otolaryngology-Head and Neck Surgery*, vol. 155, no. 1, pp. 155–159, 2016.

[6] C. M. Baldassari, R. Howell, M. Amorn, R. Budacki, S. Choi, and M. Pena, "Complications in pediatric deep neck space abscesses," *Otolaryngology-Head and Neck Surgery*, vol. 144, no. 4, pp. 592–595, 2011.

[7] N. Abdel-Haq, M. Quezada, and B. I. Asmar, "Retropharyngeal abscess in children," *The Pediatric Infectious Disease Journal*, vol. 31, no. 7, pp. 696–699, 2012.

[8] Y. Shimizu, H. Hidaka, D. Ozawa et al., "Clinical and bacteriological differences of deep neck infection in pediatric and adult patients: review of 123 cases," *International Journal of Pediatric Otorhinolaryngology*, vol. 99, pp. 95–99, 2017.

[9] W. Yang, L. Hu, Z. Wang et al., "Deep neck infection," *Medicine*, vol. 94, no. 27, p. e994, 2015.

[10] D. B. Thapa, N. H. Greene, and A. G. Udani, "Complete obstruction of endotracheal tube in an infant with a retropharyngeal and anterior mediastinal abscess," *Case Reports in Pediatrics*, vol. 2017, Article ID 1848945, 4 pages, 2017.

[11] A. Q. Al-Naami, L. Ali Khan, Y. Ali Athlawy et al., "Ochrobactrum anthropi induced retropharyngeal abscess with mediastinal extension complicating airway obstruction: a case report," *Journal of Medical Radiation Sciences*, vol. 61, pp. 126–129, 2014.

18

Vitamin B6 Neonatal Toxicity

Andrea Guala,[1] Giulia Folgori,[1,2] Micaela Silvestri,[1] Michelangelo Barbaglia,[1] and Cesare Danesino (iD)[3]

[1]SOC Pediatrics, Castelli Hospital, Verbania, Italy
[2]Post-graduate School in Pediatrics, University "Piemonte Orientale", Novara, Italy
[3]Department of Molecular Medicine, University of Pavia, Pavia, Italy

Correspondence should be addressed to Cesare Danesino; cidi@unipv.it

Academic Editor: Junji Takaya

Vitamin B6 is a micronutrient required by the body. It acts as a coenzyme in biochemical reactions. Vitamin B6 toxicity is not caused by the intake of food-based sources. The few reported cases of vitamin B6 toxicity are always caused by overdosing of nutritional supplements. Chronic toxicity typically occurs with peripheral neuropathy such as paraesthesia, ataxia, and imbalance, paradoxically mimicking vitamin B6 deficiency. However, the prognosis is favorable, and symptoms usually show improvement once excessive vitamin B6 levels return to the physiological range. We report a newborn presenting with diffuse tremor at birth, interpreted as secondary to the mother's intake of high doses of a supplement containing vitamin B6 during pregnancy and breastfeeding. As expected, the newborn's serum levels of vitamin B6 were high. The tremors disappeared when the maternal supplement was stopped.

1. Introduction

Vitamin B6 is an essential water-soluble micronutrient, and its requirement in human adults ranges from 0.4–1.3 mg/day [1] to 1.5–1.8 mg/day [2]. Vitamin B6 refers to multiple chemically similar compounds (pyridoxine, pyridoxal, and pyridoxamine), of which pyridoxine is the most common (Figure 1). Cells use pyridoxal phosphate (PLP), the co-enzymatic form of vitamin B6, in many different enzymatic reactions such as neurotransmitter production, amino acids, glucose and lipids metabolism, hemoglobin synthesis and function, and gene expression. Vitamin B6 is widely present in foods (meat, fish, poultry, cereals, vegetables, and fruit), and intake of food-based sources of pyridoxine will not usually cause toxicity. The only reported cases of vitamin B6 toxicity are from chronic supratherapeutic dosing of supplements or excessive iatrogenic assumption [3]. Toxicity typically occurs with peripheral neuropathy like paraesthesia, ataxia, and imbalance, paradoxically mimicking a vitamin B6 deficiency. This sensory neuropathy usually develops at doses of pyridoxine above 1000 mg per day in

adults, although it has been reported at doses of less than 500 mg per day in patients taking supplements for several months. None of the studies had sensory nerve damage at daily intakes below 200 mg of pyridoxine per day [4, 5]. The prognosis is usually favorable with symptoms decreasing or resolving when supratherapeutic intake of pyridoxine has been discovered and stopped [6]. We report the case of a newborn with spontaneous tremors whose pregnant and breastfeeding mother had been taking high doses of a dietary supplement containing vitamin B6. The tremors disappeared when the supplement was stopped.

2. Case Report

The patient was born after eutocic delivery at 38 weeks of gestation. Birth weight and length were 3150 g and 49 cm, with a head circumference of 33.5 cm. Apgar scores at 1–5 minutes were 9–10. Breastfeeding began approximately 30 min after birth with no formula supplementation. The pregnancy was uneventful, and maternal hypothyroidism was controlled by replacement therapy with levothyroxine

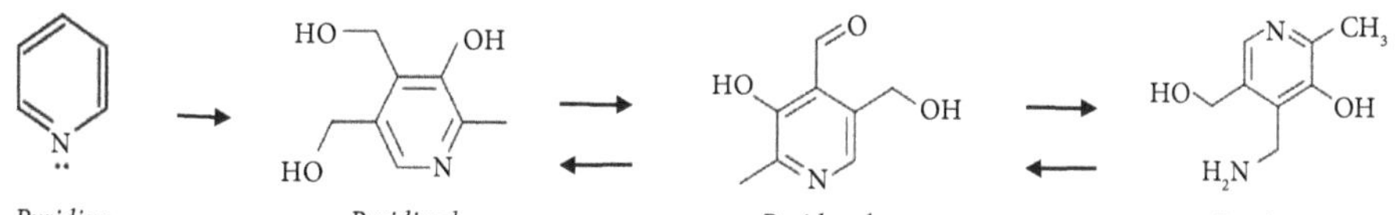

FIGURE 1: Chemical structure and derivation of the molecules with vitamin B6 action [20].

sodium, which was the only drug assumed to be under medical control. The mother reported smoking two cigarettes/day during pregnancy but denied alcohol consumption. A few hours after birth, both spontaneous and stimulated tremors involving the four limbs and the chin were noted, associated with skin redness. Tremors were also present while asleep. Clinical examination demonstrated normal vital signs and stable cardiorespiratory parameters. A blood sample revealed borderline hypoglycemia with a blood glucose concentration of 55 mg/dL (reference values 55 mg/dl-65 mg/dl). Infant formula was initiated as a supplement to breast milk to restore optimal glucose concentration.

Normalization of glycemic values was quickly obtained, but tremors persisted, prompting a more extensive evaluation of the patient with capillary hemogasanalysis, blood electrolytes, and vitamins. All results were within normal limits, except for vitamin B6 (102.7 microg/L n.v. 8.7–27.2 microg/L) and vitamin B12 (772 pg/mL n.v. 191–663 pg/mL). The presence of several drugs, such as cocaine, was also excluded.

Consultation with a childhood neuropsychiatrist excluded jitteriness [7]. Brain ultrasound and electrocardiography (ECG) did not disclose any abnormalities.

The presence of levels of vitamin B6 much higher than normal reference values was an indication to test the parents, and a clear increase in the pyridoxine values in the mother (52.1 microg/ml, n.v. 8.7–27.2) was found, while the father showed normal values.

A maternal dietary assessment disclosed a history of high-dose multivitamin supplements (2 tablets/day) available over-the-counter throughout pregnancy and into lactation (Table 1). The intake of vitamin supplements was immediately stopped, and, in the following weeks, tremors decreased together with the reduction of vitamin B6 levels both in the maternal and in the young patient serums (Table 2).

At two months of age, control electroencephalography (EEG) showed rare biphasic sharp wave anomalies in the left central parieto-temporal center, which were interpreted as a manifestation of neurovegetative hyperexcitability. At the same time, a childhood neuropsychiatric consultation described mild autonomic instability in an infant with age-appropriate neuromotor development.

Control EEG and ECG at 6 months of age were normal, and all parameters of physical growth were age-appropriate.

3. Discussion

In general, vitamin and mineral supplementation are common habits, aiming to prevent cardiovascular and oncologic diseases and, potentially, obtain mental and physical

TABLE 1: Vitamin content of 2 tablets (dose taken by the mother of the over-the counter supplement during pregnancy); *NRV = Nutritional Reference Values.

Vitamin	Two tablet content	*NRV%
Vitamin B6	4 mg	286%
Folic acid	400 mcg	200%
Vitamin B12	6 mcg	240%

benefits [8–11], but their true efficacy is still not evident or well demonstrated. Similarly, supplementation during pregnancy has been studied in relation to both maternal and fetal wellness [12, 13].

The only clear evidence for vitamin supplementation, based on its efficacy in the prevention of neural tube defects, has been obtained for folic acid in the periconceptional period.

Maternal diet, vitamin, and mineral supplementation in the postpartum maternal diet can modify the nutrient composition of colostrum and breast milk [14, 15].

Vitamin B6, an essential water-soluble vitamin that acts as a coenzyme in many biochemical reactions, a chronic iatrogenic overdose of vitamin B6, can cause neurological toxicity. The mechanism and specific contribution of the various B6 vitamins to neurological toxicity are largely unknown, but it is likely that they are mediated by inhibition of pyridoxal-5-phosphate-dependent enzymes [3].

Pyridoxine, the inactive form of B6, competitively inhibits pyridoxal-5′-phosphate, leading to symptoms of toxicity that mimic those of vitamin B6 deficiency [4]. Clinical history and physical examination are essential to identify patients in whom a potential drug toxicity is present [16], thus directing towards specific blood tests, including vitamin B6. In case of confirmation of vitamin B6 level well above reference values, the intake of drugs or supplements, identified as the cause of neurological symptoms, must be immediately stopped. Consequently, in the following weeks, the toxicity levels of vitamin B6 will progressively decrease with the complete normalization of the clinical picture.

For the patient we report, anamnestic data suggest that the high levels of vitamin B6 in the fetus are more likely due to transfer in the womb. In fact, the mother referred to a prolonged assumption of dietary supplements (as self-medication), continuing after delivery, which stopped only after the identification of an increased level of the nutrient. The transfer of vitamin B6 from mother to fetus during pregnancy has been known for a long time, as has a possible maternal vitamin B6 deficiency related to the active diaplacental transport and the request for vitamin B6 supplementation [17]. Similarly, several authors studied the relation between Vitamin B6 intake in the mother, the levels

TABLE 2: Vitamin B6 serum levels found in patient and mother. *serum normal levels (n.v. 8.7–27.2 micrograms/L).

	October 2020	November 2020	December 2020	April 2021
Newborn, serum B6 micrograms/L	102.7*	30.8*	59.1*	24.6*
Mother, serum B6 micrograms/L	400 mcg	52.1	22.1*	20.6*

in breast milk, and the effects on some behavioral abnormalities in children [18, 19].

In our case, vitamin B6 levels, although clearly higher than normal values, were below the levels previously reported as being able to induce clinically evident toxicity [4, 5].

Available evidence and the list of supplements that the mother has assumed suggest that vitamin B6 is reasonably the only nutrient that could be related to the clinical symptoms observed.

Hadtsteinand and Vrolijk [2] hypothesize that PDXK (pyridoxal kinase) inhibition, among others, by vitamin B6 availability results in GABA neurotransmission disruption and could be *the most plausible mechanism of B6 toxicity.*

The occurrence of vitamin B6 toxicity because of its supraphysiological supplementation might, of course, be associated with the presence of rare genetic variants, and PDXK might be a candidate gene to be investigated.

Our speculation is that some alleles in genes encoding proteins of vitamin B6 metabolism and/or excretion might promote in some subjects an accumulation of vitamin B6 or a greater cellular sensitivity to its action. This would lead to pyridoxine accumulation in the body, with a consequent toxic effect and the development of neurological manifestations.

The limitations of this report are mainly related to the fact that our data were obtained from a single case.

We believe in the importance of this study, which underlines that a widespread assumption of apparently harmless supplements without medical control may cause relevant clinical problems.

The "take home message" is that (i) it is important to remind doctors and nurses caring for pregnant women to inform their patients about the possible existence of clinical risks even in assuming "over the counter" products; (ii) toxic effects of self-medication may be transferred to the fetus; and (iii) information about possible, even if rare, toxic effects should be always plainly reported in the accompanying leaflet.

References

[1] Italian Society of Human Nutrition and L. A. R. N. Sinu, "Nutritional Reference Levels for Italian Population," 2014, https://www.sinu.it/tabelle-larn-2014.

[2] F. Hadtstein and M. Vrolijk, "Vitamin B-6-Induced neuropathy: exploring the mechanisms of pyridoxine toxicity," *Advanced Nutrition*, vol. 12, pp. 1911–1929, 2021.

[3] M. F. Vrolijk, A. Opperhuizen, E. H. J. M. Jansen, G. J. Hageman, A. Bast, and G. R. M. M. Haenen, "The vitamin B6 paradox: supplementation with high concentrations of pyridoxine leads to decreased vitamin B6 function," *Toxicology in Vitro*, vol. 44, pp. 206–212, 2017.

[4] D. A. Bender, "Non-nutritional uses of vitamin B6," *British Journal of Nutrition*, vol. 81, no. 1, pp. 7–20, 1999.

[5] M. P. Wilson, B. Plecko, P. B. Mills, and P. T. Clayton, "Disorders affecting vitamin B6 metabolism," *Journal of Inherited Metabolic Disease*, vol. 42, no. 4, pp. 629–646, 2019.

[6] A. Hemminger and B. K. Wills, *Vitamin B6 Toxicity*", StatPearls Publishing, Treasure Island (FL), 2020.

[7] D. C. Armentrout and J. Caple, "The jittery newborn," *Journal of Pediatric Health Care*, vol. 15, no. 3, pp. 147–149, 2001.

[8] D. P. Ingles, J. B. Cruz Rodriguez, and H. Garcia, "Supplemental vitamins and minerals for cardiovascular disease prevention and treatment," *Current Cardiology Reports*, vol. 22, no. 4, pp. 22–26, 2020.

[9] C. M. Mangione, M. J. Barry, W. K. Nicholson et al., "Vitamin, mineral, and multivitamin supplementation to prevent cardiovascular disease and cancer," *JAMA*, vol. 327, no. 23, pp. 2326–2333, 2022.

[10] J. Sarris, B. Mehta, V. Ovari, and I. Ferreres Gimenez, "Potential mental and physical benefits of supplementation with a high-dose, B-complex multivitamin/mineral supplement: what is the evidence?" *Nutrition Hospital*, vol. 38, pp. 1277–1286, 2021.

[11] L. D. Baker, J. E. Manson, S. R. Rapp et al., *Effects of cocoa Extract and a Multivitamin on Cognitive Function: A Randomized Clinical Trial*, Alzheimer's & Dementia, 2022.

[12] M. Li, E. Francis, S. N. hinkle, A. S. Ajjarapu, and C. Zhang, "Preconception and prenatal nutrition and neurodevelopmental disorders: a systematic review and meta-analysis," *Nutrients*, vol. 11, no. 7, pp. 1628–1632, 2019.

[13] M. Taagaard, H. Trap Wolf, A. Pinborg et al., "Multivitamin intake and the risk of congenital heart defects: a cohort study," *European Journal of Obstetrics & Gynecology and Reproductive Biology*, vol. 278, pp. 90–94, 2022.

[14] M. Keikha, R. Shayan-Moghadam, M. Bahreynian, and R. Kelishadi, "Nutritional supplements and mother's milk composition: a systematic review of interventional studies," *International Breastfeeding Journal*, vol. 16, pp. 1–7, 2021.

[15] E. Spigolon, I. Cimolato, E. Priante et al., "Diet in pregnant women that delivered prematurely and preterm newborn's bone status," *Journal of Maternal-Fetal and Neonatal Medicine*, vol. 35, no. 15, pp. 2859–2866, 2022.

[16] S. Keller and L. S. Dure, "Tremor in childhood," *Seminars in Pediatric Neurology*, vol. 16, pp. 60–70, 2001.

[17] L. Reinken and O. Dapunt, "Vitamin B6 nutriture during pregnancy," *International Journal for Vitamin and Nutrition Research*, vol. 48, no. 4, pp. 341–347, 1978.

[18] L. Boylan, S. Hart, K. B. Porter, and J. A. Driskell, "Vitamin B-6 content of breast milk and neonatal behavioral functioning," *Journal of the American Dietetic Association*, vol. 102, no. 10, pp. 1433–1438, 2002.

[19] A. L. McCullough, A. Kirksey, T. D. Wachs et al., "Vitamin B-6 status of Egyptian mothers: relation to infant behavior and maternal-infant interactions," *The American Journal of Clinical Nutrition*, vol. 51, no. 6, pp. 1067–1074, 1990.

[20] A. L. Lehninger, D. L. Nelson, and M. M. Cox, *Principles of Biochemistry*, Worth Publishers Inc, New York, NY USA, 2006.

19

Mimic for Child Physical Abuse: Biochemical and Genetic Evidence of Hypophosphatasia without Classic Radiologic Findings

Kasra Zarei ⓘ, John A. Bernat, Yutaka Sato, Rachel Segal, and Guru Bhoojhawon

University of Iowa, Carver College of Medicine, 200 Hawkins Drive, Iowa City, IA 52242, USA

Correspondence should be addressed to Kasra Zarei; kasra-zarei@uiowa.edu

Academic Editor: Juan Mejía-Aranguré

Infants presenting with multiple fractures without a plausible accident history need to be evaluated for child abuse or underlying predisposing conditions such as osteogenesis imperfecta and hypophosphatasia. We present a case of infantile hypophosphatasia with multiple unexplained fractures but otherwise normal radiographs in the setting of biochemical and genetic evidence of hypophosphatasia. Standard screening tests for hypophosphatasia include serum alkaline phosphatase level and genetic testing. Despite the presented case's positive biochemical and genetic testing, the case did not have any other radiologic finding suggesting infantile hypophosphatasia, such as severe bone mineralization deficits and rickets. While patients with hypophosphatasia can have increased bone fragility, this has been reported in the context of radiologic abnormalities of the skeleton. Thus, this case is potentially the first reported infantile hypophosphatasia case presenting with no findings of rickets on radiographs, raising concern that the fractures and especially the radius head dislocation might be due to physical abuse.

1. Introduction

Unexplained fractures in young children raise concern for child abuse. Although rare, fractures occur in numerous medical conditions. One such condition is hypophosphatasia, a genetic condition caused by mutations in the *ALPL* gene which encodes tissue-nonspecific alkaline phosphatase, leading to defective bone and teeth mineralization. Hypophosphatasia spans a multitude of clinical manifestations from before birth to early adulthood, and the diagnosis is often delayed. To our knowledge, this case is the first reported case of an infant with biochemical and genetic evidence of hypophosphatasia without classic radiological findings, which was the subject of child abuse evaluation.

2. Case Presentation

A previously healthy full-term 6-month-old male infant was brought to the Emergency Department (ED) with an 8-hour history of not moving his right arm and marked fussiness.

He had been behaving normally until a brief period when he was left unsupervised with two toddlers as the babysitter went to the kitchen to wash a bottle. Upon arrival, he had tachycardia (169 beats/minute). The rest of his vitals were normal. He could move all his extremities except the right upper extremity. He had a visible deformity of the right arm, and his neurological exam was normal.

Radiographs of the right upper extremity revealed an acute spiral right humeral fracture and healed fracture of the right mid-radius and ulna. This prompted a comprehensive child abuse workup. A skeletal survey showed thickened cortex in the mid-shaft of left humerus, radius, and ulna with subtle cortical irregularity, suggestive of healed fractures (Figure 1). The computed tomography (CT) scan of the head was negative (not shown). The dilated fundus examination was negative for retinal hemorrhages. The patient's arm was placed in a sling, and he was admitted for further management.

Upon further history, the caretakers reported that four days prior, the patient fell out of bed onto carpeted flooring.

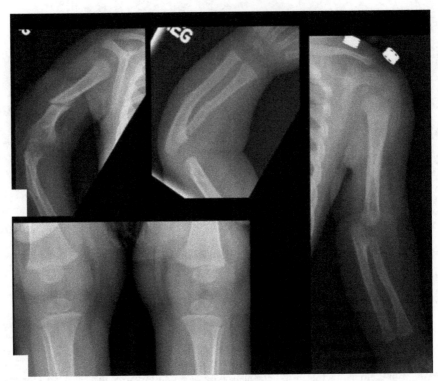

FIGURE 1: Spiral fracture of the right humerus is present (a). A right forearm radiograph shows healed midshaft fractures of the radius and ulna (b). The left upper extremity radiograph shows midshaft sclerosis and subtle cortical irregularity of the humerus, radius, and ulna, suggestive of healed fractures (c). The bone density is normal and no rarefaction of the zones of provisional calcification is present in the wrist and knees (b–d).

He was initially upset but was nursed back to sleep and was at baseline after he woke up. A similar fall happened several months ago, but the patient had returned to his baseline quickly without signs of injury. Developmental history was normal. There was no family history of unexplained or infantile fractures, bone disorders, connective tissue disorders, or bleeding disorders. There was no history of domestic violence in the home. Laboratory evaluation included normal calcium, phosphorus, magnesium, copper, ceruloplasmin, parathyroid hormone, 25-hydroxy vitamin D levels, free T4, and thyroid stimulating hormone (TSH). Urine drug screen was negative for illicit substances. Genetics consultation was conducted with subsequent *COL1A1* and *COL1A2* gene testing to evaluate for osteogenesis imperfecta (OI). A next-generation sequencing panel of OI-related genes was performed by an external genetic testing laboratory. The patient was discharged to the parents on hospital day 4, per child protective services (CPS) recommendations.

OI genetic testing returned negative, but the testing laboratory reported two variants in the *ALPL* gene, a pathogenic variant (c.526G > A, p.Ala176Thr), and a likely pathogenic variant (c.119C > T, p.Ala40Val). To confirm the diagnosis of hypophosphatasia, additional testing was sent and revealed low serum alkaline phosphatase (46 U/L; normal: 122–469 U/L), high serum pyridoxal 5′-phosphate (476 mcg/L; reference range: 5–50 mcg/L), and high urine phosphoethanolamine (850 nmol/mg; reference range: 15–341 nmol/mg). Parental site-specific testing for the two

ALPL variants revealed that the patient's mother had the p.Ala40Val variant and his father had the p.Ala176Thr variant. Based on his clinical history and laboratory findings despite the absence of classical radiographic findings, our patient was diagnosed with hypophosphatasia. On subsequent follow-up 10 weeks after discharge, he was growing well and had no new fractures. Enzyme replacement therapy was considered but ultimately not started.

3. Discussion

Hypophosphatasia is a rare (~1 in 100,000) inherited disorder of bone development caused by deficiency of serum alkaline phosphatase, leading to defective bone mineralization. The clinical presentation of hypophosphatasia is variable with multiple subtypes based on timing of onset of symptoms and presentation: (1) perinatal-onset: infant is born with symptoms, (2) infantile-onset: before six months of age, (3) childhood-onset: between six months of age to less than 18 years of age, (4) adult-onset: over 18 years of age, and (5) odonto-hypophosphatasia: presents at any age with only dental manifestations [1]. Recently, a mild prenatal form has been described as a sixth subtype [2]. The severity ranges from stillbirth without mineralized bone to pathologic fractures of the lower extremities in later adulthood.

While there are many clinical, biochemical, and radiographic features suggestive of hypophosphatasia, there are no formal criteria for diagnosis [3–5]. Furthermore, clinical features seen in one subtype may overlap with other subtypes. Patients with infantile hypophosphatasia often have severe bone mineralization deficit with bowing of the limbs and small thorax and pulmonary hypoplasia or rickets [3, 4]. Childhood hypophosphatasia may present with limited mobility, chronic pain, short stature, rickets, long bone deformity, and nontraumatic fractures [6]. However, marked bone fragility during childhood is rare [2]. All types display low serum alkaline phosphatase and the presence of one or two pathogenic variants in the *ALPL* gene [7]. The presented case did have one pathogenic variant and one likely pathogenic variant in the *ALPL* gene, allowing a diagnosis giving the clinical and biochemical findings.

There is one case describing an older child with unexplained fractures and otherwise normal radiographs who was found to have biochemical evidence of hypophosphatasia [2]: this case report described a 9-year-old female with a fracture of the right tibia from jumping, unexplained fracture of the right femoral neck, and unexplained fracture of the metaphysis of the right femur [2]. There were no reported cases of infants with biochemical and/or genetic evidence of hypophosphatasia without classic radiologic findings. The patient in this case we present had biochemical and genetic evidence of hypophosphatasia and otherwise normal radiographs except for mild osteopenia with no evidence of rickets despite multiple fractures. More apparent radiographic abnormalities in hypophosphatasia include bowing deformity of the long bones, severe osteopenia, and generalized metaphyseal rickets-like changes [4]. Less apparent cases pose challenges in differentiating from nonaccidental trauma like the current case.

Bone diseases, including osteogenesis imperfecta and hypophosphatasia, can be frequently confused with child physical abuse [7, 8]. Patient history, clinical course, family history, physical examination, routine laboratory tests, and radiographic imaging all contribute to distinguishing hypophosphatasia and bone diseases from child physical abuse [8]. Multiple fractures are less typical of hypophosphatasia, but hypophosphatasia cannot be excluded from the differential diagnostic list until biochemical testing is done as illustrated in this case. Serial measurement of serum alkaline phosphatase activity is usually sufficient to identify hypophosphatasia [7].

It is also important to consider child physical abuse when hypophosphatasia is the working diagnosis, which is not always the practice [4, 5, 9]. Systematic reviews of the literature only identified a handful of studies that directly compared and contrasted child abuse with metabolic or genetic bone disease in the same study [8, 10–15]. Of the five studies identified, four of them focused on cases of osteogenesis imperfecta [11–14]. To our knowledge, only one study directly mentioned the consideration of child abuse in the differential diagnosis of hypophosphatasia [8, 10]. Infants presenting with multiple fractures without a plausible accident history need to be evaluated for child physical abuse first and foremost while considering underlying predisposing conditions such as hypophosphatasia and osteogenesis imperfecta. It should also be kept in mind that children with a medical condition may also be abused or abuse cannot be ruled out [8, 11]. The healing fractures of the left and right radius and ulna on the patient's radiographs are not typical findings in hypophosphatasia but more consistent with healing traumatic fractures rather than pathologic fractures. In addition, the bending deformities of the upper and lower extremities could be due to normal variant of neonatal period or hypophosphatasia causing a delayed resolution or due to healing inflicted fractures.

As a result of these factors, diagnostic considerations in this case may include the following: hypophosphatasia leading to decreased bone mineralization might have caused bone weakness and multiple fractures with minimal trauma. However, the literature shows that asymptomatic children with hypophosphatasia and normal-appearing bones experience fractures anywhere between the ages of 6 months and 18 years of age (anecdotally often around 8-9 years of age) [3]. All infants with the infantile form of hypophosphatasia on the other hand present with overt findings of rickets and abnormal bones that explain the bone fragility [3, 7]. Lastly, radial head dislocation observed in this child cannot be explained by hypophosphatasia alone and may be due to physical abuse. Thus, physical abuse in the context of hypophosphatasia cannot be ruled out for this child, who has at least two sets of fractures from two different timeframes involving his right arm as well as a chronic-appearing radial head dislocation of the same arm. It is also possible that the incidental diagnosis of hypophosphatasia is a mild form of the disease with little or no impact on bone fragility. Unfortunately, there is no gold standard test for diagnosing child abuse, as the diagnosis is often determined by some combination of the patient's history, physical exam findings, radiographic findings, and an investigation by a state agency.

Thus, this case is the first report of infantile hypophosphatasia presenting with no findings of rickets on radiographs, raising concern that his fractures and especially radius head dislocation might be due to physical abuse.

References

[1] S. Simon, H. Resch, K. Klaushofer, P. Roschger, J. Zwerina, and R. Kocijan, "Hypophosphatasia: from diagnosis to treatment," *Current Rheumatology Reports*, vol. 20, no. 11, p. 69, 2018.

[2] P. Moulin, F. Vaysse, E. Bieth et al., "Hypophosphatasia may lead to bone fragility: don't miss it," *European Journal of Pediatrics*, vol. 168, no. 7, pp. 783–788, 2009.

[3] J. H. Simmons, "Best practices in: recognizing and diagnosing hypophosphatasia," *Clinical Endocrinology News*, vol. 8, no. 11, 2013.

[4] K. Kozlowski, J. Sutcliffe, A. Barylak et al., "Hypophosphatasia. Review of 24 cases," *Pediatric Radiology*, vol. 5, no. 2, pp. 103–117, 1976.

[5] M. P. Whyte, F. Zhang, D. Wenkert et al., "Hypophosphatasia: validation and expansion of the clinical nosology for children from 25 years experience with 173 pediatric patients," *Bone*, vol. 75, pp. 229–239, 2015.

[6] E. T. Rush, "Childhood hypophosphatasia: to treat or not to treat," *Orphanet Journal of Rare Diseases*, vol. 13, no. 1, p. 116, 2018.

[7] E. Mornet and M. E. Nunes, "Hypophosphatasia," in *GeneReviews*, M. P. Adam, H. H. Ardinger, R. A. Pagon et al., Eds., University of Washington, Seattle, WA, USA, 1993.

[8] N. K. Pandya, K. Baldwin, A. F. Kamath, D. R. Wenger, and H. S. Hosalkar, "Unexplained fractures: child abuse or bone disease? A systematic review," *Clinical Orthopaedics and Related Research*, vol. 469, no. 3, pp. 805–812, 2011.

[9] D. Wenkert, W. H. McAlister, S. P. Coburn et al., "Hypophosphatasia: nonlethal disease despite skeletal presentation in utero (17 new cases and literature review)," *Journal of Bone and Mineral Research*, vol. 26, no. 10, pp. 2389–2398, 2011.

[10] F. Horan and P. Beighton, "Infantile metaphysial dysplasia or "battered babies"? A reassessment of material in the fairbank collection," *The Journal of Bone and Joint Surgery*, vol. 62-B, no. 2, pp. 243–247, 1980.

[11] C. R. Paterson and S. J. McAllion, "Osteogenesis imperfecta in the differential diagnosis of child abuse," *BMJ*, vol. 299, no. 6713, pp. 1451–1454, 1989.

[12] C. R. Paterson and S. J. McAllion, "Classical osteogenesis imperfecta and allegations of nonaccidental injury," *Clinical Orthopaedics and Related Research*, vol. 452, pp. 260–264, 2006.

[13] C. R. Paterson, J. Burns, and S. J. McAllion, "Osteogenesis imperfecta: the distinction from child abuse and the recognition of a variant form," *American Journal of Medical Genetics*, vol. 45, no. 2, pp. 187–192, 1993.

[14] R. D. Steiner, M. Pepin, and P. H. Byers, "Studies of collagen synthesis and structure in the differentiation of child abuse from osteogenesis imperfecta," *The Journal of Pediatrics*, vol. 128, no. 4, pp. 542–547, 1996.

[15] L. S. Taitz, "Child abuse and metabolic bone disease: are they often confused?" *BMJ*, vol. 302, no. 6787, p. 1244, 1991.

20

Recurrent Pneumonia due to Fibrosing Mediastinitis in a Teenage Girl: A Case Report with Long-Term Follow-Up

Avigdor Hevroni [iD],[1] **Chaim Springer,**[1] **Oren Wasser,**[1] **Avraham Avital,**[1] **and Benjamin Z. Koplewitz**[2]

[1]*Institute of Pulmonology, Hadassah-Hebrew University Medical Center, Jerusalem, Israel*
[2]*Department of Radiology, Hadassah-Hebrew University Medical Center, Jerusalem, Israel*

Correspondence should be addressed to Avigdor Hevroni; avigdor@hadassah.org.il

Academic Editor: Amalia Schiavetti

A teenage girl was evaluated for recurrent right pneumonia. The evaluation revealed a calcified mediastinal mass that compressed the right intermediate and middle lobar bronchi, as well as the right pulmonary artery and veins. The clinical picture together with imaging studies and borderline positive serology testing suggested a diagnosis of fibrosing mediastinitis associated with histoplasmosis. This rare condition is characterized by the local proliferation of invasive fibrous tissue within the mediastinum due to a hyperimmune reaction to *Histoplasma capsulatum*. Antifungal and anti-inflammatory therapies are usually ineffective, and surgical intervention contains a high morbidity risk. Palliative surgery and stenting of the compressed airway have been suggested. In the past, the prognosis was thought to be poor, but recent studies demonstrate a more positive outcome. Our patient had been radiologically and functionally stable under follow-up for over thirteen years and has married and delivered two healthy children, both following an uneventful pregnancy.

1. Introduction

Fibrosing mediastinitis (FM) is a rare disorder characterized by the proliferation of locally invasive fibrous tissue within the mediastinum. Affected patients suffer from signs and symptoms related to the compression of vital organs located within the mediastinum. Although the etiology of FM remains unclear, most cases have been related to immune-mediated hypersensitivity reactions to antigens from the fungus *Histoplasma capsulatum*, which is endemic to North and Central America [1–3]. In the past, the prognosis was considered poor [1]; however, our case and other recent reports suggest a more favorable prognosis [2]. Here, we will present the evaluation and follow-up of a teenage girl presented with recurrent right lobe pneumonia which was finally diagnosed as FM.

2. Case Report

A thirteen-year-old girl was admitted to our hospital due to recurrent right pneumonia throughout the previous three years. She lost 3 kg in body weight in the preceding weeks but did not have fever or night sweats. She was born in Israel to parents of North African descent, with her mother completing treatment for Hodgkin's lymphoma 1.5 years before the girl's admission. During the years 1997–1999, when the patient was between six and eight years old, the family lived in Panama, Mexico and Florida.

Upon physical examination, she appeared well and had no signs of respiratory distress. Lung auscultation revealed decreased breath sounds over the right lung. There was no clubbing, and the rest of the exam was unremarkable. The basic laboratory results were insignificantly remarkable with no significant elevation of inflammatory markers.

A chest radiograph showed consolidation in the right lower lobe (RLL), with pleural thickening and effusion, and with resultant marked right lower lobe volume loss (Figure 1).

The recurrence of pneumonia focusing in the areas of the right middle and lower lobes (RML & RLL), demanded elimination of an anatomical disorder of the airways or

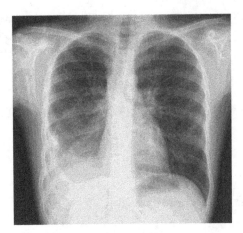

FIGURE 1: Posteroanterior chest radiography at presentation showing right lower lobe consolidation with pleural thickening and effusion, resulting in marked right lower lobe volume loss.

foreign body aspiration; therefore, a direct anatomical investigation was accomplished by bronchoscopy. The bronchoscopy revealed severe obstruction of the right bronchus intermedious and a complete obstruction of the bronchus to the RML due to external compression.

Bronchoalveolar lavage (BAL) sampling was done to look for relevant infectious etiologies. Bacterial cultures, acid-fast staining, and silver staining were all negative for bacteria, tuberculosis, or fungus.

A chest computed tomography (CT) was done for assessing the external compression shown by bronchoscopy and for ruling out additional relevant, though less probable, etiologies for recurrent right pneumonia. Additional etiologies for recurrent right pneumonia include some congenital anomalies such as congenital pulmonary airway malformation or a diaphragmatic hernia. The chest CT showed subcarinal and right hilar masses (3.6 and 2 cm, resp.) with prominent calcifications. These calcifications severely compressed the right bronchial tree, right pulmonary artery, and right inferior pulmonary vein (RPA and RPV), causing complete atelectasis of the RML (Figure 2).

In the differential diagnosis of the calcified mass, the first to be considered were tuberculosis, fungal infection, and a malignancy. Other options included nodule calcification due to a granuloma formation in response to a healed infection, for example, a healed varicella pneumonia [4]. It may have also represented the noncaseating granulomatous disease such as sarcoidosis or primary pulmonary amyloidosis. Another rare nonmalignant tumor to be considered was pulmonary chondroma as a part of the Carney triad which typically affects young females [5]. Last but not the least, calcification of the lung parenchyma may be present secondary to calcium and phosphate metabolism abnormalities [6] or to a benign inflammatory stimulus leading to calcifying fibrous pseudotumour (CFPT) of the lung [7].

An elaborated series of tests were completed due to suspected tuberculosis. PPD (Mantoux test) was negative as was the mother's (as a possible source). A quantiferon test and gastric fluid culture yielded the same results. Specimens of bronchoalveolar lavage fluid, pleural fluid, and pleural

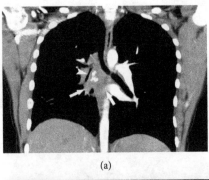

(a)

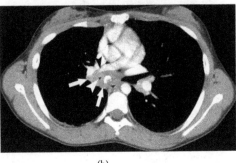

(b)

FIGURE 2: Axial (a) and coronal (b) reformats of the chest CT following a contrast injection, showing a subcarinal and right hilar ill-defined soft tissue mass (white arrows) with prominent interior calcifications causing marked compression on the bronchus intermedius, right middle lobe bronchus (white arrowhead), and right inferior pulmonary vein (black arrowhead).

biopsy all came back negative for TB as well as for malignancy, granulomas, fungi, or other pathologies. In addition to a pleural biopsy, a biopsy from the calcified mass was also obtained by a transbronchial biopsy. Though the biopsy detected a few inflammatory cells alongside fibrous tissue, it did not reveal any infectious pathogens, granulomas, or other specific pathologies.

Extensive evaluation showed negative results for other relevant infectious etiologies (except for what will be mentioned below), immune deficiencies, and autoimmune diseases. Serum angiotensin-converting enzyme activity was also within normal limits.

The patient's previous residence in areas endemic for histoplasmosis (U.S. and Mexico) gave us a clue to histoplasmosis infection as a possible source for our findings. Histoplasmosis antibody tests (performed by the Centers for Disease Control and Prevention (CDC) in Atlanta, Georgia, United States) were weakly positive with regard to the complement fixation test (titer of 1:8) and negative for the immunodiffusion test.

The clinical picture, imaging studies [8], serology results (although borderline), and past residence in areas endemic for histoplasmosis together with negative findings of other possible etiologies, all pointed to the diagnosis of histoplasmosis-related FM.

A series of complementary tests were done to better demonstrate the compression, to evaluate the severity of the lung disease, and for quantitative follow-up.

Cardiac magnetic resonance imaging (MRI) demonstrated normal ventricular function and narrowing of the RPA and RPV (Figure 3). Pulmonary function testing (PFT) revealed a mildly restrictive pattern with normal CO diffusion to alveolar gas (DL_{CO}/VA). On a perfusion/ventilation scan (V/Q), the ventilation scan showed a mild ventilation defect at the RT lower lobe, while the perfusion scan showed a severe perfusion defect in the middle and lower RT lobes. Cardiopulmonary exercise test (CPET) results displayed suboptimal peak O_2 consumption with a normal respiratory reserve.

2.1. Treatment. After ruling out a malignancy, but before TB test results returned, antitubercular treatment was commenced along with prednisone for two weeks due to the pleural involvement and the bronchial obstruction. As soon as the TB test results were found to be negative, the patient was slowly weaned off this treatment.

After the diagnosis of histoplasmosis-related FM became the most probable diagnosis, we started treatment with itraconazole (200 mg twice a day) for three months. In addition, several trials of bronchoscopic balloon dilatation of the right intermedious bronchus were performed but achieved only transient relief.

2.2. Follow-Up. Presently, after 13 years of follow-up, the patient functions normally regarding daily tasks but experiences some limitations during strenuous physical activity. She experiences annual or sometimes biannual symptoms of a chest infection which are treated with antibiotics.

Upon physical examination, she shows no signs of respiratory distress, with an SpO_2 of 100% on room air and good air entry to both lungs.

Throughout the follow-up period, no significant changes in the classified mass's size or impact were documented on CT scans. MRI images also showed no change. Lung function tests and physiologic respiration abilities on CPET remain intact compared to baseline.

The patient is now married and has delivered two healthy children, both with regular vaginal deliveries following an uncomplicated pregnancy, under tight multidisciplinal supervision.

3. Discussion

Histoplasmosis is a fungal infection resulting from the inhalation of spores of the fungus *Histoplasma capsulatum* which is endemic to the Ohio and Mississippi river valleys in the United States and also to Mexico and Central and South America. An estimated 40 million people in the United States have been infected with *H. capsulatum*, with 500,000 new cases occurring each year. Still, even in these localities, FM is relatively rare.

Transmission occurs by the mycelial form of *H. capsulatum* which is found in the soil. When spores produced by the mycelial form of *H. capsulatum* become airborne, they are inhaled and are deposited in the alveoli. At normal body temperature (37°C), the spores germinate into the yeast form

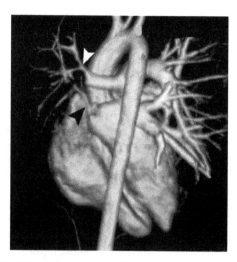

FIGURE 3: 3D reconstruction of the cardiac MRI demonstrates marked narrowing of the right pulmonary artery (black arrowhead) and the right inferior pulmonary veins (white arrowhead).

of this dimorphic fungus and are ingested by pulmonary macrophages. The yeasts become parasitic, multiply within these cells, and travel to hilar and mediastinal lymph nodes where they gain access to the blood circulation and are disseminated to various organs.

The diagnosis is easier by visualizing the yeast in tissue or by culture. The majority of infected persons is asymptomatic or has mildly symptomatic, self-limiting illnesses. However, in some situations significant manifestations may develop [9].

There are several types of serious histoplasmosis-related pulmonary conditions. The first is *acute diffuse pulmonary histoplasmosis* which occurs in patients exposed to a large number of infectious spores. The symptoms develop within a week or two and can progress to respiratory failure or progressive extrapulmonary dissemination. Most patients recover without treatment, but some of them remain dyspneic and fatigued for months. Conversely, *chronic pulmonary histoplasmosis* follows exposure in patients with underlying lung diseases. The clinical and radiographic findings resemble those of reactivated tuberculosis. The progressive disease process that ends in necrosis and loss of lung tissue results from a hyperimmune reaction to fungal antigens rather than from the infection itself. The symptoms can progress to cavities, formation of bronchopleural fistula, aspergilloma, atypical mycobacterial infections, chronic or recurrent pneumonia in areas of lung damage, and concurrent neoplasms in 5% of cases [2]. The third type, *disseminated pulmonary histoplasmosis*, is a rare disease which occurs primarily in immunocompromised patients [9], especially in patients with HIV infections. The spectrum of this illness is variable and ranges from a chronic, intermittent course in immunocompetent persons to an acute and rapidly fatal infection in infants and severely immunosuppressed people. In the fourth type, *granulomatous mediastinitis*, the mediastinal lymph nodes are enlarged, encapsulated, and caseous, following a direct infection by *H. capsulatum*. The last condition, *fibrosing mediastinitis* (FM), is also known as sclerosing mediastinitis. This is a benign but often progressive and potentially lethal disorder, characterized by infiltration of dense fibrous tissue into mediastinal fat [2].

A small number of patients with histoplasmosis develop FM. The average interval separating the initial symptoms from diagnosis is 3.5 years although in most cases the acute episode of histoplasmosis is not identified. Affected patients suffer from signs and symptoms related to the compression of the vital organs located within the mediastinum such as the superior vena cava (SVC), pulmonary veins, and arteries, trachea, bronchi, or esophagus. CT scans show a localized, calcified mass in the paratracheal or subcarinal regions of the mediastinum or the pulmonary hila. This mass may represent an idiosyncratic fibroinflammatory reaction to previous *H. capsulatum* infection. FM is also attributed to tuberculosis, sarcoidosis, autoimmune diseases, and radiation therapy. It may also be idiopathic. However, due to different clinical courses and the pathology itself, the aforementioned causes of FM are considered a different disease type than FM of histoplasmosis origin.

Diagnosis is usually based on the clinical picture and on characteristic imaging studies. Serologic studies are of limited diagnostic value. A biopsy can be hazardous, and when achievable, it is not always diagnostic. Therefore, it is usually reserved for excluding other diagnoses.

There is probably no curative therapy for FM to date. Antifungal and anti-inflammatory treatments such as glucocorticoids are generally ineffective, with only few reports suggesting benefits [10]. Surgical treatment presents a high risk of morbidity and mortality due to the hard fibrous mass caused by FM which consolidates the vital mediastinal structures. Lobectomy, pneumonectomy, stenotic airway resection, reconstruction, or bypass of involved arteries and veins may be offered to relieve symptoms. Bronchoscopic stent placement in the airways or percutaneous stent placement in blood vessels such as the SVC and pulmonary arteries or veins allow symptomatic relief but often necessitate reintervention [11]. Recently, reports from the Mayo Clinic demonstrated improvement in progressive FM following treatment with rituximab. After the researchers had reported accumulation of CD20-positive B lymphocytes in FM tissue, they considered treatment with rituximab, a monoclonal antibody targeted against CD20. Twelve patients with FM complicated by vascular or airway compromise along with increased metabolic activity by positron emission tomography with fluoro-D-glucose (FDG PET) test were treated with rituximab. All of them demonstrated symptomatic and radiologic improvement following this treatment, as predicted [12, 13].

Previous case reports and case series of FM reported a poor prognosis with a high mortality rate [1]. However, in a recent publication describing the course of 80 adult patients with FM, with an average follow-up of 41 months, the mortality rate was similar to the age-matched controls [2].

Presently, 13 years since the primary diagnosis, our patient is under no specific treatment; her mediastinal mass is stable, and she has only minor limitations with regard to exercise. She is married, has given birth to two healthy children, and lives a relatively normal life.

References

[1] J. E. Loyd, B. F. Tillman, J. B. Atkinson, and R. M. Desprez, "Mediastinal fibrosis complicating histoplasmosis," *Medicine*, vol. 67, no. 5, pp. 295–310, 1998.

[2] T. Peikert, T. V. Colby, D. E. Midthun et al., "Fibrosing mediastinitis: clinical presentation, therapeutic outcomes, and adaptive immune response," *Medicine*, vol. 90, no. 6, pp. 412–423, 2011.

[3] M. A. Schade and N. M. Mirani, "Fibrosing mediastinitis: an unusual cause of pulmonary symptoms," *Journal of General Internal Medicine*, vol. 28, no. 12, pp. 1677–1681, 2013.

[4] A. N. Khan, H. H. Al-Jahdali, C. M. Allen, K. L. Irion, S. Al Ghanem, and S. S. Koteyar, "The calcified lung nodule: what does it mean?," *Annals of Thoracic Medicine*, vol. 5, no. 2, p. 67, 2010.

[5] F. J. Rodriguez, M. C. Aubry, H. D. Tazelaar, J. Slezak, and J. Aidan Carney, "Pulmonary chondroma: a tumor associated with Carney triad and different from pulmonary hamartoma," *American Journal of Surgical Pathology*, vol. 31, no. 12, pp. 1844–1852, 2007.

[6] L. Camara Belém, G. Zanetti, A. Soares Souza Jr. et al., "Metastatic pulmonary calcification: state-of-the-art review focused on imaging findings," *Respiratory Medicine*, vol. 108, no. 5, pp. 668–676, 2014.

[7] M Peachell, J Mayo, and S Kalloger, "Calcifying fibrous pseudotumour of the lung," *BMJ*, vol. 58, no. 12, pp. 1018-1019, 2003.

[8] S. E. Rossi, H. P. McAdams, M. L. Rosado-de-Christenson, T. J. Franks, and J. R. Galvin, "Fibrosing mediastinitis," *RadioGraphics*, vol. 21, no. 3, pp. 737–757, 2001.

[9] R. Kurowski and M. Ostapchuk, "Overview of histoplasmosis," *American Family Physician*, vol. 66, no. 12, pp. 2247–2252, 2002.

[10] J. Wheat, G. Sarosi, D. McKinsey et al., "Practice guidelines for the management of patients with histoplasmosis," *Clinical Infectious Diseases*, vol. 30, no. 4, pp. 688–695, 2000.

[11] S. P. Ponamgi, C. V. DeSimone, C. J. Lenz et al., "Catheter-based intervention for pulmonary vein stenosis due to fibrosing mediastinitis: the Mayo Clinic experience," *International journal of cardiology. Heart & vasculature*, vol. 8, pp. 103–107, 2015.

[12] B. D. Westerly, G. B. Johnson, F. Maldonado, J. P. Utz, U. Specks, and T. Peikert, "Targeting B lymphocytes in progressive fibrosing mediastinitis," *American Journal of Respiratory and Critical Care Medicine*, vol. 190, no. 9, pp. 1069–1071, 2014.

[13] S. Mirza, U. Specks, K. Keogh, and T. Peikert, "Rituximab in the management of complicated fibrosing mediastinitis: the Mayo Clinic Experience," *American Thoracic Society International Conference Washington*, vol. 195, p. A7121, 2017.

21

An Unusual Diagnosis of Sporadic Type III Osteogenesis Imperfecta in the First Day of Life

Shreeja Shikhrakar,[1] **Sujit Kumar Mandal** ⓓ,[2] **Pradeep Sharma,**[1] **Sneha Shrestha,**[1] **and Sanket Bhattarai**[3]

[1]Department of Pediatrics, Kathmandu University School of Medical Sciences, Dhulikhel, Nepal
[2]Kakani Primary Health Center, Nuwakot, Nepal
[3]Paanchkhal Primary Health Center, Kavre, Nepal

Correspondence should be addressed to Sujit Kumar Mandal; sujeetmandal4888@gmail.com

Academic Editor: Maria Moschovi

Osteogenesis imperfecta (OI) is a group of rare, permanent genetic bone disorders resulting from the mutations in genes encoding type 1 collagen. It usually is inherited by an autosomal dominant pattern, but it can sometimes occur sporadically. Among the four main types, type III is the most severe type which presents with multiple bone fractures, skeletal deformities, blue sclera, hearing, and dental abnormalities. It is estimated that only 1 in 20,000 cases of OI are detected during infancy, and the diagnosis carries a poor prognosis. This case is reported for the rarity of sporadic OI diagnosis in neonates. We present a case of a 1-day-old neonate following a normal vaginal delivery referred to our center in the view of low birth weight and multiple bony deformities. Physical examination revealed an ill-looking child with poor suckling, gross bony deformities in upper and lower limbs, and blue sclera. X-ray showed thin gracile bones with multiple bone fractures. Echocardiography revealed a 4 mm patent ductus arteriosus. The patient was diagnosed with type III OI with patent ductus arteriosus. Though OI is rare in neonates and infants, it should be considered in the differentials in a newborn presenting with multiple bony deformities regardless of family history, history of trauma, or physical abuse. OI is also associated with cardiac anomalies such as the atrial septal defect and patent ductus arteriosus for which echocardiography is recommended routinely.

1. Background

Osteogenesis imperfecta (OI) is a group of rare genetic bone disorders affecting 1 in 13500–15000 births [1]. It results from the mutations in several genes including COL1A1 and COL1A2 genes encoding $\alpha 1$ and $\alpha 2$ chains of type 1 collagen [1–3]. Around 85%–90% of the cases are inherited by an autosomal dominant pattern and the rest can occur sporadically. Osteogenesis imperfecta (OI) is classified into four types, where type I is the least severe, type II is the lethal type perinatally, type III is the most severe one among survivors, and type IV is of intermediate severity [1, 4]. Type III OI presents with multiple bone fractures, skeletal deformities, blue sclera, hearing, and dental abnormalities [5]. Even though patients with type III OI are thought to have numerous fractures in the fetal and perinatal stages, the findings are often missed in antenatal ultrasonography [2, 5]. Here, we describe a rare case of osteogenesis imperfecta type III with PDA with radiographic findings of diffuse osteopenic changes, multiple fractures, and bone deformities in a newborn. In addition to the rarity of type III OI, only approximately 1 in 20000 cases of OI are detected during infancy [5]. This case is reported for the diagnosis of sporadic type III OI in a 1-day-old newborn.

2. Case Presentation

A 1-day-old newborn male born to a 24-year-old primigravida lady was referred to our center with complaints of multiple bony deformities and low birth weight. The baby did not cry immediately after birth and cried only after oronasal suctioning and tactile stimulation. The mother denied a history of trauma or any kind of physical abuse. Mother had regular antenatal visits, but prenatal anomaly scans were not done. There was no significant family history and consanguineous marriage.

On physical examination, the baby was ill-looking, and his vitals were stable. He had a blue sclera but no pallor or icterus. His anterior fontanelle was at level. His tone was normal. He had an ill-sustained and poor suckling. Gross bony deformities were present over bilateral upper and lower extremities (Figure 1). No abnormal findings were noted on systemic examination. He had a low birth weight of 2100 grams and was small for gestational age. His length was 37 cm, which was below the 3rd percentile. The ponderal index was calculated to be 4.

Investigations revealed significantly raised white cells (17300 per mm^3) and differential counts were neutrophil 80 and lymphocytes 12. His platelets were 183000 per mm^3. His hemoglobin was 15.9 g/dL, and his peripheral blood smear was normal. Serum calcium was 9.1, inorganic phosphorus 7.3 mg/dL, sodium 137 mEq/L, potassium 4.6 mEq/L, urea 30 mg/dL, and creatinine 0.6 mg/dL. He was severely hypoglycemic with random blood sugar less than 20 mg/dL. His total bilirubin was 8.9 mg/dL, and direct bilirubin was 0.8 mg/dL. The X-ray revealed thin gracile bones with multiple fractures including bilateral clavicles, left humeral diaphysis, bilateral lower limbs, and bilateral ribs which were marked in the left hemithorax (Figure 2). Diffuse osteopenic changes and marked bone deformities were seen as incurvation of the bilateral humerus and left radius and ulna suggestive of osteogenesis imperfecta type III (Figure 3). Echocardiography revealed a patent ductus arteriosus (PDA) of about 4 mm.

Based on clinical and radiographic findings, the child was primarily diagnosed as OI type III. The patient was treated with administration of intravenous fluids, ampicillin, and amikacin for 4 days. Oral cholecalciferol 100 IU twice a day and multivitamins once a day were continued along with oxygen supplementation via facemask. On the 1st day of admission, oxygen saturation was maintained in room air and feeding was started. No active intervention was advised, and the patient was discharged on oral cholecalciferol supplementation twice a day to continue along with oral multivitamin once a day to continue. The parents were advised to immunize the child as per Nepal's immunization schedule, provide adequate sun exposure, and breastfeed exclusively for 6 months along with the medications prescribed. At the time of discharge, the child was afebrile, clinically stable, and feeding well. Mother was counseled regarding the proper handling of the baby to minimize fractures and the incurable nature of the disease. She was also advised for a multidisciplinary consultation approach for better management of the condition.

The management was done by a consultant pediatrician with the assistance of pediatric residents at a tertiary care hospital in Nepal. The patient died at the age of 4 months at home which was confirmed via teleconsultation.

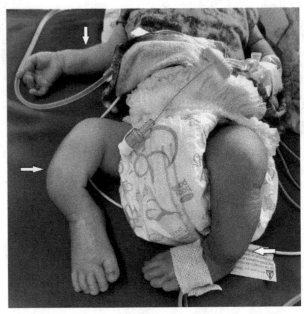

FIGURE 1: Gross bony deformities present over bilateral upper and lower extremities (shown by arrow head).

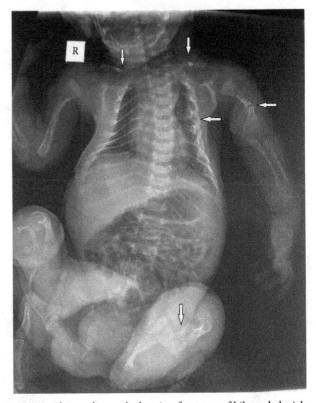

FIGURE 2: Plain radiograph showing fractures of bilateral clavicles, left humeral diaphysis, bilateral lower limbs, and bilateral ribs which were marked in the left hemithorax (fracture lines shown by arrowhead).

3. Discussion

Type 1 collagen is the most abundant collagen which consists of two α1 chains and one α2 chain that are important for maintaining bone strength and is encoded by COL1A1 gene

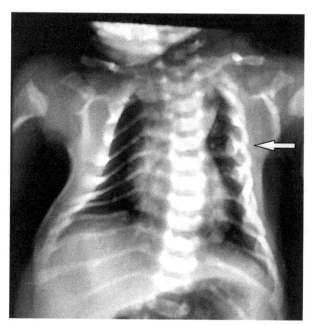

FIGURE 3: Diffuse osteopenic changes and fractures of ribs (marked more on left hemithorax shown by arrowhead).

and COL1A2 genes, respectively. Their mutation causes quantitative and qualitative defects of type 1 collagen and noncollagenous matrix proteins resulting in impaired bone strength. In addition, mutations in several genes including IFITM5, SERPINF1, CRTAP, LEPRE1, PPIB, BMP1, SERPINH1, FKBP10, SP7, TMEM38B, SEC24D, CREB3L1, PLOD2, and WNT1 have been implicated in pathogenesis of OI [1, 2]. These genetic defects can be either a quantitative defect presenting with a milder presentation or a qualitative defect presenting with a more severe manifestation [1].

OI is characterized by the triad of fragile bones, blue sclera, and deafness [5]. Owing to the widespread role of type I collagen, the clinical manifestations of OI vary from mild phenotype which is diagnosed later in life to lethal form, which may be diagnosed perinatally [1–3]. The skeletal manifestations also vary with the severity of the disease and include brittle bones, low bone density, multiple fractures, bowing of the extremities, and deformities of the spine which include scoliosis, spondylolisthesis, and vertebral compression fractures. The extraskeletal manifestations may include blue sclera, hydrocephalus, deafness, dentinogenesis imperfecta, dental malocclusion, and pulmonary, cardiac, or gastrointestinal anomalies [1, 3]. Cardiovascular and respiratory manifestations are the leading cause of death in patients with OI. Among the varied cardiac abnormalities such as atrial septal defects (ASD), mitral insufficiency, aortic root dilation, and septal and posterior left ventricular wall thickening, ASD and PDA were the commonest as stated by ElAbd and Moghazy [6].

Furthermore, multiple bone fractures and bone deformities are the predominant skeletal manifestations in OI type III present in the perinatal stages and are fairly uncommon after adolescence [2].

The type III and type II OI can be diagnosed with prenatal ultrasonography revealing bone fractures. In

contrast, to type II OI which can be detected as early as 14 weeks of gestation, type III OI is usually detected after 18 weeks of gestation exhibiting severe shortening of the long bones, hypoplastic thorax, marked bowing, fracture, and femur length to abdominal circumference ratio measuring less than 0.16. However, the diagnosis is often missed during prenatal ultrasonography. In a case series reported by John et al. [5], no significant anomaly suggesting OI was seen in 3 out of 3 reported cases in prenatal ultrasonography. These findings can also be confirmed with biochemical analysis such as collagen analysis of skin fibroblast culture or blood deoxyribonucleic acid analysis [5, 7, 8].

Moreover, diagnosis of various forms of OI can also be possible prenatally via gene mutation analysis in the second trimester of pregnancy [9]. The positive family history strongly supports the diagnosis of OI; however, the type of OI may vary in offspring. In addition, the reports of the sporadic occurrence of OI have been reported [2]. In distinction, type IV may occasionally be detected and diagnosis of OI type I is unreliable by prenatal ultrasonography [8].

Since there is no definitive cure to this disease, the management focused on preventing physical disability and improving physical activity [2]. Few management options are available to reduce the manifestations of this disease. There are shreds of evidence suggesting the role of bisphosphonate therapy in increasing the bone mineral density, cortical thickness, and trabecular bone volume and reducing the fracture rate of the long bones in young children with OI [10]. Bisphosphonate therapy is usually initiated after bone density scan [10]. Despite evidences, bisphosphonates could not be initiated in our patient due to various constraints including inaccessibility of the drug amidst COVID-19 pandemic and patient parties' refusal for further treatment in the ground of poor prognosis. Moreover, proper nutrition and activity are the mainstays of treatment of OI including calcium and vitamin D supplementation [3]. In our case, the child was conservatively managed with oral cholecalciferol and adequate sun exposure. Nowadays, bone deformities are treated with surgical osteotomies by drilling small holes in the cortices, and later, minimally invasive nailing is done [2]. However, the child in our case did not undergo any surgery owing to his small age and low birth weight.

The prognosis of OI is seen in terms of patients' ability to walk in later life which is dependent on the type of OI. It has been shown that patients with type III and type IV OI have a lower chance of ultimately walking compared to type I [11]. Babies born with OI type III possess a very bad prognosis. These patients sustain severe disability due to multiple fractures and bone deformities. Since patients with type III OI can have as many as 200 fractures in their lifetime, orthopedic management even with intramedullary nails is difficult. These individuals rarely live past 30 years of age even with proper management [12].

4. Conclusion

Though rare, the diagnosis of osteogenesis imperfecta should be kept in the differentials regardless of the family history in a newborn presenting with multiple bony deformities, low birth weight, and low anthropometric measures in the absence of trauma and physical abuse. Prenatal ultrasonography though helpful may not be entirely dependable in diagnosing OI prenatally. Echocardiography should be done routinely in OI for detection of associated cardiac anomalies such as ASD and PDA to increase the survival of the cases.

Authors' Contributions

Shreeja Shikhrakar and Sujit Kumar Mandal wrote,reviewed, and edited the article. Sneha Shrestha and Sanket Bhattarai collected data and edited the article. Pradeep Sharma contributed to patient management and critically reviewed the manuscript for intellectual content.

References

[1] S. Tournis and A. D. Dede, "Osteogenesis imperfecta - a clinical update," *Metabolism*, vol. 80, pp. 27–37, 2018.

[2] J.-J. Sinikumpu, M. Ojaniemi, P. Lehenkari, and W. Serlo, "Severe osteogenesis imperfecta Type-III and its challenging treatment in newborn and preschool children. A systematic review," *Injury*, vol. 46, no. 8, pp. 1440–1446, 2015.

[3] J. M. Franzone, S. A. Shah, M. J. Wallace, and R. W. Kruse, "Osteogenesis imperfecta: a pediatric orthopedic perspective," *Orthopedic Clinics of North America*, vol. 50, no. 2, pp. 193–209, 2019.

[4] D. O. Sillence, A. Senn, D. M. Danks, and A. Senn, "Genetic heterogeneity in osteogenesis imperfecta," *Journal of Medical Genetics*, vol. 16, no. 2, pp. 101–116, 1979.

[5] B. M. John, S. K. Patnaik, and R. W. Thergaonkar, "Multiple fractures in neonates and osteogenesis imperfecta," *Medical Journal Armed Forces India*, vol. 62, no. 1, pp. 73-74, 2006.

[6] H. S. A. ElAbd and M. Moghazy, "Cardiological assessment of a cohort of Egyptian patients with osteogenesis imperfecta type III," *Egyptian Journal of Medical Human Genetics*, vol. 17, no. 2, pp. 197–200, 2016.

[7] B. Edelu, I. Ndu, I. Asinobi, H. Obu, and G. Adimora, "Osteogenesis imperfecta: a case report and review of literature," *Annals of Medical and Health Sciences Research*, vol. 4, no. 7, 2014.

[8] F. S. van Dijk, J. M. Cobben, A. Kariminejad et al., "Osteogenesis imperfecta: a review with clinical examples," *Molecular Syndromology*, vol. 2, no. 1, pp. 1-20, 2011.

[9] A. Renaud, J. Aucourt, J. Weill et al., "Radiographic features of osteogenesis imperfecta," *Insights Imaging*, vol. 4, no. 4, pp. 417–429, 2013.

[10] T. Palomo, F. Fassier, J. Ouellet et al., "Intravenous bisphosphonate therapy of young children with osteogenesis imperfecta: skeletal findings during follow up throughout the growing years," *Journal of Bone and Mineral Research*, vol. 30, no. 12, pp. 2150–2157, 2015.

[11] R. H. Engelbert, C. S. Uiterwaal, V. A. Gulmans, H. Pruijs, and P. J. Helders, "Osteogenesis imperfecta in childhood: prognosis for walking," *The Journal of Pediatrics*, vol. 137, no. 3, pp. 397–402, 2000.

[12] L. Hackley and L. Merritt, "Osteogenesis imperfecta in the neonate," *Advances in Neonatal Care*, vol. 8, no. 1, pp. 21–30, 2008.

22

Symptomatic Internal Carotid Agenesis in Children

Abdullah Alhaizaey [ID],[1] **Ibrahim Alhelali** [ID],[2] **Musaed Alghamdi**,[3] **Ahmed Azazy**,[1] **and Mohammed A. Samir**[4]

[1]*Division of Vascular Surgery, Aseer Central Hospital, Abha Maternity and Children Hospital, Abha, Saudi Arabia*
[2]*Pediatric Intensive Care, Abha Maternity and Children Hospital, Abha, Saudi Arabia*
[3]*Department of Pediatrics, Menoufia University, Shibin Al Kawm, Egypt*
[4]*Aseer Central Hospital, Abha, Saudi Arabia*

Correspondence should be addressed to Abdullah Alhaizaey; aalhizaey@hotmail.com

Academic Editor: Sathyaprasad Burjonrappa

Carotid artery agenesis is a rare congenital anomaly, and there are controversies in the leading cause for it. We present a 6-year-old girl with resolved focal neurological ischemic stroke that showed bilateral internal carotid artery (ICA) agenesis. Through this paper, we highlight the carotid canal congenital obliteration hypothesis as it may be a risk for such finding.

1. Introduction

Agenesis of the internal carotid artery (ICA) is defined as the congenital absence of the internal carotid artery. It is rare, occurring in less than 0.01% of the population and is often an incidental finding [1, 2]. Bilateral ICA agenesis with patent common and external carotid arteries is extremely rare [3]. There is not yet an established hypothesis regarding the congenital and embryological anomalies that may lead to such agenesis. In this paper, we support the hypothesis that the embryological origin of the ICA differs from that of the common and external carotid arteries. The embryological development of the basal skull is important because the petrous bone carotid canal congenital diminution may lead to such anomalies [4]. Consent was taken for publishing such clinical finding.

2. Case Presentation

A six-year-old girl without any known illnesses was admitted to a pediatric hospital with sudden hemiplegia of the right upper and lower limbs. On clinical assessment, she was drowsy and her blood pressure was within the normal range, but she had sinus tachycardia (heart rate of 140 beats per minute) and her oxygen saturation was >96% in room air. She demonstrated total right-sided hemiplegia with power grade zero of four, loss of sensation with hypertonia, and exaggerated deep tendon reflexes.

Family history was negative for similar conditions. The patient was delivered normally at 36 weeks of gestation; however, her mother had not followed prenatal and postnatal care advice. The patient was admitted and was resuscitated, which normalized her vital signs to 120/68 mm Hg for blood pressure and 90 heart beats/minute. Urgent radiological investigation including brain and neck computed tomography with and without arterial phase contrast was performed. A bilateral absence of the internal carotid arteries was seen with a complete bilateral obliteration of the petrous bone carotid canals. Multiple collaterals were seen communicating with the anterior cerebral circulation that was supplied by an enlarged posterior communicating artery (POCMA) from a basilar artery (BA) and carotid rete mirabile from the external carotid artery (Figures 1 and 2). Further radiological workup including magnetic resonance imaging with arterial (MRA) and venous (MRV) contrast enhancement of the brain and neck showed infarction of the left cortical area at the region of the central sulcus. No intracranial or extracranial aneurysms were seen, the flow to condition with oral aspirin. She has been followed up regularly for 6 months without any complaints.

3. Discussion

Agenesis of the ICA is rare. There is controversy regarding whether the common and external carotid arteries (CCA and ECA) have the same embryological origin as that of the ICA (3, 4, and 6). Few reported cases show bilateral agenesis of the ICA with patent ECA and CCA [4, 5] as in our case. This may support the hypothesis that the embryological origin of the ICA differs from that of the ECA and CCA. Carotid canal diminution or obliteration is usually associated with carotid artery agenesis rather than aplasia or hypoplasia. [6, 7] In our case, both ICA orifices were obliterated congenitally. Most reported cases were asymptomatic and were discovered incidentally during routine radiological examinations [4, 5], but a transient ischemic attack (TIA) causing a focal neurological lesion could occur. Therefore, carotid agenesis could be a differential diagnosis for TIA, especially in younger patients. Radiological examination using computed tomography with arterial and venous phase contrast or MRI and MRV for the brain and neck including the skull base may provide clues regarding the deferential diagnosis including such congenital agenesis, mainly focusing on basal skull canals as the occlusion of carotid canal may lead to obliteration of the internal carotid arteries [6]. In such cases, the brain blood supply is maintained through the collaterals; for example, in our patient, the posterior circulation enabled the blood supply.

4. Conclusion

ICA agenesis is considered a differential diagnosis for childhood ischemic brain stroke. ICA agenesis with a patent ECA and CCA may support the hypothesis of a separate embryological origin for the ICA. Bilateral agenesis highlights the importance of radiological review for skull base bone anatomy. Diminution or obliteration of the carotid canal increases the possibility that such agenesis is related to embryological skull base bony canal changes.

References

[1] K. Suyama, S. Mizota, T. Minagawa, K. Hayashi, H. Miyazaki, and I. Nagata, "A ruptured anterior communicating artery aneurysm associated with internal carotid artery agenesis and a middle cerebral artery anomaly," *Journal of Clinical Neuroscience*, vol. 16, no. 4, pp. 585-586, 2009.

[2] F. perla, g. carbotta, D. Di nardo et al., "Agenesis of the internal carotid artery: a family pathology?" *Giornale di Chirurgia—Journal of Surgery*, vol. 38, no. 1, pp. 46–49, 2017.

[3] M. Orakdöğen, Z. Berkman, M. Erşahin, N. Biber, and H. Somay, "Agenesis of the left internal carotid artery associated with anterior communicating artery aneurysm: case report," *Turkish Neurosurgery*, vol. 17, pp. 273–276, 2007.

[4] C. A. Given II, F. Huang-Hellinger, M. D. Baker, N. B. Chepuri, and P. P. Morris, "Congenital absence of the internal carotid artery: case reports and review of the collateral circulation," *American Journal of Neuroradiology*, vol. 22, pp. 1935–1939, 2001.

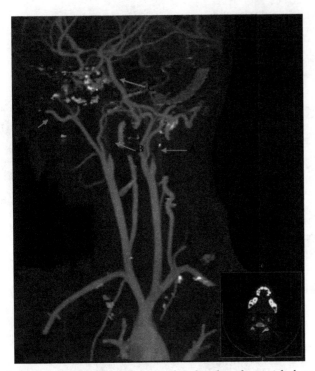

FIGURE 1: Sagittal view for CT head and neck with arterial phase contrast showed bilateral internal carotid artery (ICA) agenesis as shown by arrows A and B. Arrow C shows collaterals communicating with cerebral circulation that was supplied by an enlarged posterior communicating artery (POCMA) from a basilar artery (BA) and arrow D shows carotid rete mirabile from the external carotid artery.

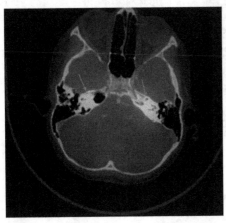

FIGURE 2: Skull base bone view with arrow showing obliteration for petrous bone carotid canal in the 6-year-old patient with bilateral ICA agenesis.

the superior sagittal sinus was normal, and there was no evidence of venous flow attenuation, thrombi, or venous occlusions. Echocardiography, hemoglobin electrophoresis, and a thrombophilia profile showed normal results.

The patient was started on 1 mg/kg of subcutaneous enoxaparin every 12 hours as an anticoagulant along with 5 mg/kg oral aspirin. She improved within 72 hours, and her weakness resolved completely, with a normal range of movement and sensation. She was discharged in good

[5] D. J. Quint, R. S. Boulos, and T. D. Spera, "Congenital absence of the cervical and petrous internal carotid artery with inter-cavernous anastomosis," *American Journal of Neuroradiology*, vol. 10, pp. 435–439, 1989.

[6] A. Di Ieva, E. Bruner, T. Haider et al., "Skull base embryology: a multidisciplinary review," *Child's Nervous System*, vol. 30, no. 6, pp. 991–1000, 2014.

[7] P. De Wals, F. Tairou, M. I. Van Allen et al., "Reduction in neural-tube defects after folic acid fortification in Canada," *New England Journal of Medicine*, vol. 357, no. 2, pp. 135–142, 2007.

23

Hirschsprung's Associated Enterocolitis (HAEC) Personalized Treatment with Probiotics Based on Gene Sequencing Analysis of the Fecal Microbiome

Georg Singer ⓘ,[1] Karl Kashofer,[2] Christoph Castellani ⓘ,[1] and Holger Till[1]

[1]Department of Paediatric and Adolescent Surgery, Medical University of Graz, Graz, Austria
[2]Institute of Pathology, Medical University of Graz, Graz, Austria

Correspondence should be addressed to Christoph Castellani; christoph.castellani@medunigraz.at

Academic Editor: Piero Pavone

Approximately 40% of children with Hirschsprung's disease (HD) suffer from Hirschsprung's associated enterocolitis (HAEC) despite correct surgery. Disturbances of the intestinal microbiome may play a role. Treatment with probiotics based on individual analyses of the fecal microbiome has not been published for HD patients with recurrent HAEC yet. A boy with trisomy 21 received transanal pull-through at the age of 6 months for rectosigmoid HD. With four years, he suffered from recurrent episodes of HAEC. The fecal microbiome was measured during three healthy and three HAEC episodes by next-generation sequencing. The patient was started on daily probiotics for 3 months; the fecal microbiome was measured weekly. The fecal microbiome differed significantly between healthy and HAEC episodes. HAEC episodes were associated with significant decreases of Actinobacteria and significant increases of Bacteroidetes and Proteobacteria. Probiotic treatment led to a significant increase of alpha diversity and a significant increase of *Bifidobacterium* and *Streptococcus* as well as decreases of *Rikenellaceae*, *Pseudobutyrivibrio*, *Blautia*, and *Lachnospiraceae*. A longitudinal observation of the microbiome has never been performed following correction of Hirschsprung's disease. Probiotic treatment significantly changed the fecal microbiome; the alterations were not limited to strains contained in the administered probiotics.

1. Introduction

Hirschsprung's disease (HD) is represented by a congenital segmental absence of the enteral nervous system in both the myenteric and submucosal plexus with variable proximal expression due to a failure of migration of neural crest cells during embryonic development [1]. The resulting intestinal obstruction is usually treated by surgical removal of the aganglionic bowel and a pull-through of unaffected ganglionic bowel.

Despite correct endorectal pull-through for HD, up to 40% of the patients continue to suffer from Hirschsprung's associated enterocolitis (HAEC) defined as a clinical condition with diarrhea, abdominal discomfort, fever, and eventually subsequent septic shock [2]. Nevertheless, the exact pathogenesis of HAEC still remains unclear.

Considering the complex interrelation between the epithelium, the immune system, and the microbiome of the intestine, disturbances of the intestinal microbial composition may predispose a patient to develop HAEC independent of correct surgical treatment.

Currently, next-generation sequencing is widely applied in gastrointestinal studies and facilitates the comprehensive description of the whole genome of the intestinal microbiota. With reference to Hirschsprung's disease, however, there are a limited number of reports describing disruptions of the intestinal microbiome in patients suffering from HAEC when compared to healthy Hirschsprung's disease patients [3–5]. Additionally, it has been shown that treatment with probiotics not only significantly diminishes the incidence but also decreases the severity of HAEC [6]. These two findings support the hypothesis that disruptions of the intestinal microbiome may be associated with the development of HAEC.

Nevertheless, the available evidence is based on interindividual comparisons of the intestinal microbiome including patients with or without enterocolitis, respectively. An intraindividual comparison of the intestinal microbiome during episodes with and without enterocolitis has not been performed yet. Neither has been studied whether or not treatment of Hirschsprung's disease patients with probiotics alters the intestinal microbiome.

Therefore, the aim of the present report was to describe the intestinal microbiome of a patient suffering from Hirschsprung's disease during episodes with and without enterocolitis and during treatment with probiotics applying 16S rRNA gene next-generation sequencing.

2. Case Presentation

A three-year-old boy with a rectosigmoidal Hirschsprung's disease and trisomy 21 received laparoscopically assisted Georgeson pull-through operation at the age of six months. Histology confirmed normal ganglion cells at the site of the anastomosis. The initial postoperative course was unremarkable; especially, the anastomosis healed with neither stricture nor dehiscence. Nevertheless, the boy suffered from recurrent episodes of HAEC with diarrhea, abdominal distention, pain, and alterations of the general condition classified as grade I according to the APSA criteria [7].

2.1. Healthy and HAEC Episodes. Stool samples were taken for microbial assessment during three healthy episodes and three HAEC episodes, sampled to PSP spin stool DNA sample kits (Stratec Molecular GmbH, Berlin, Germany), and stored at −21°C until measurement. The microbiome analysis was performed in duplicates as already published [8]. Statistical analysis was performed using the compare_categories.py and the group_significance.py scripts of QIIME 1.8. These scripts implement several statistical methods for the analysis of strength and statistical significance of sample groupings or OTUs via the vegan and ape R packages. Category significance was calculated using the Adonis and ANOSIM tests, while OTU significance was calculated using the Kruskal–Wallis test.

Alpha diversity between healthy and HAEC episodes was not significantly different (Chao 1 Index: mean healthy episode 967, SD 94; mean HAEC episode 1,009, SD 72; $p = 0.432$).

To assess beta diversity, a community analysis was performed by using principal coordinate analysis (PCoA) plots and Adonis and ANOSIM tests. A statistically significant difference in the composition of the fecal microbiome between healthy and HAEC episodes was found (Figure 1).

Taxonomic analysis revealed a statistically significant decrease of the relative abundances of Actinobacteria and significant increases of Bacteroidetes, Proteobacteria, and Cyanobacteria on the phylum level during HAEC episodes (Figure 2). A detailed overview of the statistically significant

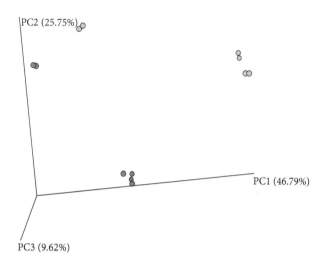

FIGURE 1: Principal coordinate analysis (PCoA, Bray–Curtis) plots of each sample as a point in a multidimensional space based on the composition of the bacterial population in each sample. Closeness of two points indicates similar bacterial population composition between the samples. PCoA plot of the fecal microbiome of three separate healthy episodes (green dots) and three HAEC episodes (red dots) with measurements performed in duplicate is given. Adonis and ANOSIM tests revealed statistically significant differences in the composition of the intestinal microbiome between healthy and HAEC episodes (Adonis: $p = 0.009$, $R^2 = 0.31$; ANOSIM: $p = 0.007$, $R^2 = 0.52$).

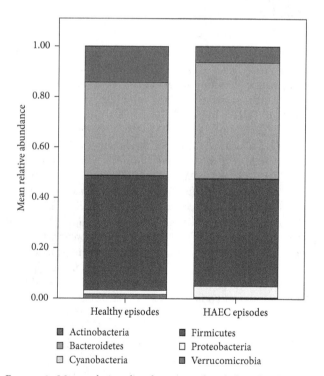

FIGURE 2: Mean relative abundances on the phylum levels comparing three healthy episodes and three HAEC episodes. Statistically significant changes were found for the phyla Actinobacteria, Bacteroidetes, Proteobacteria, and Cyanobacteria.

differences of the relative abundances on the remaining levels comparing healthy and HAEC episodes is given in Table 1. One of the most striking changes was seen for the

TABLE 1: Relative bacterial abundances (%) on the different levels of the different episodes (n = 3 healthy and n = 3 HAEC). From the class level downstream, only germs with statistically significant differences ($p < 0.05$) are listed.

Phylum	Class	Order	Family	Genus	Healthy	HAEC	p value
Actinobacteria					14.09	6.25	0.004
	Actinobacteria	Bifidobacteriales	Bifidobacteriaceae	Bifidobacterium	12.94	5.50	0.004
Bacteroidetes					37.47	46.30	0.003
	Bacteroidia	Bacteroidales			37.50	46.30	0.003
			Bacteroidaceae	Bacteroides	29.90	33.70	0.02
			Rikenellaceae		1.70	4.20	0.02
Cyanobacteria					0.03	0.29	0.02
	4C0d-2				0.03	0.29	0.02
		YS2			0.03	0.30	0.02
Firmicutes					44.90	42.10	0.2
	Bacilli	Lactobacillales			2.84	0.24	0.02
	Clostridia	Clostridiales	Lachnospiraceae	Dorea	1.70	0.60	0.004
				Lachnospira	0.50	1.60	0.02
			Ruminococcaceae	Oscillospira	0.40	0.80	0.006
				Ruminococcus	2.40	1.40	0.01
			Veillonellaceae	Veillonella	0.03	0.14	0.04
Proteobacteria					1.60	4.52	0.01
	Alphaproteobacteria				0.48	1.71	0.01
		RF32			0.48	1.70	0.01
	Deltaproteobacteria	Desulfovibrionales	Desulfovibrionaceae	Bilophila	0.12	0.46	0.004
	Gammaproteobacteria	Pasteurellales	Pasteurellaceae	Haemophilus	0.18	0.50	0.025
Verrucomicrobia					1.79	0.48	0.14

genus Bifidobacterium which was reduced from 13% to 5% during HAEC episodes.

2.2. Probiotic Treatment. The patient was started on continuous treatment with probiotics for three months. In detail, he received one sachet of OMNi-BiOTiC® PANDA (Institut Allergosan, Graz, Austria) in the morning and one sachet of OMNI-BiOTiC® 10 AAD (Institut Allergosan, Graz, Austria) in the evening. OMNi-BiOTiC® PANDA contains Lactococcus lactis W58, Bifidobacterium bifidum W23, and Bifidobacterium lactis W52 (total of 3×10^9 CFU/sachet). OMNi-BiOTiC® 10 AAD contains Lactobacillus acidophilus W55, Lactobacillus acidophilus W37, Lactobacillus paracasei W72, Lactobacillus rhamnosus W71, Lactobacillus salivarius W24, Lactobacillus plantarum W62, Bifidobacterium bifidum W23, Bifidobacterium lactis W18, Bifidobacterium longum W51, and Enterococcus faecium W54 (total of 5×10^9 CFU/sachet). During these 3 months of treatment, fecal samples were taken weekly (as described above) adding to a total number of 14 samples.

During the observation period, the patient had episodes of diarrhea on 18% of the days (7 out of 39 days) without probiotic treatment and on 14% of the days under probiotic treatment (13 out of 90 days).

In the period of probiotic treatment, six stool samples were taken for microbiome analysis during diarrhea episodes and eight during healthy episodes. Probiotic treatment led to a significantly increased alpha diversity (Chao 1 Index) irrespective of healthy or HAEC episodes (mean healthy episode with probiotics 1,269, SD 111; mean HAEC episode with probiotics 1,274, SD 91; mean healthy episode without probiotics 967, SD 94; mean HAEC episode without

probiotics 1,009, SD 72; $p < 0.05$ vs. their corresponding episode without probiotics).

Community analysis of the samples taken before and under probiotics is depicted in Figure 3. Statistically significant differences of the composition of the fecal microbiome were found between healthy and HAEC episodes and under probiotic treatment.

Mean relative abundances on the phylum and genus levels are depicted in Figure 4. On the phylum level, the most striking findings were that, during HAEC episodes under probiotic treatment, the significant increase of Bacteroidetes and the decrease of Actinobacteria were not encountered (compare Figure 4). On the genus level, Bifidobacterium and Streptococcus were significantly increased during probiotic treatment. Additionally, probiotic treatment led to significant decreases of Rikenellaceae, Pseudobutyrivibrio, Blautia, and Lachnospiraceae.

3. Discussion

In a corrected HD patient, HAEC led to significant alterations of the fecal microbiome when compared to healthy episodes. Additionally, we were able to show that treatment with probiotics significantly alters the intestinal microbiome with the most striking changes observed comparing probiotic therapy to HAEC episodes. Moreover, these changes were not limited to the strains contained in the administered probiotics.

Even though a variety of different hypotheses have been formulated, the exact pathophysiology of HAEC still remains unclear. Recent studies have shown that a disruption of the intestinal mucosal barrier ("leaky gut"), an increase of

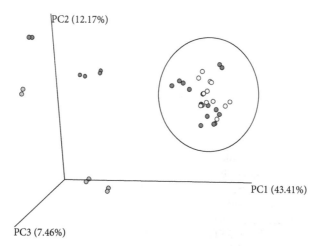

FIGURE 3: Principal coordinate analysis (PCoA, Bray–Curtis) of the fecal microbiome of healthy episodes (green dots) and HAEC episodes (red dots) before probiotic treatment and under probiotic treatment (healthy: blue dots, HAEC: yellow dots). Adonis and ANOSIM tests revealed statistically significant differences in the composition of the fecal microbiome between these episodes (Adonis: $p = 0.001$, $R^2 = 0.49$; ANOSIM: $p = 0.001$, $R^2 = 0.98$). Measurements were performed in duplicates.

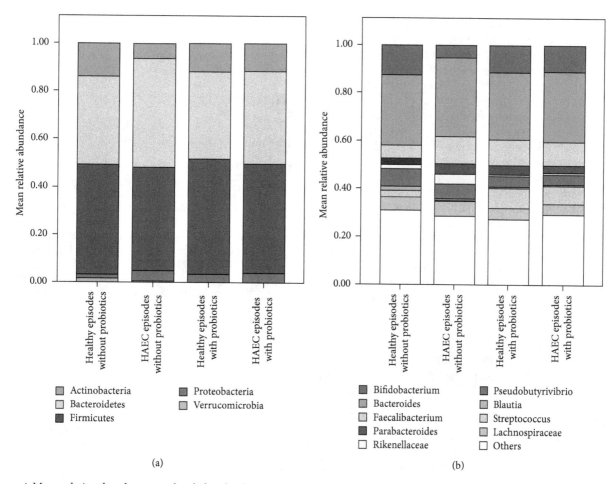

FIGURE 4: Mean relative abundances on the phylum levels (a) and genus level (b) before and under probiotic treatment in healthy and HAEC episodes. Note that on the genus level, only genera with more than 5% relative abundance are depicted.

inflammatory parameters, an abnormal immune response of the intestinal tract, and infection due to specific pathogens like *Clostridium difficile* may play pivotal roles in the development of HAEC [9]. However, both experimental and clinical studies recently have given a first insight into an altered intestinal microbiome in Hirschsprung's disease and HAEC and have revealed conflicting findings. For instance, Yan and coworkers have assessed the microbial signature of intestinal contents taken during surgery from different sections along the intestinal tract in a study population consisting of four patients (two patients with HAEC and two patients with Hirschsprung's disease) [5]. Bacteroidetes and Proteobacteria accounted for the highest proportion among the intestinal flora in Hirschsprung's disease patients. In contrary, Proteobacteria and Firmicutes were the most common microbes in HAEC patients. Comparing these results to those of the present study, we were able to find significant increases of Bacteroidetes and Proteobacteria during HAEC episodes. Nevertheless, changes of Firmicutes were not encountered in our patient (compare Figure 2). In another multicentric study consisting of patients suffering from Hirschsprung's disease, 9 with a history of HAEC and 9 without, the bacterial composition of the HAEC group showed a modest reduction in Firmicutes and Verrucomicrobia with increased Bacteroidetes and Proteobacteria compared to the group without HAEC [3]. Although these changes did not reach statistical significance, they are similar to the alterations found in our patient. However, all of the abovementioned studies were performed as interindividual comparisons, and therefore, biases influencing the intestinal microbiome caused by differences concerning geography, nutrition, and age cannot be ruled out. The present study reveals significant alterations of the fecal microbiome during HAEC episodes in an intraindividual comparison for the first time.

The fecal microbiome of the present patient during HAEC episodes indicates a proinflammatory state of the intestine. For instance, it has been proposed that an increased prevalence of Proteobacteria is a potential diagnostic signature of dysbiosis and risk of disease [10]. Other microbial diversity studies have also continually demonstrated an expansion of the Proteobacteria phylum in patients with inflammatory bowel disease [11]. It also has been shown that Actinobacteria can produce antibacterial agents [12]. Therefore, the decrease of their relative abundance during HAEC episodes most likely is associated with decreased levels of these agents fueling the proinflammatory intestinal state. However, it remains unknown whether these changes are a cause or a consequence of HAEC.

Treatment with probiotics was shown to be beneficial in a variety of diseases including acute infectious diarrhea, antibiotic-associated diarrhea, Clostridium difficile-associated diarrhea, hepatic encephalopathy, ulcerative colitis, irritable bowel syndrome, and necrotizing enterocolitis [13]. Regarding HAEC, however, the available reports are contradictory. While some studies have described that probiotics not only significantly diminish the incidence but also decrease the severity of HAEC [6], others did not confirm these findings [14]. Whether or not probiotic treatment can influence the occurrence of HAEC was not the focus of the present study, and answering this question would need prospective randomized trials. Nevertheless, analyses of the fecal microbiome of Hirschsprung's disease patients during probiotic treatment have not been performed yet. While the defecation pattern was not changed in our patient, we were able to describe alterations of the fecal microbiome during probiotic treatment with the most profound changes compared to HAEC episodes without probiotics. It is not surprising that the DNA of the applied probiotics can be detected in the feces of the treated patients. However, the fact that also other genera such as Streptococcus, Rikenellaceae, and Blautia were affected by probiotic treatment supports a broader influence of oral probiotic treatment on the gastrointestinal microbiome.

The main limitation of the present study remains the fact that it only presents data of one case. Nevertheless, we were able to compare within this patient three separate episodes of HAEC (APSA grade I) versus three healthy episodes. Additionally, a total of 14 investigations of the fecal microbiome during a three-month probiotic treatment period are included. Thus, this manuscript presents an innovative and important clinical concept inviting future studies including more patients. In conclusion, for the first time, this case presents the effective treatment of a child with HD and postoperative episodes of HAEC. Additionally, profound changes of the microbial composition during three months of probiotic treatment were found.

Acknowledgments

We thank the Institut Allergosan pharm. Produkte Forschungs- u. Vertriebs GmbH for providing the probiotics.

References

[1] V. Sasselli, V. Pachnis, and A. J. Burns, "The enteric nervous system," Developmental Biology, vol. 366, no. 1, pp. 64–73, 2012.

[2] K. M. Austin, "The pathogenesis of Hirschsprung's disease-associated enterocolitis," Seminars in Pediatric Surgery, vol. 21, no. 4, pp. 319–327, 2012.

[3] P. K. Frykman, A. Nordenskjold, A. Kawaguchi et al., "Characterization of bacterial and fungal microbiome in children with Hirschsprung disease with and without a history of enterocolitis: a multicenter study," PLos One, vol. 10, no. 4, Article ID e0124172, 2015.

[4] Y. Li, V. Poroyko, Z. Yan et al., "Characterization of intestinal microbiomes of hirschsprung's disease patients with or without enterocolitis using illumina-MiSeq high-throughput sequencing," PLos One, vol. 11, no. 9, Article ID e0162079, 2016.

[5] Z. Yan, V. Poroyko, S. Gu et al., "Characterization of the intestinal microbiome of Hirschsprung's disease with and without enterocolitis," Biochemical and Biophysical Research Communications, vol. 445, no. 2, pp. 269–274, 2014.

[6] X. Wang, Z. Li, Z. Xu, Z. Wang, and J. Feng, "Probiotics prevent Hirschsprung's disease-associated enterocolitis: a prospective multicenter randomized controlled trial," International Journal of Colorectal Disease, vol. 30, no. 1, pp. 105–110, 2015.

[7] A. Gosain, P. K. Frykman, R. A. Cowles et al., "Guidelines for the diagnosis and management of Hirschsprung-associated enterocolitis," Pediatric Surgery International, vol. 33, no. 5, pp. 517–521, 2017.

[8] G. Gorkiewicz, G. G. Thallinger, S. Trajanoski et al., "Alterations in the colonic microbiota in response to osmotic diarrhea," PLos One, vol. 8, no. 2, Article ID e55817, 2013.

[9] L. Hong and V. Poroyko, "Hirschsprung's disease and the intestinal microbiome," Clinical Microbiology: Open Access, vol. 3, no. 5, 2014.

[10] N. R. Shin, T. W. Whon, and J. W. Bae, "Proteobacteria: microbial signature of dysbiosis in gut microbiota," *Trends in biotechnology*, vol. 33, no. 9, pp. 496–503, 2015.

[11] I. Mukhopadhya, R. Hansen, E. M. El-Omar, and G. L. Hold, "IBD-what role do Proteobacteria play?," *Nature Reviews Gastroenterology and Hepatology*, vol. 9, no. 4, pp. 219–230, 2012.

[12] G. B. Mahajan and L. Balachandran, "Antibacterial agents from actinomycetes-a review," *Frontiers in Bioscience*, vol. 4, no. 1, pp. 240–253, 2012.

[13] T. Wilkins and J. Sequoia, "Probiotics for gastrointestinal conditions: a summary of the evidence," *American Family Physician*, vol. 96, no. 3, pp. 170–178, 2017.

[14] M. El-Sawaf, S. Siddiqui, M. Mahmoud, R. Drongowski, and D. H. Teitelbaum, "Probiotic prophylaxis after pullthrough for Hirschsprung disease to reduce incidence of enterocolitis: a prospective, randomized, double-blind, placebo-controlled, multicenter trial," *Journal of Pediatric Surgery*, vol. 48, no. 1, pp. 111–117, 2013.

24

Unique Mutation in SP110 Resulting in Hepatic Veno-Occlusive Disease with Immunodeficiency

Osama Hamdoun,[1] **Asia Al Mulla,**[1] **Shamma Al Zaabi,**[1] **Hiba Shendi,**[2]
Sharifa Al Ghamdi,[2] **Jozef Hertecant,**[2] **and Amar Al-Shibli**[2]

[1]*Department of Academic Affairs, Tawam Hospital, Al-Ain, UAE*
[2]*Department of Pediatrics, Tawam Hospital, Al-Ain, UAE*

Correspondence should be addressed to Osama Hamdoun; osamahamdoun@hotmail.com

Academic Editor: Amalia Schiavetti

Familial hepatic veno-occlusive disease with immunodeficiency (VODI, OMIM: 235550) is a rare form of combined immune deficiency (CID) that presents in the first few months of life with failure to thrive, recurrent infections, opportunistic infections along with liver impairment. Herein, we are describing a Pakistani patient with a homozygous novel variant in the *SP110* gene, presenting with classical phenotypic manifestations of VODI. He presented at the age of 3 months with opportunistic infections and later developed liver failure. *Conclusion.* Hepatic veno-occlusive disease with immunodeficiency is a rare cause of immunodeficiency, and this is the first case report from the Middle East in a patient of Pakistani origin. It is important to have a high suspicion for this disease, in patients presenting early life with a picture of CID and deranged liver function, as the earlier the diagnosis and treatment, the better the prognosis.

1. Introduction

Familial veno-occlusive disease with immunodeficiency syndrome (VODI; Online Mendelian Inheritance in Man (OMIM) 235550) is an autosomal recessive immunodeficiency syndrome [1]. The key features of VODI include: (1) immunodeficiency (usually combined affecting the cellular and humoral function) and (2) liver involvement in the form of hepatomegaly with/without hepatic failure or histologically proved hepatic veno-occlusive disease (hVOD). Mutations in Sp110 gene leads to SP110 protein deficiency and the clinical manifestations of VODI [2].

Patients with VODI usually show manifestations early in life with repeated bacterial, viral, and fungal infections. These infections are usually serious and may be life-threatening. Herein, we are describing a case with homozygous novel variant in the *SP110* gene with classical phenotypic manifestations of VODI.

2. Case Presentation

This is a 3 month-old-male of Pakistani origin. He was delivered by normal vaginal delivery at term with an uncomplicated perinatal course. Parents are second degree relatives. He first presented initially to hospital at the age of 3 months with fever, oral thrush resistant to topical antifungal gels, and diarrhea.

Laboratory workup showed significant pan-hypogammaglobulinaemia with derangement of liver function test. Lymphocyte subset analysis showed moderate T-cell lymphopenia mainly affecting the CD4 population but was otherwise unremarkable (Table 1).

During his hospital stay, he suddenly developed acute respiratory failure, which required resuscitation and intubation. At that time, CXR showed bilateral ground glass appearance, which was suggestive of pneumocystis pneumonia (PCP) or cytomegalovirus (CMV) infection. CMV viral load was elevated of 39000; as a result, he was diagnosed with

TABLE 1: Investigations at 3 months of age.

Investigation at age of 2-3 months	Result	Reference range
IgM	<0.25 g/l	0.15–0.70 g/l
IgG	<2.0 g/l	2.1–7.7 g/l
IgA	<0.06 g/l	0.05–0.40 g/l
CD3	1.404 cells/Micro/L	3.5–5 cells/Micro/L
CD4	0.744 cells/Micro/L	2.8–3.9 cell/Micro/L
CD8	0.637 cells/Micro/L	0.637 cells/Micro/L
CD19	0.581 cells/Micro/L	0.581 cells/Micro/L
NK cells	0.037 cells/Micro/L	0.1–1.3 cell/Micro/L
CD4/CD8	1.168 cells/Micro/L	0.9–3.6 cell/Micro/L
CMV quantitative	166,250	<490 cp/ml
WBC	17.5×10^9	$5–10 \times 10^9$
Hgb	12.5	11–13 g/l
Platelet	67×10^9	$140–400 \times 10^9$
Hepatitis B s Ab	Negative	
Hepatitis C Ab	Negative	
Hepatitis A IgM	Negative	
HIV	Negative	
BAL	Negative	
Karyotyping	46 + XY	
Liver enzymes		
Albumin	22 g/dl	
AST	217	22–58 IU/l
ALT	96	11–39 IU/l
Total bilirubin	22	5–22 micromol/l
PT	19.7	Seconds
PTT	46.9	Seconds

disseminated CMV infection and was treated with ganciclovir with excellent response; repeated CMV viral load after treatment is less than 5780 copies, which is undetectable. He had bronchoalveolar lavage which showed mixed upper respiratory flora. His lymphocyte subsets normalized with CD4 count of 1,800 cells Micro/L. In spite of normal lymphocyte subsets, the presence of disseminated CMV and pan-hypogammaglobulinaemia was highly suspicious of severe combined immunodeficiency (SCID). Unfortunately, lymphocyte proliferation studies were not available. The patient was therefore commenced on antimicrobial prophylaxis and immunoglobulin replacement therapy, and currently patient is not having any new infections.

Moreover, the patient developed recurrent ascitic fluid accumulation, hypoalbuminemia, and further derangement of liver enzymes. Investigations ruled out protein losing enteropathy and nephropathy.

Abdominal ultrasound showed slightly enlarged liver and moderate amount of ascites. Peritoneal fluid analysis was normal. Liver biopsy showed sinusoidal obstructive syndrome (veno-occlusive disease), portal and lobular eosinophils, and noncaseating granulomas. Currently, his liver disease is static, but it is expected to worsen overtime.

Table 1 shows the laboratory data of the patient at the time of the presentation.

Whole exome sequencing (WES) was suggestive of the hepatic veno-occlusive disease with immunodeficiency as it confirmed *SP110* (NM_080424.2) homozygous variant c.691 C > T p (Gln231∗). Null Mutation is expected to result in absent protein expression, and the disease is most likely from consanguineous parents Table 2.

3. Discussion

VODI was described originally in Australians of Lebanese origin by Mellis and Bale in 1976 [3]. A majority of children reported with VODI have been of Lebanese origin with prevalence of one in 2,500 [1].

There were other reports afterwards from different regions of the world with novel mutations from families of Italian, Hispanic, and Arabic ethnic origins [2, 4] (Figure 1).

The age of presentation is around 4 months (usually before 12 months) with respiratory distress, fever, failure to thrive and diarrhea, as well as disseminated CMV infection, rotavirus-related gastroenteritis, and respiratory *Pneumocystis jiroveci*. Our patient presented at the age of 3 months with recurrent oral thrush and failure to thrive. At 4 months, he developed disseminated CMV infection with hepatitis and pneumonitis. In a group of 16 patients with VODI, clinical hepatosplenomegaly was detected in 12 patients at presentation [3, 4]. Ninety percent of the children with VODI present with either hepatomegaly (83% with preceding infection) or hepatic failure (53% with preceding infection) [2].

Neurological manifestations (occur in up to 30%) of cases are due to the veno-occlusive disease of the brain which may manifest as cerebral necrosis. Some of the patients described in the literature had cerebral leukodystrophy.

Thrombocytopenia and syndrome of inappropriate antidiuretic hormone secretion also have been described [5].

VODI is associated with 100% mortality in the first year of life if unrecognized and untreated with immunoglobulin replacement and *Pneumocystis jirovecii* prophylaxis, and a

TABLE 2: Result of WES showing the defect of the *SP110*.

Gene	Variant coordinates	In silico parameters*	Allele frequencies**	Type and classification***
SP110	Chr2(GRCh37):g.231076245G>A NM_080424.2:c.691C>T p.(Gln231*)	PolyPhen: N/A Align-GVGD: N/A SIFT: N/A Mutation taster: N/A Conservation: nt weak	gnomAD :- ESP :- 1000 G :- CentoMD :-	Stop gain Likely pathogenic (class 2)

Variant description based on Alamut Batch 1.7 (latest database available). *Align-GVD: C0: least likely to interfere with function; C65: most likely to interfere with function; splice prediction tools: SSF, MaxEnt, and HSF. **Exome Aggregation Consortium (ExAC) database, Exome Sequencing Project (ESP), 1000Genome project (1000G), and CentoMD 4.0. ***Based on ACMG recommendations.

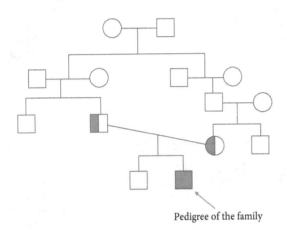

Pedigree of the family

FIGURE 1: Pedigree of the family.

90% mortality overall by the midteenage years if not treated with bone marrow transplant [5].

The immunodeficiency is characterized by severe hypogammaglobulinemia, clinical evidence of T-cell immunodeficiency with normal numbers of circulating T and B cells, absent lymph node germinal centres, and absent tissue plasma cells. Bacterial and opportunistic infections including *Pneumocystis jirovecii* infection, mucocutaneous candidiasis, and enterovirus or cytomegalovirus infections occur [1].

VODI is inherited in an autosomal recessive manner. Carrier testing for at-risk relatives and prenatal diagnosis for pregnancies at increased risk are possible if both pathogenic variants in a family are known [5, 6].

The *SP110* protein plays a crucial role in shaping the inflammatory milieu that supports host protection during infection by fine-tuning of NF-κB activity which is required for normal T and B cell responses. A range of mutations in *SP110* causes decreased *SP110* protein levels and clinical disease. [7, 8] Some of the acquired immune deficiencies have been associated with veno-occlusive disease as well [9].

It is important to diagnose VODI in the first year of life as it is associated with 100% mortality if missed and untreated. There are reports of successful treatment of VODI with hematopoietic stem cell transplantation in few patients [10].

4. Conclusion

Hepatic veno-occlusive disease with immunodeficiency is a rare cause of immunodeficiency. To the best of our knowledge, this is the first report on a Pakistani patient with a novel homozygous mutation in *SP110* (NM_080424.2)

homozygous variant c.691 C > T p. (Gln231*) [11]. The patient was presented with classical presentation of liver impairment with immune deficiency.

References

[1] T. Roscioli, S. T. Cliffe, D. B. Bloch et al., "Mutations in the gene encoding the PML nuclear body protein Sp110 are associated with immunodeficiency and hepatic veno-occlusive disease," *Nature Genetics*, vol. 38, no. 6, pp. 620–622, 2006.

[2] F. A. Marquardsen, F. Baldin, F. Wunderer et al., "Detection of Sp110 by flow cytometry and application to screening patients for veno-occlusive disease with immunodeficiency," *Journal of Clinical Immunology*, vol. 37, no. 7, pp. 707–714, 2017.

[3] C. Mellis and P. M. Bale, "Familial hepatic venoocclusive disease with probable immune deficiency," *The Journal of Pediatrics*, vol. 88, no. 2, pp. 236–242, 1976.

[4] S. T. Cliffe, D. B. Bloch, S. Suryani et al., "Clinical, molecular, and cellular immunologic findings in patients with SP110-associated veno-occlusive disease with immunodeficiency syndrome," *Journal of Allergy and Clinical Immunology*, vol. 130, no. 3, pp. 735–742, 2012.

[5] Tony Roscioli, J. B. Ziegler, M. Buckley, and M. Wong, "Hepatic veno-occlusive disease with immunodeficiency," *GeneReviews*, 2018.

[6] E. L. Ivansson, K. Megquier, S. V. Kozyrev et al., "Variants within the SP110 nuclear body protein modify risk of canine degenerative myelopathy," *Proceedings of the National Academy of Sciences of the United States of America*, vol. 113, no. 22, 2016.

[7] T. Wang, P. Ong, T. Roscioli, S. T. Cliffe, and J. A. Church, "Hepatic veno-occlusive disease with immunodeficiency (VODI): first reported case in the U.S. and identification of a unique mutation in Sp110," *Clinical Immunology*, vol. 145, no. 2, pp. 102–107, 2012.

[8] T. Roscioli, J. B. Ziegler, M. Buckley, and M. Wong, "The responsible gene is SP110 required for its transcriptional regulatory function and cellular translocation," *Journal of Biomedical Science*, vol. 25, p. 34, 2018.

[9] J. A. Buckley and G. M. Hutchins, "Association of hepatic veno-occlusive disease with the acquired immunodeficiency syndrome," *Modern Pathology*, vol. 8, no. 4, pp. 398–401, 1995.

[10] H. Ganaiem, E. M. Eisenstein, A. Tenenbaum et al., "The role of hematopoietic stem cell transplantation in SP110 associated veno-occlusive disease with immunodeficiency syndrome," *Pediatric Allergy and Immunology*, vol. 24, no. 3, pp. 250–256, 2013.

[11] J.-S. Leu, S.-Y. Chang, C.-Y. Mu, M.-L. Chen, and B.-S. Yan, "Functional domains of SP110 that modulate its transcriptional regulatory function and cellular translocation," *Journal of Biomedical Science*, vol. 25, no. 1, p. 34, 2018.

25

Infantile Myofibroma Presenting as a Large Ulcerative Nodule in a Newborn

Farooq Shahzad [1,2] **Ava G. Chappell,**[2] **Chad A. Purnell,**[2] **Monica Aldulescu,**[1] **and Sarah Chamlin**[1,2]

[1]Ann & Robert H. Lurie Children's Hospital, Chicago, Illinois, USA
[2]Northwestern University Feinberg School of Medicine, Chicago, Illinois, USA

Correspondence should be addressed to Farooq Shahzad; fooqs@hotmail.com

Academic Editor: Christophe Chantrain

The differential diagnosis of a congenital cutaneous vascular-appearing mass in a newborn is broad and includes both benign and malignant tumors. We report the case of a newborn who presented with an erythematous exophytic skin nodule on the right upper leg. Excision was performed due to ulceration, concern for bleeding, and for diagnosis. Pathology revealed the mass to be an infantile myofibroma. This case highlights the importance of considering a broad differential diagnosis in a newborn with a cutaneous mass. While history, physical exam, and imaging can help diagnose some cases, a biopsy or excision is often needed to distinguish benign lesions from more concerning lesions.

1. Introduction

The diagnosis of vascular-appearing cutaneous masses in an infant can be challenging. We present a neonate with a vascular-appearing ulcerated skin lesion that was presumed to be a hemangioma by the referring primary care provider, and pathology later revealed it to be an infantile myofibroma (IM). A brief review of the differential diagnoses considered for this case is provided, along with the suggested management of infantile myofibroma.

2. Case Presentation

An 11-day-old male was referred for evaluation of a cutaneous mass of the right upper lateral thigh (Figure 1). The child had an uncomplicated full-term birth. The parents reported that the lesion looked like a "red ball" at birth, but over several days the surface became darker in color. The mass was nontender. His parents also noticed some blood on the diaper near the mass. On exam, the child had an exophytic erythematous nodule with overlying eschar and friable surface measuring 2×2 cm on the right upper lateral

thigh. The appearance was not typical of a congenital hemangioma. Due to concerns about bleeding, the possibility that this might develop into a difficult-to-manage open wound, and the need for a diagnosis, the entire lesion was excised at 14 days of life. Primary closure was performed after undermining with recruitment of local tissue (Figure 2). The final pathology revealed the diagnosis of infantile myofibroma (Figures 3–7). The child's postoperative course was uneventful with no tumor recurrence at 6-month follow-up.

3. Discussion

Clinical diagnosis of vascular-appearing congenital skin nodules can be difficult, and often a tissue diagnosis is required. The differential diagnosis in this child included: congenital hemangioma, juvenile xanthogranuloma, pilomatrixoma, myofibroma, and fibrosarcoma.

Congenital hemangiomas are fully formed at birth, and then either undergo rapid involution (rapidly involuting congenital hemangioma or RICH), fail to involute (non-involuting congenital hemangioma or NICH), or undergo

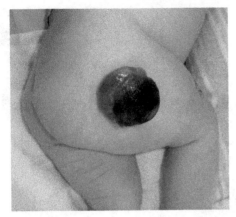

FIGURE 1: Cutaneous mass of the right thigh.

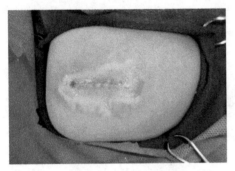

FIGURE 2: Excision of mass and primary closure.

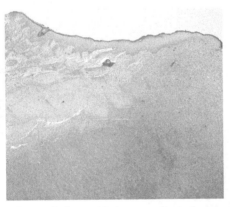

FIGURE 3: Histopathology with hematoxylin and eosin staining. Scanning view (1x magnification) shows a dermal proliferation of spindled cells with lighter and darker areas.

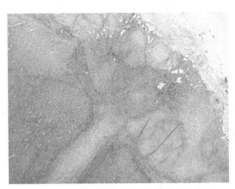

FIGURE 4: Low power view (5x magnification) shows a nodular/multinodular tumor with a zonal appearance of hypercellular areas in the center and hypocellular areas at the periphery.

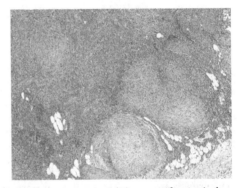

FIGURE 5: Higher power view (10x magnification) shows a multinodular, biphasic tumor with alternating hyper and hypocellular areas.

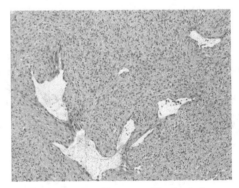

FIGURE 6: High-power view (20x magnification) shows numerous hemangiopericytoid slit-like vessels in the center of the tumor.

initial rapid involution that then stops at some point (partially involuting congenital hemangioma or PICH). They often have a rim of pallor and coarse overlying blood vessels and may ulcerate, as a rare complication. Juvenile xanthogranulomas are yellow, red, or purple colored nodules that are present at birth or appear in the first year of life. They are usually solitary but can be multiple and undergo growth and ulceration. Their natural history is spontaneous regression [1]. Pilomatrixomas are common but frequently misdiagnosed [2]. They are benign tumors of the hair matrix cells that grow slowly and calcify. They appear as raised subcutaneous nodules that are skin colored, red, or blue.

Usually arising in childhood, they can occasionally appear in infancy [3]. Treatment is surgical excision. Congenital fibrosarcomas are firm round skin lesions present at birth. They are slow growing, red to purple in color, fixed to deep structures and may have superficial telangiectasias or ulcerate. Biopsy provides a definitive diagnosis [4].

Of note, although neuroblastoma and nasal glioma were not included in the differential diagnosis in this case, they can present as a cutaneous, vascular-appearing masses in neonates. Nasal gliomas are frequently misdiagnosed as

FIGURE 7: Staining for smooth muscle actin shows that myofibroblastic areas (myoid component) are positive while the fibroblastic areas (nonmyoid areas) are negative (10x magnification).

hemangiomas, especially by nonpediatric providers. They are collections of heterotopic neuroglial tissue that present as raised red masses on the nasal dorsum. Any midline nasal mass should raise the suspicion for a glioma or encephalocele, and CT or MRI is frequently obtained for further evaluation of the lesion and possible intracranial extension. Neuroblastoma is the most common neonatal malignant tumor, with 2/3 having metastases [5]. Cutaneous metastasis can be initial presentation of this disease with blue or purple nodules. Biopsy provides the diagnosis, which prompts a metastatic workup.

Infantile myofibromas, although rare, are the most common fibrous tumors of infancy [6]. They can arise in any part of the body, but are most commonly found in the skin and subcutaneous tissue. The majority are present at birth or arise within the first 2 years of life with a male to female ratio of 2 : 1 [7, 8]. Occasionally, they are present in adulthood [9]. Infantile myofibroma may be solitary (70 to 80%) or multicentric (20 to 30%) [8, 10]. The most common location of a solitary IM is the head and neck, followed by the trunk and extremities [8, 10]. They present as nontender, rubbery, subcutaneous, or dermal nodules of 0.5 to 7 cm in diameter that are dusky-red to purple in color [10]. Surface telangiectasias may be noted, and ulceration occurs rarely. Their appearance frequently leads to confusion in distinguishing them from congenital hemangiomas [10]. The multicentric form IM can have from a few to up to 100 lesions [11], and occasionally a large lesion is surrounded by multiple smaller lesions [8]. Important for physicians to keep in mind, approximately one third of multicentric myofibromas have visceral involvement [12].

Most cases of IM are thought to be sporadic. Familial forms of IM have been reported with autosomal dominant and recessive inheritance patterns [13, 14]. Mutations in the PDGFRB (platelet-derived growth factor receptor beta) and NOTCH3 gene have been identified in the autosomal dominant forms of the disease [15, 16]. Genetic counseling should be considered in familial cases, as future offspring may be affected.

Histopathology can provide a definitive diagnosis. IM have a characteristic histological pattern with an outer zone of spindle-shaped myofibroblasts arranged in fascicles and an inner zone of round cells with enlarged hyperchromatic nuclei surrounding thin walled hemangiopericytoma-like blood vessels. Necrosis, calcification, and vascular extension may be present in the central area. Immunohistochemical stains provide definitive diagnosis with the smooth muscle stains actin and vimentin being positive and S100 (positive in neurofibroma) and GLUT-1 (positive in infantile hemangioma) being negative.

The natural history of IM is of gradual regression, possibly due to apoptosis, over the first few years of life, although some lesions exhibit an initial phase of rapid growth [17]. Of note, bony involvement can result in pathological fractures [11]. Visceral IM portends a poor prognosis with a 33 to 75% mortality rate, primarily due to mass effect on the organs [7, 12]. Tumors have been reported to involve the pulmonary, cardiac, gastrointestinal, and central nervous systems, although they can affect virtually any organ [18–22]. The prognosis is worst with pulmonary involvement. Evaluation of visceral involvement in multicentric IM can be performed with imaging such as a skeletal survey, chest X-ray, echocardiogram, ultrasound, and CT scans [22], and whole body MRI can be performed in infants which gives an excellent evaluation of the tumors and avoids radiation [23]. Management of visceral IM is surgical excision for solitary symptomatic lesions, and recurrence rate after excision is 7 to 10% [8, 12]. Multiple lesions, unresectable lesions, and recurrences can be treated with chemotherapy ± radiation [24]. The chemotherapeutic agents that have been used include alkylating agents (cyclophosphamide and ifosfamide), vinca alkaloids (vincristine, vinblastine, and vinorelbine), doxorubicin, actinomycin-D, and methotrexate [25]. Targeted inhibitors like sunitinib [25] and crizotinib [26] are showing promise as a treatment strategy for aggressive cases.

4. Conclusion

This case highlights a common clinical scenario faced by pediatricians caring for newborns: accurately diagnosing a congenital vascular skin nodule. When the diagnosis of a vascular-appearing pediatric mass is not clear, further workup includes imaging studies such as ultrasound and MRI and is done by an experienced radiologist who may differentiate a solid tumor with vascularity from a congenital hemangioma. An incisional or excisional biopsy is often performed with specific immunohistochemical stains for precise diagnosis. If there is concern for systemic disease, appropriate workup should be performed. Prompt referral to an experienced pediatric dermatologist or pediatric plastic surgeon is crucial for the best plan of care.

Abbreviations

IM: Infantile myofibroma.

Authors' Contributions

Dr. Shahzad conceptualized and designed the study, collected the data, performed the literature review, and reviewed and revised the manuscript. Dr. Chappell performed the literature review and drafted the initial manuscript. Dr. Purnell collected the data and critically reviewed the manuscript. Dr. Aldulescu critically reviewed and revised the manuscript. Dr. Chamlin critically reviewed and revised the manuscript. All authors approved the final manuscript as submitted and agreed to be accountable for all aspects of the work.

References

[1] M. W. Chang, "Update on juvenile xanthogranuloma: unusual cutaneous and systemic variants," *Seminars in Cutaneous Medicine and Surgery*, vol. 18, no. 3, pp. 195–205, 1999.

[2] A. Pirouzmanesh, J. F. Reinisch, I. Gonzalez-Gomez, E. M. Smith, and J. G. Meara, "Pilomatrixoma: a review of 346 cases," *Plastic and Reconstructive Surgery*, vol. 112, no. 7, pp. 1784–1789, 2003.

[3] R. Méndez-Gallart, M. G. Tellado, J. Del Pozo-Losada, and J. M. Rois, "A rapid onset erythematous facial lesion in a neonatal patient," *Pediatric Dermatology*, vol. 26, no. 2, pp. 195-196, 2009.

[4] T. Enos, G. A. Hosler, N. Uddin, and A. Mir, "Congenital infantile fibrosarcoma mimicking a cutaneous vascular lesion: a case report and review of the literature," *Journal of Cutaneous Pathology*, vol. 44, no. 2, pp. 193–200, 2017.

[5] A. S. Alfaar, W. M. Hassan, M. S. Bakry, and I. Qaddoumi, "Neonates with cancer and causes of death; lessons from 615 cases in the SEER databases," *Cancer Medicine*, vol. 6, no. 7, pp. 1817–1826, 2017.

[6] T. E. Wiswell, J. Davis, B. E. Cunningham, R. Solenberger, and P. J. Thomas, "Infantile myofibromatosis: the most common fibrous tumor of infancy," *Journal of Pediatric Surgery*, vol. 23, no. 4, pp. 315–318, 1988.

[7] J. Mashiah, S. Hadj-Rabia, A. Dompmartin et al., "Infantile myofibromatosis: a series of 28 cases," *Journal of the American Academy of Dermatology*, vol. 71, no. 2, pp. 264–270, 2014.

[8] E. B. Chung and F. M. Enzinger, "Infantile myofibromatosis," *Cancer*, vol. 48, no. 8, pp. 1807–1818, 1981.

[9] A. Beham, S. Badve, S. Suster, and C. D. M. Fletcher, "Solitary myofibroma in adults: clinicopathological analysis of a series," *Histopathology*, vol. 22, no. 4, pp. 335–341, 1993.

[10] D. Stanford and M. Rogers, "Dermatological presentations of infantile myofibromatosis: a review of 27 cases," *Australasian Journal of Dermatology*, vol. 41, no. 3, pp. 156–161, 2000.

[11] P. W. Brill, D. R. Yandow, L. O. Langer, A. L. Breed, R. Laxova, and E. F. Gilbert, "Congenital generalized fibromatosis: case report and literature review," *Pediatric Radiology*, vol. 12, no. 6, pp. 269–278, 1982.

[12] T. E. Wiswell, E. L. Sakas, S. R. Stephenson, J. J. Lesica, and S. R. Reddoch, "Infantile myofibromatosis," *Pediatrics*, vol. 76, no. 6, pp. 981–984, 1985.

[13] D. J. Zand, D. Huff, D. Everman et al., "Autosomal dominant inheritance of infantile myofibromatosis," *American Journal of Medical Genetics*, vol. 126A, no. 3, pp. 261–266, 2004.

[14] H. Narchi, "Four half-siblings with infantile myrofibromatosis: a case for autosomal-recessive inheritance," *Clinical Genetics*, vol. 59, no. 2, pp. 134-135, 2001.

[15] J. A. Martignetti, L. Tian, D. Li et al., "Mutations in PDGFRB cause autosomal-dominant infantile myofibromatosis," *The American Journal of Human Genetics*, vol. 92, no. 6, pp. 1001–1007, 2013.

[16] Y. H. Cheung, T. Gayden, P. M. Campeau et al., "A recurrent PDGFRB mutation causes familial infantile myofibromatosis," *The American Journal of Human Genetics*, vol. 92, no. 6, pp. 996–1000, 2013.

[17] Y. Fukasawa, H. Ishikura, A. Takada et al., "Massive apoptosis in infantile myofibromatosis: a putative mechanism of tumor regression," *The American Journal of Pathology*, vol. 144, no. 3, pp. 480–485, 1994.

[18] M. Short, A. Dramis, P. Ramani, and D. H. Parikh, "Mediastinal and pulmonary infantile myofibromatosis: an unusual surgical presentation," *Journal of Pediatric Surgery*, vol. 43, no. 11, pp. e29–e31, 2008.

[19] V. T. de Montpréville, A. Serraf, H. Aznag, N. Nashashibi, C. Planché, and E. Dulmet, "Fibroma and inflammatory myofibroblastic tumor of the heart," *Annals of Diagnostic Pathology*, vol. 5, no. 6, pp. 335–342, 2001.

[20] T. Newson, R. Cerio, I. Leigh, and D. Jaywardhene, "Infantile myofibromatosis: a rare presentation with intussusception," *Pediatric Surgery International*, vol. 13, no. 5-6, pp. 447-448, 1998.

[21] S. S. Kaplan, J. G. Ojemann, D. K. Grange, C. Fuller, and T. S. Park, "Intracranial infantile myofibromatosis with intraparenchymal involvement," *Pediatric Neurosurgery*, vol. 36, no. 4, pp. 214–217, 2002.

[22] M. Gopal, G. Chahal, Z. Al-Rifai, B. Eradi, G. Ninan, and S. Nour, "Infantile myofibromatosis," *Pediatric Surgery International*, vol. 24, no. 3, pp. 287–291, 2008.

[23] S. Salerno, M. C. Terranova, M. Rossello, M. Piccione, O. Ziino, and G. L. Re, "Whole-body magnetic resonance imaging in the diagnosis and follow-up of multicentric infantile myofibromatosis: a case report," *Molecular and Clinical Oncology*, vol. 6, no. 4, pp. 579–582, 2017.

[24] B. Raney, A. Evans, L. Granowetter, L. Schnaufer, A. Uri, and P. Littman, "Nonsurgical management of children with recurrent or unresectable fibromatosis," *Pediatrics*, vol. 79, no. 3, pp. 394–398, 1987.

[25] P. Mudry, O. Slaby, J. Neradil et al., "Case report: rapid and durable response to PDGFR targeted therapy in a child with refractory multiple infantile myofibromatosis and a heterozygous germline mutation of the PDGFRB gene," *BMC Cancer*, vol. 17, no. 1, p. 119, 2017.

[26] J. E. Butrynski, D. R. D'Adamo, J. L. Hornick et al., "Crizotinib in ALK-rearranged inflammatory myofibroblastic tumor," *New England Journal of Medicine*, vol. 363, no. 18, pp. 1727–1733, 2010.

26

Trichophyton as a Rare Cause of Postoperative Wound Infection Resistant to Standard Empiric Antimicrobial Therapy

Sheema Gaffar (ID),[1] **John K. Birknes,**[2] **and Kenji M. Cunnion** (ID)[1,3,4]

[1]*Department of Pediatrics, Eastern Virginia Medical School, 700 West Olney Road, Norfolk, VA 23507, USA*
[2]*Division of Pediatric Neurosurgery, Children's Hospital of the King's Daughters, 601 Children's Lane, Norfolk, VA 23507, USA*
[3]*Division of Infectious Diseases, Children's Hospital of the King's Daughters, 601 Children's Lane, Norfolk, VA 23507, USA*
[4]*Children's Specialty Group, 811 Redgate Avenue, Norfolk, VA 23507, USA*

Correspondence should be addressed to Kenji M. Cunnion; cunniokm@evms.edu

Academic Editor: Paul A. Rufo

Fungal infections are rare causes of acute surgical wound infections, but *Candida* is not an infrequent etiology in chronic wound infections. *Trichophyton* species is a common cause of tinea capitis but has not been reported as a cause of neurosurgical wound infection. We report a case of *Trichophyton tonsurans* causing a nonhealing surgical wound infection in a 14-year-old male after hemicraniectomy. His wound infection was notable for production of purulent exudate from the wound and lack of clinical improvement despite empiric treatment with multiple broad-spectrum antibiotics targeting typical bacterial causes of wound infection. Multiple wound cultures consistently grew *Trichophyton* fungus, and his wound infection clinically improved rapidly after starting terbinafine and discontinuing antibiotics.

1. Introduction

Trichophyton fungi are a common cause of tinea capitis but have not been reported as a cause of postsurgical scalp wound infection [1]. Here, we report a 14-year-old male with a chronic wound infection after hemicraniectomy that was eventually determined to be caused by *Trichophyton*.

2. Case Report

This case report was reviewed by the local IRB at Eastern Virginia Medical School (18-09-NH-0217) and deemed "not human subjects research."

A 14-year-old male with a past medical history of mild intermittent asthma presented in December 2017 with a subdural empyema resulting from direct extension from frontal sinusitis. His intracranial abscess was surgically drained as part of a hemicraniectomy procedure. Cultures of his intracranial abscess grew *Streptococcus intermedius*, and he was treated with antibiotics for 2 months. His craniectomy plate was reimplanted in June 2018. Two and a half weeks later, he presented with pain and mild wound dehiscence. Several patches of alopecia along the edges of the wound were noted. A culture of purulent material expressed from the wound grew rare *Pseudomonas aeruginosa*. Despite appropriate antibiotics, there was no clinical improvement in drainage or pain, leading to surgical removal of the reimplanted bone in July 2018. One week postoperatively, he reported increasing pain along the incision while being treated with ceftazidime. There were fluctuance and profound tenderness to palpation along the incision site (Figure 1(a)), and a new thick purulent discharge was expressible from the wound. There were a few patchy areas of alopecia along the wound edges, which at the time were attributed to preoperative shaving, frequent wound cleaning, and removal of dressings and tape. The skin in the areas of alopecia was not scaly. Expressed purulent drainage was cultured, and his antibiotics were switched to vancomycin and meropenem. The new wound culture grew hyphal fungus on a blood agar plate after 4 days. In total, six wound cultures of the expressed purulent material from the wound were performed over two weeks, and all grew colonies with

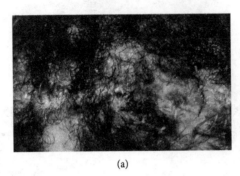
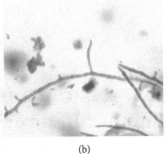

(a)   (b)

FIGURE 1: (a) Scalp wound appearance at the time first culture was obtained that grew *Trichophyton*. (b) Lactophenol cotton blue stain of the colony material showing hyphae and budding.

branched hyphae morphologically consistent with *Trichophyton* (Figure 1(b)). Once identification of *Trichophyton* was made, he was started on oral terbinafine and his antibiotics were discontinued. His wound infection improved rapidly thereafter with decreasing amounts of purulent drainage, fluctuance, pain, and tenderness. After three weeks of terbinafine treatment, all discharge and tenderness had resolved. Follow-up after 6.5 weeks of terbinafine treatment demonstrated an optimal response, including patchy regrowth of hair, and terbinafine was discontinued.

University of Texas Health San Antonio (UTHSA) identified the fungal species as T. tonsurans. Fungal susceptibility testing was also performed by UTHSA. Identification included phenotypic characterization and DNA sequencing of the following targets: ITS, D1/D2, and TUB. This isolate was susceptible to terbinafine (MIC = 0.008 mcg/ml) and griseofulvin (MIC = 1 mcg/ml).

3. Discussion

Chronic wounds can be categorized into progressive ulcerative wounds (e.g., diabetic foot ulcers, decubitus ulcers, and venous stasis ulcers), slow healing wounds that require debridement (e.g., burns), and nonhealing incisions [2]. Chronic wound studies typically focus on adult patients. One study of 915 chronic surgical wounds over 4 months reported a 23% incidence of fungal infection [2], while another study of 824 nonchronic surgical wounds reported a 2% incidence [3]. In another survey of polymicrobial chronic wound infections, *Candida albicans* was implicated as the most common contributor [4]. Thus, the risk of fungal wound infection appears to be much greater for chronic as compared to nonchronic wounds. The vast majority of postoperative fungal wound infections are caused by *Candida*. Risk factors for delayed wound healing from *Candida* wound infections included occlusive dressings and treatment with antibacterial ointments [4, 5]. *Aspergillus* has been reported to cause fungal endophthalmitis after ophthalmologic surgery, while *Trichophyton* has been reported to cause fungal keratitis after cataract surgery [6]. Cases of postoperative infection from *Trichophyton* have also been reported after hair transplantation [7].

Tinea capitis caused by *Trichophyton* is common in pediatrics. Clinical manifestations of tinea capitis can be categorized into alopecic and inflammatory [8]. Tinea capitis causing alopecia appears as a few large-diameter lesions, called microsporosis, or as many small alopecic lesions, called trichophytosis [9]. Inflammatory tinea capitis has a similar divergence per wound characteristic. Yellow crusts with associated odor are characteristic of favus reaction, while suppurative exudate and edema with associated pain are characteristic of kerion [9]. The crusting and spongy subcutaneous edema, which is sometimes accompanied by a thick white exudate, in kerion-specific inflammatory tinea capitis results from a T cell-mediated hypersensitivity reaction to *Trichophyton*, rather than subcutaneous infection [10]. The patient we describe had a chronic wound infection at his hemicraniectomy incision site with significant incisional pain, progressive scalp edema with purulent exudate, and wound dehiscence. The symptomatic characteristics are consistent with kerion. However, the consistent growth of *Trichophyton* from the purulent exudate is not typical for kerion and is more suggestive of a true wound infection rather than allergic reaction to superficial tinea capitis.

The lack of clinical response by this wound infection in the face of multiple broad-spectrum antibiotic regimens was worrisome, leading to concern for potentially unrecognized chronic osteomyelitis of the skull, a retained foreign body, or a multidrug resistant organism. The possibility of a fungal wound infection should also be included in this differential diagnosis. For chronic wound infections, the literature consistently recommends obtaining fungal cultures to isolate the agent [9, 11, 12] because fungal culture is known to have higher sensitivity than fungal microscopy [13, 14]. To our knowledge, *Trichophyton* has not been reported as a primary pathogen in surgical wound infections. In this instance, treatment with terbinafine, an optimal antimicrobial to treat *Trichophyton*, led to clinical improvement in a few days. *Trichophyton* appears to be an exceptionally rare [13] but potential cause of chronic fungal wound infection.

Acknowledgments

Thanks are due to Ferne Elsass for her help with wound care and to Suzanne Quesnel for her help in the Clinical Microbiology Laboratory.

References

[1] M. Schmidt, "Boric acid inhibition of *Trichophyton rubrum*

growth and conidia formation," *Biological Trace Element Research*, vol. 180, no. 2, pp. 349–354, 2017.

[2] S. E. Dowd, J. D. Hanson, E. Rees et al., "Survey of fungi and yeast in polymicrobial infections in chronic wounds," *Journal of Wound Care*, vol. 20, no. 1, pp. 40–47, 2013.

[3] D. Kaya, C. Aldirmaz Agartan, and M. Yucel, "Fungal agents as a cause of surgical wound infections: an overview of host factors," *Wounds*, vol. 19, no. 8, pp. 218–222, 2007.

[4] M. B. Giandoni and W. J. Grabski, "Cutaneous candidiasis as a cause of delayed surgical wound healing," *Journal of the American Academy of Dermatology*, vol. 30, no. 6, pp. 981–984, 1994.

[5] F. A. Paskiabi, S. Bonakdar, M. A. Shokrgozar et al., "Terbinafine-loaded wound dressing for chronic superficial fungal infections," *Materials Science and Engineering: C*, vol. 73, pp. 130–136, 2017.

[6] C. M. Lin, S. I. Pao, Y. H. Chen, J. T. Chen, D. W. Lu, and C. L. Chen, "Fungal endophthalmitis caused by Trichophyton spp. after cataract surgery," *Clinical and Experimental Ophthalmology*, vol. 42, no. 7, pp. 696-697, 2014.

[7] P. Colli, A. Fellas, and R. M. Trueb, "*Staphylococcus Iugdunensis* and *Trichophyton tonsurans* infection in synthetic hair implants," *International Journal of Trichology*, vol. 9, no. 2, pp. 82–86, 2017.

[8] J. V. Veasey, B. A. F. Miguel, S. A. S. Mayor, C. Zaitz, L. H. Muramatu, and J. A. Serrano, "Epidemiological profile of tinea capitis in São Paulo City," *Anais Brasileiros de Dermatologia*, vol. 92, no. 2, pp. 283-284, 2017.

[9] J. V. Veasey and G. D. S. C. Muzy, "*Tinea capitis*: correlation of clinical presentations to agents identified in mycological culture," *Anais Brasileiros de Dermatologia*, vol. 93, no. 3, pp. 465-466, 2018.

[10] I. Zaraa, A. Hawilo, A. Aounallah et al., "InflammatoryTinea capitis: a 12-year study and a review of the literature," *Mycoses*, vol. 56, no. 2, pp. 110–116, 2012.

[11] C. T. Stankey, A. B. Spaulding, A. Doucette et al., "Blood culture and pleural fluid culture yields in pediatric empyema patients," *Pediatric Infectious Disease Journal*, vol. 37, no. 9, pp. 952–954, 2018.

[12] S. P. Sheth, P. Ilkanich, and C. Blaise, "Complicated *fusobacterium* sinusitis: a case report," *Pediatric Infectious Disease Journal*, vol. 37, no. 9, pp. 246–248, 2018.

[13] C. C. Ang and Y. K. Tay, "Inflammatory *tinea capitis*: non-healing plaque on the occiput of a 4-year-old child," *Annals, Academy of Medicine, Singapore*, vol. 39, no. 5, pp. 412–414, 2010.

[14] E. M. Higgins, L. C. Fuller, and C. H. Smith, "Guidelines for the management of tinea capitis," *British Journal of Dermatology*, vol. 143, no. 1, pp. 53–58, 2000.

27

Tocilizumab for the Treatment of Mevalonate Kinase Deficiency

Nadia K. Rafiq ⓘ,[1] Helen Lachmann,[2] Frodi Joensen,[3] Troels Herlin ⓘ,[4] and Paul A. Brogan[1]

[1]*Infection and Inflammation and Rheumatology Section, University College London Great Ormond Street Institute of Child Health, 30 Guilford Street, London WC1 E1H, UK*
[2]*National Amyloidosis Centre, University College London Division of Medicine, London, UK*
[3]*National Hospital of the Faroe Islands, J. C. Svabos Gøta, Tórshavn 100, Faroe Islands*
[4]*Department of Paediatrics, Pediatric Rheumatology Clinic, Palle Juul-Jensens Boulevard 99, 8200 Aarhus N, Denmark*

Correspondence should be addressed to Nadia K. Rafiq; n.rafiq@nhs.net

Academic Editor: Ozgur Cogulu

Mevalonate kinase deficiency (MKD) is a severe autoinflammatory disease caused by recessive mutations in MVK resulting in reduced function of the enzyme mevalonate kinase, involved in the cholesterol/isoprenoid pathway. MKD presents with periodic episodes of severe systemic inflammation, poor quality of life, and life-threatening sequelae if inadequately treated. We report the case of a 12-year-old girl with MKD and severe autoinflammation that was resistant to IL-1 and TNF-α blockade. In view of this, she commenced intravenous tocilizumab (8 mg/kg every 2 weeks), a humanised monoclonal antibody targeting the IL-6 receptor (IL-6R) that binds to membrane and soluble IL-6R, inhibiting IL-6-mediated signaling. She reported immediate cessation of fever and marked improvement in her energy levels following the first infusion; after the fifth dose, she was in complete clinical and serological remission, now sustained for 24 months. This is one of the first reported cases of a child with MKD treated successfully with tocilizumab and adds to the very limited experience of this treatment for MKD. IL-6 blockade could therefore be an important addition to the armamentarium for the treatment of this rare monogenic autoinflammatory disease.

1. Introduction

Mevalonate kinase deficiency (MKD) is a rare autosomal recessive autoinflammatory disease caused by mutations in MVK, causing loss of function of the enzyme mevalonate kinase (MVK). Broadly, two clinical phenotypes are recognized that vary in severity as determined by the level of residual enzyme activity. The milder phenotype of MKD is a periodic fever syndrome characterized by frequent episodes of fever typically lasting 3–7 days, abdominal pain, lymphadenopathy, inflammatory eye disease, rashes, and arthralgia [1] and typically associated with intracellular MVK activity greater than 1% [2]. The more severe phenotype is mevalonic aciduria (MA), usually associated with MVK enzyme activity less than 0.5%. MA may result in a high rate of stillbirth; survivors present soon after birth with severe systemic inflammation, facial dysmorphism, severe failure to thrive, developmental delay, seizures, and hepatic involvement [3]. Worldwide, approximately only

300 patients with MKD have been reported [4], including a recent large series from Europe [1].

The pathophysiology of autoinflammation in MKD is poorly understood and is suggested to occur as a result of loss of synthesis of isoprenoid lipids downstream of MVK [5], in particular geranylgeranyl diphosphate. This latter is necessary for prenylation (the addition of a hydrophobic compound) of small GTPases, the loss of which causes activation of the inflammasome and release of IL-1β [6]. More recent studies have indicated a central role for the pyrin inflammasome as the driver of autoinflammation in MKD [7]. There is an inverse relationship between RhoA activation and activation of the pyrin inflammasome: RhoA activation induces downstream kinases, pyrin phosphorylation, and inhibitory binding of phosphorylated pyrin by 14-3-3 proteins [7]. In MKD, deficient geranylgeranylation of RhoA renders it inactive. This is because RhoA activation is dependent on its translocation to the plasma membrane, and this membrane targeting of RhoA is dependent on geranylgeranylation at its C-terminus [7]. Since geranylgeranyl pyrophosphate, the substrate of geranylgeranylation, is a product of the mevalonate pathway, loss-of-function mutations of MVK results in depletion of geranylgeranyl pyrophosphate, failure of Rho membrane binding, and thus persistent RhoA inactivation and consequently pyrin activation which induces IL-1β overproduction in myeloid cells [7, 8]. Thus mutations of MVK lead to release of the normal, constitutive tonic inhibition of the pyrin inflammasome and excess IL-1 production [7].

Consequently, attempts to treat MKD have mainly focused on IL-1 blockade, as reflected in recent international expert consensus guidance [9]. In fact, therapeutic success with IL-1 blockade is at best modest. For anakinra (recombinant interleukin-1 receptor antagonist, blocking IL-1β and IL-1α), a retrospective series [10] reported only 30% complete remission, and 70% partial remission in patients with MKD treated with daily anakinra. Canakinumab, a monoclonal antibody against IL-1β, appears to have superior efficacy to anakinra in retrospective studies, with up to half of patients achieving complete response [10–12]. A major prospective randomised controlled trial of canakinumab (150 mg monthly) for MKD has reported that 35% met a definition of response at 16 weeks; and 45% had a physician global assessment of <2/10 [13]. Since it is now increasingly apparent that MKD is in fact a multicytokine-driven disease, with involvement of other proinflammatory cytokines including IL-6 and tumour necrosis factor-α (TNF-α) [14, 15], this somewhat limited efficacy of IL-1 blockade is perhaps unsurprising. It is thus clear that whilst IL-1 blockade may be useful in some patients with MKD, alternative treatments for those who fail to respond adequately to IL-1 blockade are urgently required.

Tocilizumab is a humanised, monoclonal, antihuman IL-6 receptor (IL-6R) antibody that binds to membrane and soluble IL-6R, inhibiting IL-6-mediated signaling [16]. Tocilizumab binds to soluble IL-6R present in serum and joint fluid as well as membrane-bound IL-6R expressed on the surface of cells, leading to inhibition of receptor-mediated IL-6 signaling and suppression of several physiological roles of IL-6 [16, 17]. Experience of using tocilizumab for the treatment of MKD is limited, with (to date) only six cases reported. We therefore add to these limited data describing a child with MKD who was successfully treated with tocilizumab having failed other treatments and review the literature regarding IL-6 blockade in MKD.

2. Case Presentation

We present the case of a twelve-year-old girl originally from the Faroe Islands with compound heterozygotic MKD (p. V377I/c.417insC), who first presented with symptomatic periodic fever attacks from the age of 3 months. These presented as recurrent episodes of fever (39–41°C) without infectious cause, occurring once or twice monthly, associated with rigors, pallor, fatigue, lymphadenopathy (inguinal, axillary, and intra-abdominal), abdominal pain, oral ulceration, and arthralgia/myalgia of the lower limbs. Attacks lasted between 3 and 7 days and were accompanied by very high acute phase responses (C reactive protein [CRP] typically greater than 100 mg/L). Attacks were also triggered by vaccinations. Her past medical history included an episode of Stevens–Johnson syndrome in response to penicillin at the age of three years and appendectomy aged 7 years of a normal appendix. She was referred to us in London at the age of 12 years. At that time, she was receiving the anti-TNFα agent etanercept, which she had been on for the previous 34 months. She had at best only partial response to etanercept in terms of attack severity and duration, but was still missing 100 days per year of school because of attacks which occurred twice a month, lasting for 3 days. In addition, despite etanercept, her inflammatory markers remained significantly raised between attacks: CRP 82 mg/L (reference range [RR] < 10); serum amyloid A (SAA) 1310 mg/L (RR < 10), indicative of severe systemic inflammation in-between attacks and significant risk of reactive AA amyloidosis. Anakinra (2 mg/kg/day; recombinant interleukin-1 receptor antagonist) had also been tried previously, but was complicated both by a severe skin rash and also by the worst disease flare she had ever experienced; hence after four weeks, this was discontinued. Following a six-week washout period from the etanercept (during which she suffered one severe attack), in December 2015 she started intravenous tocilizumab 8 mg/kg every 2 weeks.

After one dose of tocilizumab, her CRP and ESR both rapidly normalised (Figure 1(a)). She had one minor attack with minor, short-lived fleeting rash, but no fever after the first dose. Since normalisation of CRP is a well-known effect of tocilizumab and may occur without necessarily any true improvement in clinical disease activity, we also prospectively used a physician global assessment of disease activity using a 0 to 10 scale, 0 indicating no disease activity and 10 indicating severe disease activity (Figure 1(a)), and change in haemoglobin, white cell count, and platelets (Figure 1(b)) as adjunctive laboratory indicators of successful treatment. In addition, the patient reported significant improvement even after a single dose of tocilizumab, with improved energy levels, reduction in pain, and improvement in oral ulceration. She was also able to return to full-time school.

This excellent clinical and serological response has been sustained for more than 24 months. There have been no reported adverse events. The patient was switched to weekly subcutaneous tocilizumab at 162 mg in June 2016 for ease of administration and reduction in hospital attendances. A year since that change, the patient has had several short-lived flares lasting 1–3 days associated with fever, adenitis, and mouth blistering, but she has not required prednisolone as before and overall expressed a preference for the subcutaneous route as it was associated with improved quality of life despite the breakthrough fever attacks.

3. Discussion

There is no definitive treatment for MKD, and the current rationale for treatment is based on anecdotal case reports, retrospective series, and a limited (albeit increasing)

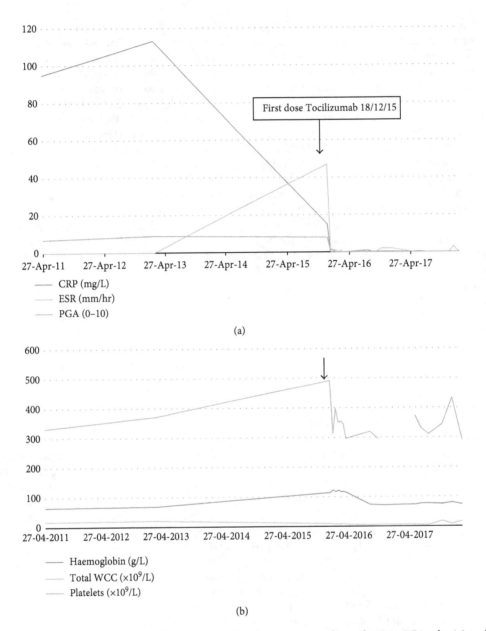

(a)

(b)

FIGURE 1: (a) Change in clinical disease activity inflammatory markers in response tocilizumab. *Note.* PGA: physician global assessment, 0–10, 0 indicating absence of disease activity and 10 indicating severe disease. ESR: erythrocyte sedimentation rate. CRP: C reactive protein. PGA fell from 8/10 immediately before the first tocilizumab infusion to 1/10 when assessed immediately prior to the next infusion 2 weeks later. This excellent clinical and serological response has been sustained for 24 months. (b) Change in haemoglobin, total white cell count, and platelet count in response to tocilizumab. Black arrow shows date of first dose of tocilizumab.

knowledge regarding the pathogenesis of autoinflammation in MKD. The European project, Single Hub and Access point for pediatric Rheumatology in Europe (SHARE), was launched to address this important unmet clinical need and provided a systematic literature review and expert consensus for the treatment of MKD and other autoinflammatory diseases [9]. It is currently suggested that patients with MKD may benefit from treatment with NSAIDs, steroids, and biologics, particularly IL-1 blockade or etanercept. Furthermore, the SHARE guidance emphasizes that statins and colchicine are not effective in MKD [9]. Upon failure of IL-1 blockade and etanercept, IL-6 blockade should be the next

biologic instigated, before considering haematopoietic stem cell transplantation (HSCT) [9], although data supporting the use of tocilizumab in MKD are very limited. As such, our case represents (to the best of our knowledge) only the seventh subject with MKD treated with tocilizumab. The efficacy we observed was immediate, dramatic, and sustained over 24 months. This suggests that IL-6 blockade should be given more consideration in patients with MKD, especially after failure of IL-1 blockade is demonstrated.

The biggest series of patients with MKD was recently described from the Eurofever registry [1] providing additional, albeit retrospective data regarding the treatment of

TABLE 1: Previous reports of tocilizumab for the treatment of MKD.

	Shendi et al. ($n = 1$) [19]	Stoffels et al. ($n = 2$) [15]		Lane et al. ($n = 2$) [20]		Muster et al. ($n = 1$) [21]
Patient	1	2	3	4	5	6
TOC dose (mg/kg) and route of administration	7 IV	8 IV	8 IV	8 IV	8 IV	8 IV
Frequency of administration (weeks)	4	4	4	4	4	4
Age (range), years at onset of TOC	13	Not described	Not described	24	13	36
Treatment prior to TOC	COL PRED ETA ANA	ANA	ANA	ANA ETA	ETA	NSAID SIMVA ANA
Duration of treatment (months)	20	5	5	24	13	48–60
Outcome Clinical	CR	CR	CR	CR		PR
Serological	CR	Not described	PR	CR		—
Adverse events	URTI	Not described	Not described	Not described		Not described
Comments	·CR at dose of 8 mg/kg but due to adverse events dose reduced, ultimately with stable clinical and serological status on 7 mg/kg IV every 4 weeks	—	—	MKD complicated by AA amyloidosis. Remained on therapy with PRED 0.5 mg/kg/day	Stabilized on monotherapy with TOC	After starting TOC, average hospital admissions dropped 11/yr to 3/yr TOC given in combination with IVMP for first 3 yrs then as monotherapy

IV: intravenous; COL: colchicine; PRED: prednisolone; ETA: etanercept; ANA: anakinra; NSAID: nonsteroidal anti-inflammatory drug; SIMVA: simvastatin; CR: complete response; PR: partial response; URTI: upper respiratory tract infection; TOC: tocilizumab; yrs: years.

MKD. Of note, in that series, 27/114 patients received anakinra: 6/28 (22%) were reported as complete responders; 18/27 (67%) were partial responders; and 11% had no response to anakinra. Anakinra doses are not described in detail in this report, but are likely to be an important factor influencing this (at best) modest efficacy [18]. Canakinumab was given to 5/114 patients and resulted in complete remission in 4/5, with a partial response in the remaining subject [10]. Etanercept was used in 27/114 patients and had a beneficial effect in 16/27 patients (59%), of whom only two (7%) had a complete response [10]. Eleven/27 patients (41%) failed to respond to etanercept [10]. Of note, only 2 patients with severe MKD received tocilizumab, but the treatment responses are not described in any detail in this series [10]. Whilst expert consensus places tocilizumab as an important third-line biologic treatment for MKD [9], there have only been six MKD cases treated with this agent reported worldwide [15,19–21]. The details of these reports are summarized in Table 1.

The pathogenesis of autoinflammation in MKD is poorly understood although recent studies have emphasized that, unlike cryopyrin-associated periodic fever syndromes (CAPS; a purely IL-1-driven autoinflammatory disease), MKD is probably a multicytokine-driven monogenic autoinflammatory disease [2, 5, 15]. One mechanistic model of inflammation in MKD is that of enhanced IL-1β release as a result of decreased Rho/Rac GTPase prenylation, particularly in hyperthermic conditions [5]. Stoffels et al., however, observed an increased cytokine response from cells from MKD patients specific for TLR4, TLR2, and NOD2 stimulation, which included not only IL-1β, but also IL-1α, TNFα, and IL-6 [15]. Based on this observation, they questioned whether or not IL-1β is the central driving cytokine in the pathogenesis of MKD. Since they also observed excessive caspase-1 protein in leucocytes from MKD patients, they postulated that this could provide an explanation as to why these cells are more easily triggered to secrete IL-1β, but emphasized also that other proinflammatory cytokines are involved. They concluded that this could account for the fact that not all patients respond to blockade of IL-1, as emphasized by the aforementioned results of the only randomised controlled trial published to date [13]. These observations, and the emerging (albeit limited) clinical experience of IL-6 blockade in MKD (Table 1), argue strongly for consideration of IL-6 blockade in MKD, particularly for those who fail to respond adequately to IL-1 blockade [15], but perhaps also for a clinical trial exploring dosing and efficacy of tocilizumab as first-line choice of biologic for

MKD. From a practical perspective, tocilizumab is significantly cheaper than canakinumab and avoids the need for daily injections as is the case of anakinra.

The dose and route of administration of tocilizumab for MKD has varied across the published reports (Table 1). Shendi et al. [19] used tocilizumab at an intravenous dose of 8 mg/kg, every four weeks. This is the NICE approved dose for the treatment of rheumatoid arthritis [22] and for some forms of JIA in children weighing ≥30 kg [23]. This patient went into remission with normalisation of inflammatory markers, but had recurrent upper respiratory tract infections (well described with tocilizumab) [24] necessitating a 50% dose reduction. This lower dose was inadequate to control the MKD however, and was therefore increased again to 7 mg/kg four weekly, with reasonable disease control [19]. We did not observe any infections in our patient, who was treated with 8 mg/kg tocilizumab every two weeks (as per a typical systemic JIA dosing regimen [25]), or latterly whilst on weekly subcutaneous tocilizumab. Regarding this latter point, there are no data that suggest any benefit over intravenous or subcutaneous administration; clearly subcutaneous administration has potential practical advantages, such as avoiding the need for hospital admission for intravenous administration as was the case for a patient.

In conclusion, we report a dramatic and sustained (24 months) clinical and serological response to tocilizumab in a 12-year-old child with MKD, which to the best of our knowledge represents only the seventh patient reported. Since a recent randomised placebo-controlled clinical trial of IL-1 blockade has suggested that more than 50% of patients may fail to respond adequately, we suggest that further consideration should be given to alternative approaches such as IL-6 blockade, particularly for those individuals who fail IL-1 blockade, and especially before considering haematopoietic stem cell transplantation as a therapeutic option.

References

[1] N. M. Ter Haar, J. Jeyaratnam, H. J. Lachmann et al., "The phenotype and genotype of mevalonate kinase deficiency: a series of 114 cases from the Eurofever Registry," *Arthritis and Rheumatology*, vol. 68, no. 11, pp. 2795–2805, 2016.

[2] L. A. Favier and G. S. Schulert, "Mevalonate kinase deficiency: current perspectives," *Application of Clinical Genetics*, vol. 9, pp. 101–10, 2016.

[3] D. Haas and G. F. Hoffmann, "Mevalonate kinase deficiencies: from mevalonic aciduria to hyperimmunoglobulinemia D syndrome," *Orphanet Journal of Rare Diseases*, vol. 1, no. 1, p. 13, 2006.

[4] S. Zhang, "Natural history of mevalonate kinase deficiency: a literature review," *Pediatric Rheumatology*, vol. 14, no. 1, p. 30, 2016.

[5] J. Jurczyluk, M. A. Munoz, O. P Skinner et al., "Mevalonate kinase deficiency leads to decreased prenylation of Rab GTPases," *Immunology and Cell Biology*, vol. 94, no. 10, pp. 994–999, 2015.

[6] B. Massonnet, S. Normand, R. Moschitz et al., "Pharmacological inhibitors of the mevalonate pathway activate pro-IL-1 processing and IL-1 release by human monocytes," *European Cytokine Network*, vol. 20, no. 3, pp. 112–120, 2009.

[7] Y. H. Park, G. Wood, D. L. Kastner, and J. J. Chae, "Pyrin inflammasome activation and RhoA signaling in the autoinflammatory diseases FMF and HIDS," *Nature Immunology*, vol. 17, no. 8, pp. 914–921, 2016.

[8] S. Normand, B. Massonnet, A. Delwail et al., "Specific increase in caspase-1 activity and secretion of IL-1 family cytokines: a putative link between mevalonate kinase deficiency and inflammation," *European Cytokine Network*, vol. 20, no. 3, pp. 101–107, 2009.

[9] N. M. Ter Haar, M. Oswald, J. Jeyaratnam et al., "Recommendations for the management of autoinflammatory diseases," *Annals of the Rheumatic Diseases*, vol. 74, no. 9, pp. 1636–1644, 2015.

[10] L. Rossi-Semerano, B. Fautrel, D. Wendling et al., "Tolerance and efficacy of off-label anti-interleukin-1 treatments in France: a nationwide survey," *Orphanet Journal of Rare Diseases*, vol. 10, no. 1, p. 19, 2015.

[11] N. Ter Haar, H. Lachmann, S. Ozen et al., "Treatment of autoinflammatory diseases: results from the Eurofever Registry and a literature review," *Annals of the Rheumatic Diseases*, vol. 72, no. 5, pp. 678–685, 2013.

[12] C. Galeotti, U. Meinzer, P. Quartier et al., "Efficacy of interleukin-1-targeting drugs in mevalonate kinase deficiency," *Rheumatology*, vol. 51, no. 10, pp. 1855–1859, 2012.

[13] F. De Benedetti, J. Anton, M. Gattorno et al., "A Phase III pivotal umbrella trial of canakinumab in patients with autoinflammatory periodic fever syndromes (cochicene resistant FMF, HIDS/MKD and TRAPS)," *Annals of the Rheumatic Diseases*, vol. 75, no. 2, p. 615, 2016.

[14] J. P. Drenth, M. van Deuren, J. van der Ven-Jongerkrijg et al., "Cytokine activation during attacks of hyperimmunoglobulinemia D and periodic fever syndrome," *Blood*, vol. 85, no. 12, pp. 3586–3593, 1995.

[15] M. Stoffels, J. Jongekrijg, T. Remijn, N. Kok, J. W. M. van der Meer, and A. Simon, "TLR2/TL.R4-dependent exaggerated cytokine production in hyperimmunoglobulinaemia D and periodic fever syndrome," *Rheumatology*, vol. 54, no. 2, pp. 363–368, 2015.

[16] M. Mihara, K. Kasutani, M. Okazaki et al., "Tocilizumab inhibits signal transduction mediated by both mIL-6R and sIL-6R, but not by the receptors of other members of IL-6 cytokine family," *International Immunopharmacology*, vol. 5, no. 12, pp. 1731–40, 2005.

[17] N. Nishimoto and T. Kishimoto, "Humanized antihuman IL-6 receptor antibody, tocilizumab," in *Handbook of Experimental Pharmacology*, vol. 181, pp. 151–60, Springer, Berlin, Germany, 2008.

[18] R. Campanilho-Marques and P. Brogan, "Mevalonate kinase deficiency in two sisters with therapeutic response to anakinra: case report and review of the literature," *Clinical Rheumatology*, vol. 33, no. 11, pp. 1681–1684, 2014.

[19] H. M. Shendi, L. A. Devlin, and J. D. Edgar, "Interleukin 6 blockade for hyperimmunoglobulin D and periodic fever syndrome," *Journal of Clinical Rheumatology*, vol. 20, no. 2, pp. 103–105, 2014.

[20] T. Lane, J. D. Gillmore, A. D. Wechalekar, P. N. Hawkins, and H. J. Lachmann, "Therapeutic blockade of interleukin-6 by tocilizumab in the management of AA amyloidosis and chronic inflammatory disorders: a case series and review of the literature," *Clinical and Experimental Rheumatology*, vol. 33, no. 94, pp. S46–S53, 2015.

[21] A. Muster, P. P. Tak, D. L. P. Baeten, and S. W. Tas, "Anti-interleukin 6 receptor therapy for hyper-IgD syndrome," *BMJ*

Case Reports, vol. 2015, p. bcr2015210513, 2015.

[22] National Institute for Health and Care Excellence (NICE), *Adalimumab, Etanercept, Infliximab, Certolizumab Pegol, Golimumab, Tocilizumab and Abatacept for Rheumatoid Arthritis not Previously Treated with DMARDs or After Conventional DMARDs Only Have Failed*, NICE Technology Appraisal Guidance, NICE, London, UK, 2016.

[23] National Institute for Health and Care Excellence (NICE), *Abatacept, Adalimumab, Etanercept and Tocilizumab for Treating Juvenile Idiopathic Arthritis*, NICE Technology Appraisal Guidance, NICE, London, UK, 2015.

[24] F. De Benedetti, H. I. Brunner, N. Ruperto et al., "Randomized trial of tocilizumab in systemic juvenile idiopathic arthritis," *New England Journal of Medicine*, vol. 367, no. 25, pp. 2385–95, 2012.

[25] National Institute for Health and Care Excellence (NICE), *Tocilizumab for the Treatment of Systemic Juvenile Idiopathic Arthritis*, NICE Technology Appraisal Guidance, NICE, London, UK, 2011.

28

Magnetic Foreign Body Ingestion in Children: The Attractive Hazards

Anna Lin ⓘ,[1] Lawrence Chi Ngong Chan,[1] Kam Lun Ellis Hon ⓘ,[1] Siu Yan Bess Tsui,[2] Kristine Kit Yi Pang,[2] Hon Ming Cheung ⓘ,[1] and Alexander K. C. Leung ⓘ[3]

[1]*Department of Paediatrics, The Chinese University of Hong Kong, Hong Kong*
[2]*Department of Surgery, The Chinese University of Hong Kong, Hong Kong*
[3]*Department of Pediatrics, The University of Calgary, Calgary, Alberta, Canada*

Correspondence should be addressed to Kam Lun Ellis Hon; ehon@hotmail.com

Academic Editor: Larry A. Rhodes

Foreign body ingestions are frequent in the childhood population. Most foreign bodies are passed spontaneously through the gastrointestinal tract. However, on occasion, they can also be a rare cause of morbidity and even mortality, such as in the case of multiple magnetic foreign body ingestion, which can cause injury via magnetic attraction through bowel walls. We present two cases of multiple magnetic foreign body ingestion, which to our knowledge are the first ones reported in Hong Kong. One patient presented with shock and intestinal necrosis requiring extensive intestinal resection, whereas the other patient had no gastrointestinal injury but surgical removal was deemed necessary.

1. Introduction

Foreign body (FB) ingestions are frequent in childhood accidents and injuries and occur most commonly in children between 6 months and 6 years of age [1–3]. Toys not only provide enjoyment but also tend to be inherently attractive to young children; they are also essential tools for a child's learning and development. However, toys are also a form of FB that is occasionally ingested by curious young children. The increasing popularity of magnets for refrigerators, magnetic jewelry, and magnetic toy building and sculpting sets has led to the wider availability of these magnetic objects and an increased incidence of magnetic FB ingestion, necessitating endoscopic or surgical interventions being reported in the literature in recent years [4–7]. The ingestion of magnetic objects poses a significant health risk to children, especially with multiple magnetic objects ingestion, as magnetic attraction through bowel walls can cause gastrointestinal injury such as mural pressure necrosis, bowel perforation, fistula formation, or intestinal obstruction [8]. The public should be aware of the danger associated with these magnetic objects.

2. Case Reports

2.1. Case 1. A 27-month-old previously healthy boy presented to the emergency department with repeated vomiting, sweating, generalized weakness, dizziness, anxiety, and reduced consciousness. He was found to be in shock with a heart rate of 200 beats per minute, respiratory rate of 49 breaths per minute, and blood pressure of 84/43 mmHg. The abdomen was soft but grossly distended with sluggish bowel sounds. Arterial blood gas revealed metabolic acidosis with a pH of 7.12 and base excess of −14. The arterial lactate level was 5 mmol/L. Initial abdominal radiography showed diffuse bowel dilatation but no apparent air-fluid level and two circular radiopaque opacities in the bowel suggestive of metallic foreign bodies (Figure 1). The patient was admitted to the paediatric intensive care unit for resuscitation. He was stabilized with intravenous fluids and ionotropic support. Emergency laparotomy revealed small bowel obstruction with extensive necrosis. Approximately 107 cm of gangrenous small bowel was resected, and end-to-end anastomosis was performed. Two magnetic beads sized 5 mm × 5 mm were found (Figure 2), one in the small bowel and the other

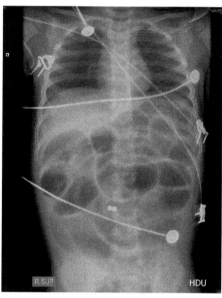

FIGURE 1: Diffuse bowel dilatation and two circular radiopaque opacities in the bowel suspicious of foreign body.

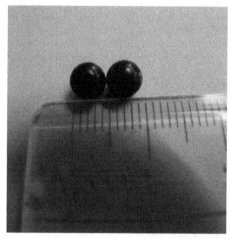

FIGURE 2: Two metallic beads were removed during surgery for gangrenous small bowel.

in the right colon. The magnetic beads were removed. Postoperative recovery was uneventful. Retrospective questioning of the parents revealed no history suspicious of FB ingestion.

2.2. Case 2. A 9-year-old boy presented to the emergency department immediately after accidental ingestion of magnetic beads. The patient was asymptomatic and vital signs were stable. There were no signs of obstruction or perforation. Initial abdominal radiography showed five round radiopaque objects in the epigastrium (Figure 3). Aggressive management was employed in view of the multiplicity of the beads ingested and potential risk of serious complications. Emergency oesophagogastroduodenoscopy showed no foreign body up to the second part of the duodenum. The beads had moved further beyond the duodenum. Laparoscopy was then performed which revealed a string of

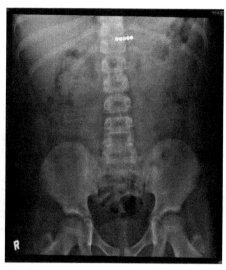

FIGURE 3: Five linear round radiopaque opacities in the epigastrium of an asymptomatic child.

five magnetic beads adhered to each other in the small bowel. The beads were removed via enterotomy. The patient remained asymptomatic and stable and made an uneventful recovery.

3. Discussion

The presentations and outcomes of these two children with multiple magnetic bead ingestion differed greatly. In the former, unwitnessed multiple magnetic bead ingestion led to a delayed presentation and complications of intestinal necrosis requiring extensive bowel resection, whereas the latter patient was brought to the emergency department immediately after accidental ingestion of multiple magnetic beads, which was likely a major factor for the better outcome.

In the former case, we postulate that the unusual mechanism of injury was due to strong magnetic forces, which adhered two different loops of bowel together during peristalsis. Despite the minimal contact surface areas between the two beads, these magnetic forces were potent enough to impair gut motility. Impaired peristalsis led to twisting, ischemia, and necrosis of the gut, resembling volvulus. The incident did not take place in the oesophagus or the stomach, which might indicate that the two beads were swallowed sequentially. Theoretically speaking, it would not have occurred if the two beads were stuck together in the early course of the transit in the gastrointestinal tract. The two beads were small and looked like candies. Curious children tend to put small items such as coins, marbles, toy parts, button batteries, bones, and pills in their mouths [9, 10]. It is the responsibility of parents and caregivers to be vigilant about possible ingestion of small items and toys in the vicinity of a child.

Based on these two cases, it follows that obstruction and ischemia in the lower intestinal tract following magnetic FB ingestion appear to be more severe and symptomatic compared to nonmagnetic FBs. This is especially true for high-powered magnets made of neodymium [9]. Clinicians should be aware that the later the initiation of treatment, the more severe the sequelae may be.

A systematic review of gastrointestinal injury caused by magnetic FB ingestions in children and adolescents found most children were younger than 6 years, magnetic FBs ingested were mainly toys, the number of FBs ranged from 2 to 100, and the majority of patients were previously healthy [4]. Delayed diagnosis and treatment existed in all of the patients to varying extents. Those who underwent exploratory laparotomy showed a wide range of bowel damage was possible, including perforation and intestinal fistula. Intestinal damage was the most common injury, followed by entero-colonic fistula. In that series, most patients required bowel resection with anastomosis or fistula repair except for two children who were managed by endoscopic removal of the FB. In a study of 72 children (mean age 6.4 years) with rare-earth magnet ingestion, the clinical outcome was specified in 93.1% (67/72) of these patients [11]. Of these 67 children, 22 (32.8%) had no adverse effects. Intervention was reported in 91.7% (66/72) of cases. Surgical intervention was required in 46 children (69.7%). Endoscopic removal was performed in 7.6% of cases. The remaining 21.2% of patients were treated conservatively with the magnets passing naturally without intervention. The number of magnets ingested ranged from 1 to 40. Ingestion of 2 to 4 magnets comprised 44.4% of the cases [11]. In general, ingesting more than one magnet can potentially lead to severe gastrointestinal injury, such as mural pressure necrosis, bowel perforation, peritonitis, intra-abdominal sepsis, fistula formation, volvulus, intestinal obstruction, ischemia, and death [5,7,12–14]. For symptomatic patients, multiple magnetic FB ingestion, or when the magnetic FB is in the stomach or the oesophagus, early surgical intervention can prevent significant morbidity and mortality [12, 15]. As with our cases, clinical vigilance should be exercised and early surgical consultation with an aggressive surgical approach is recommended. If the magnetic FB is in the oesophagus, stomach, or proximal small bowel, endoscopy should be performed to retrieve the object and to examine possible damage that might have been caused [9]. For asymptomatic patients, a conservative approach should be considered with serial abdominal radiography to monitor whether the magnetic beads remain in the same location and to wait for spontaneous passage of the magnetic FB. This is especially so if only one magnetic FB is ingested [12]. Failure of movement of the magnetic FB or development of gastrointestinal symptoms prompts reconsideration of endoscopic or surgical intervention [12]. Suffice to say that in a significant number of patients with magnetic FB ingestion, the magnetic objects pass through the gastrointestinal tract spontaneously without complications [16]. However, two or more magnetic FBs or a single magnet coingested with other metallic objects can attract each other in the gastrointestinal tract. This may cause ischemia of the bowel wall and pressure necrosis of the bowel and warrant early surgical intervention [14, 16, 17].

Parents should be warned of the danger of toys that contain metals or magnets. It is not easy to distinguish whether the ingested FB is metallic or magnetic [3]. It is recommended that young and at-risk children should not have access to toys or objects that contain small magnets or metals [18]. In this regard, the US Consumer Product Safety Commission has mandated magnet toys not to be sold to individuals under the age of 14 years [14]. Improved regulation and magnet safety standards are needed. Ideally, magnets should be large enough to decrease the chance of being ingested and the magnetic force be lowered to a flux index of 50 kG^2·mm^2, which is approximately 37 times weaker than some magnetic toys in circulation [12].

4. Conclusion

Parents and caregivers should remove high-powered small magnets from the reach of children. Physicians must be vigilant on reviewing the radiology of a child presenting with respiratory or gastrointestinal symptomatology and not to assume radiopaque objects are extracorporeal. A high index of suspicion is necessary in patients presenting with unexplained gastrointestinal symptoms, and aggressive and early removal is warranted in cases of multiple magnetic FB ingestion to reduce potential morbidity and mortality.

References

[1] K. L. E. Hon, T. F. Leung, C. W. E. Hung, K. L. Cheung, and A. K. Leung, "Ingestion - associated adverse events necessitating pediatric ICU admissions," *The Indian Journal of Pediatrics*, vol. 76, no. 3, pp. 283–286, 2009.

[2] K. L. E. Hon and A. K. C. Leung, "Childhood accidents: injuries and poisoning," *Advances in Pediatrics*, vol. 57, no. 1, pp. 33–62, 2010.

[3] J. Cho, K. Sung, and D. Lee, "Magnetic foreign body ingestion in pediatric patients: report of three cases," *BMC Surg*, vol. 17, p. 73, 2017.

[4] S. Liu, P. Lei, Y. Lv et al., "[Systematic review of gastrointestinal injury caused by magnetic foreign body ingestions in children and adolescence]," *Zhonghua Wei Chang Wai Ke Za Zhi*, vol. 14, pp. 756–761, 2011.

[5] S. Dutta and A. Barzin, "Multiple magnet ingestion as a source of severe gastrointestinal complications requiring surgical intervention," *Archives of Pediatrics & Adolescent Medicine*, vol. 162, no. 2, pp. 123–125, 2008.

[6] J. C. Brown, J. P. Otjen, and G. T. Drugas, "Too attractive," *Pediatric Emergency Care*, vol. 29, no. 11, pp. 1170–1174, 2013.

[7] M. Strickland, D. Rosenfield, and A. Fecteau, "Magnetic foreign body injuries: a large pediatric hospital experience," *The Journal of Pediatrics*, vol. 165, no. 2, pp. 332–335, 2014.

[8] E. H. Anselmi, C. G. San Román, J. E. B. Fontoba et al., "Intestinal perforation caused by magnetic toys," *Journal of Pediatric Surgery*, vol. 42, no. 3, pp. e13–e16, 2007.

[9] M. Nicoara, S. Liu, and G. Ferzli, "Laws of attraction: management of magnetic foreign body ingestion," *BMJ Case Reports*, vol. 2018, Article ID bcr-2018-2018, 2018.

[10] S. Soomro and S. A. Mughal, "Singing magnets ingestion: a rare cause of intestinal obstruction in children," *Journal of the College of Physicians and Surgeons--Pakistan*, vol. 24, no. 9, pp. 688-689, 2014.

[11] A. C. De Roo, M. C. Thompson, T. Chounthirath et al., "Rare-earth magnet ingestion–related injuries among children, 2000-2012," *Clinical Pediatrics*, vol. 52, no. 11, pp. 1006–1013, 2013.

[12] M. J. Alfonzo and C. R. Baum, "Magnetic foreign body ingestions," *Pediatric Emergency Care*, vol. 32, no. 10, pp. 698–702, 2016.

[13] H. Zheng, H. Liang, Y. Wang et al., "Altered gut microbiota composition associated with eczema in infants," *PLoS One*, vol. 11, no. 11, Article ID e0166026, 2016.

[14] M. S. Shalaby, "How dangerous a toy can be? The magnetic effect," *Archives of Disease in Childhood*, vol. 100, no. 11, pp. 1049-1050, 2015.

[15] J. Butterworth and B. Feltis, "Toy magnet ingestion in children: revising the algorithm," *Journal of Pediatric Surgery*, vol. 42, no. 12, pp. e3–e5, 2007.

[16] X. Si, B. Du, and L. Huang, "Multiple magnetic foreign bodies causing severe digestive tract injuries in a child," *Case Reports in Gastroenterology*, vol. 10, no. 3, pp. 720–727, 2016.

[17] M. Y. Othman and S. Srihari, "Multiple magnet ingestion: the attractive hazardst," *Medical Journal of Malaysia*, vol. 71, pp. 211-212, 2016.

[18] A. K. C. Leung and K. L. Hon, "Pica: a common condition that is commonly missed-an update review," *Current Pediatric Reviews*, vol. 15, 2019.

29

Fetal Gallstones in a Newborn after Maternal COVID-19 Infection

Gurleen Kaur Kahlon ⓘ, Anna Zylak ⓘ, Patrick Leblanc, and Noah Kondamudi ⓘ

Department of Pediatrics, The Brooklyn Hospital Center, 121 Dekalb Avenue, Brooklyn, NY 11201, USA

Correspondence should be addressed to Gurleen Kaur Kahlon; gurleenkahlon2012@gmail.com

Academic Editor: Denis A. Cozzi

Fetal gallstones are rare incidental findings on ultrasound during pregnancy. We describe a newborn girl with gallstones that was born to a mother who had COVID-19 infection during her last trimester. The baby remained asymptomatic, and the stones resolved spontaneously without any treatment or complications within six weeks of birth. Several conditions predispose to fetal gallstones, and it is unclear if the recent maternal COVID-19 infection had any role in the occurrence of these abnormalities or was merely coincidental. This is the first case describing an association of fetal gallstones with a COVID-19 infection in pregnancy.

1. Introduction

Fetal gallstones or sludge are uncommon and are usually an incidental sonographic finding during pregnancy [1]. There have been no reports of any association between maternal COVID-19 infection and fetal gallbladder abnormalities. COVID-19 infection can affect the gastrointestinal system, and in one study, 54% of patients with right upper quadrant ultrasound revealed a dilated sludge-filled gallbladder suggestive of biliary stasis [2]. In another report, SARS COVID-2 virus causing COVID-19 has been detected in the bile of a patient with gallbladder disease [3]. Gallbladder wall edema has been described in children affected with COVID-19-associated multisystem inflammatory syndrome [4]. Sileo et al. reported gallbladder calcification in a 38-week gestation newborn whose mother was diagnosed with COVID-19 infection at 35 weeks of gestation [5]. Presently, there is insufficient data regarding the effects of COVID-19 illness on maternal, perinatal, and neonatal outcomes. It is unclear if maternal COVID-19 infection has any role in the occurrence of gallbladder abnormalities [6].

2. Case Presentation

A 34-year-old obese G4 P1021 woman with a BMI of 32 was admitted at 38 weeks of gestation to the antenatal unit for a scheduled repeat cesarean section. Her past medical history was significant for an unspecified cardiac rhythm abnormality and well-controlled chronic hypertension on metoprolol 50 mg twice a day. The family history was significant for high cholesterol, diabetes, hypertension, gastric ulcers, cardiovascular disorders, and cancers of the breast and vagina. She initially received prenatal care at another facility and was transferred to our hospital during her last trimester. The patient reported that she developed a sore throat, cough, and body pain six weeks before and was diagnosed at the local emergency department with COVID-19 illness (PCR-positive). The patient reported that a sonogram done 3 weeks before showed a possible gallbladder abnormality. She was advised supportive care and self-quarantine for two weeks, and since then, she has made a full recovery. All prenatal lab outcomes (RPR, Hepatitis B surface antigen, HIV, QuantiFERON, Group B *Streptococcus*, and repeat COVID-19 PCR) were negative upon the present admission. The mother received cefazolin preoperatively and underwent an uneventful cesarean section. A healthy baby girl was delivered with APGAR scores of nine and nine at 1 min and 5 min, respectively. The amniotic fluid was clear with artificial rupture of membranes 2 minutes before delivery. The umbilical cord showed three vessels. The mother had a blood group of B Rh-negative, the baby's blood group was O Rh-positive, and DAT was negative. Due to Rh incompatibility, the mother received 1 gram of RhoGam postpartum. On physical examination, the baby was pink, alert, and active.

Her anthropometric measurements were as follows: birth-weight was 3227 grams (67th percentile), length was 48.26 cm (47th percentile), and head circumference was 35 cm (85th percentile). The vital signs were within the normal range for age at birth. The patient's skin exam was remarkable for erythema toxicum predominantly on the face and a lumbosacral Mongolian spot. Throughout her hospital stay, she had no visible jaundice, abdominal distention, or palpable masses. She was voiding and stooling normally. At 24 hours of life, direct bilirubin was 0.2 mg/dl, total serum bilirubin was 4.4 mg/dl, and alkaline phosphatase was 99 U/L, all within the normal range. Due to the maternal concern surrounding the previous sonogram, an abdominal ultrasound was performed soon after birth (Figures 1–3) which showed gravel of stones and sludge in the dependent aspect of the gallbladder. There was no associated gallbladder wall thickening or pericholecystic fluid to suggest acute chole-cystitis and no dilatation of the intrahepatic or extrahepatic biliary ducts. The patient was clinically stable without any evidence of hyperbilirubinemia and was discharged home on the day of life two with close outpatient follow-up. At the two-week follow-up, a cardiac murmur was detected at-tributing to hemodynamically insignificant peripheral pulmonary stenosis. At the six-week follow-up, there was complete resolution of the gallbladder abnormalities (Figure 4).

3. Discussion

The incidence of fetal gallstones of sludge can range from 5 per 1000 to 1 in 3000 live births, and the actual prevalence is estimated to be around 0.5 to 0.7/10,000 live births [7]. The frequency of diagnosis has been increasing recently due to the more ubiquitous use of ultrasound examinations. Fetal gallstones play no role in fetal or postnatal prognosis and resolve spontaneously after birth without any need for intervention [8]. The exact pathogenesis of fetal gallstones remains unknown. Various factors (Table 1) have been implicated that potentially have a role in the formation of gallstones [9–13]. There have been no previous reports regarding the association of fetal gallstones with COVID-19 infection. While it is possible that conditions listed in the table, particularly obesity, may have played a role, it is also conceivable that maternal COVID-19 infection played a significant part in the occurrence of these stones. Bhayana et al. [2] demonstrated a dilated sludge-filled gallbladder suggestive of biliary stasis in 54% of their cases. While the exact mechanism of this association remains unexplained, biliary stasis does predispose to gallstone formation.

The fetal gallbladder starts developing around the 4th week of gestation from the embryonic foregut [14]. The fetal gallbladder is commonly an oval or teardrop-shaped structure and has no active role in fetal gastrointestinal physiology [15]. The fetal gallbladder is visible on ultrasound as early as the second trimester in the form of an elliptical hypoechoic or anechogenic body, present to the right of the intrahepatic umbilical vein [16]. Because the umbilical vein and fetal gallbladder have a similar ultrasonographic appearance, prior identification of the umbilical vein is recommended. Fetal gallstones manifest as echogenic foci with acoustic shadowing compared to gallbladder sludge, which is hyperechoic without any acoustic shadowing. Gallbladder sludge is considered a precursor of fetal gallstones and is reported to occur in approximately 40% of fetal gallstone cases. It is considered a more frequent finding compared to fetal gallstones. Fetal gallstones and gallbladder sludge are mainly seen during the third trimester [11, 13, 16]. The mechanisms postulated for the occurrence of gallbladder sludge or fetal gallstones are twofold. It may be due to hematoma in the maternal placenta, which results in hemoglobin breakdown leading to bilirubin formation and eventually gallstones. The other mechanism may be related to increased maternal estrogen levels, which can depress bile acid synthesis and increase cholesterol secretion, eventually leading to gallstone formation [1, 8]. Most infants found to have gallbladder stones/biliary sludge remain asymptomatic, and the abnormalities resolve spontaneously with time. One study involving 63 infants with fetal cholelithiasis and followed with serial ultrasound examinations found that complete resolution occurred in 70% of cases within two months and greater than 90% of cases within six months. Only two patients had persistent fetal cholelithiasis beyond 12 months. Schwab et al. followed a subset of 17 patients for a 3–20-year duration and found no complications or sequelae related to fetal gallstones [11, 17]. Therapeutic interventions described in the literature include the use of ursodeoxycholic acid and laparoscopic cholecystectomy. There is presently no evidence that therapeutic interventions are superior to observations awaiting spontaneous resolution. Medical treatment or cholecystectomy should be considered for rare persistent cases, symptomatic cases, or those with related complications [9–11, 13, 18]. There appears to be no difference in resolution time between sonogram-detected fetal gallstones and biliary sludge detection during pregnancy, and both scenarios have no impact on the obstetrical management or the delivery process [1, 9, 11]. Persistent fetal cholelithiasis/biliary sludge beyond one year of age may indicate a worse prognosis [19]. Associated anomalies can influence prognosis. These are reported in 20–30% of cases and include primary pulmonary hypertension, hydronephrosis, renal ectopia, hemivertebra syndrome, and hydrocephalus. Thus, for patients identified prenatally with gallstones and biliary sludge, a careful evaluation to detect associated abnormalities is prudent [12, 20].

4. Summary

We report an asymptomatic newborn with gallstones and biliary sludge detected on abdominal ultrasound soon after birth, which was entirely resolved by six weeks of age. It is unclear if the recent maternal COVID-19 infection had any role in the occurrence of these abnormalities or was merely coincidental. Fetal gallstones are rare and mostly resolve without any medical or surgical intervention.

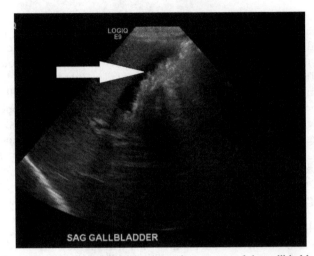

FIGURE 1: Biliary sludge in the dependent aspect of the gallbladder.

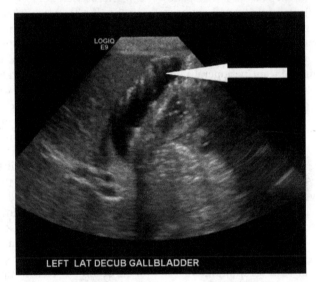

FIGURE 2: Biliary sludge and gravel of stones.

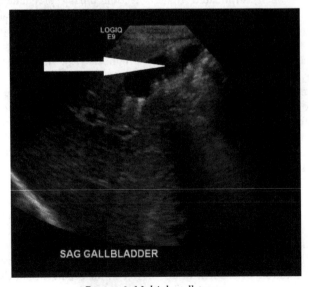

FIGURE 3: Multiple gallstones.

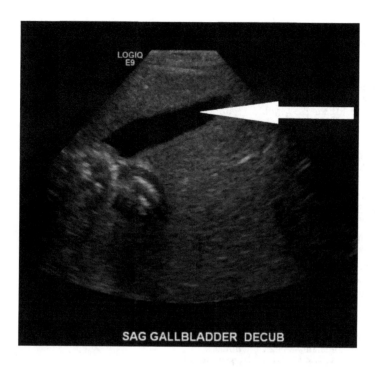

FIGURE 4: Normal gallbladder with complete resolution of the initial finding.

TABLE 1: Maternal and fetal causes associated with fetal cholelithiasis [4, 9–12].

Maternal causes	Fetal causes
(1) Hemolytic diseases (spherocytosis, sickle cell anemia, thalassemia)	(1) Hemolytic diseases (spherocytosis, sickle cell anemia, thalassemia)
(2) History of cholelithiasis	(2) Congenital malformation (CVS, GI, urologic, and skeletal)
(3) Intrahepatic cholestasis of pregnancy	(3) Anomalies of biliary tract or biliary obstruction
(4) Intestinal malabsorption	(4) Chromosome anomalies (trisomy 21; translocation 10, 11)
(5) Chronic liver disease	(5) Congenital malabsorption syndrome
(6) Hypercholesterolemia	(6) Pancreatic cystic fibrosis
(7) Increased estrogen and progesterone levels	(7) IUGR
(8) All types of diabetes	(8) Fetal obesity or macrosomia
(9) Obesity	(9) Oligohydramnios
(10) Narcotic use (methadone)	(10) Polyhydramnios
(11) Ceftriaxone treatment	(11) Prematurity
(12) Anticancer drug treatment	(12) Prenatal leukemoid reaction
(13) Prostaglandin E2 treatment	(13) Hepatitis
(14) Furosemide treatment	(14) Fetal- maternal blood group incompatibility (rhesus or ABO blood group incompatibility)
(15) Prolonged fasting	(15) Idiopathic
(16) Dehydration	
(17) Enteral nutrition	
(18) Intoxication with denatured oil treated with steroid	
(19) Twin pregnancy	
(20) Twin pregnancy with fetal demise of one twin	
(21) Placental abruption	
(22) Sepsis	

Consent

No written consent has been obtained from the patient as there is no patient-identifiable data included in this case report.

References

[1] B. Petrikovsky, R. Victor, M. D. Klein, and N. Holsten, RDMS: Gallstones. 1994-12-10-21 Gallstones © Petrikovskywww.-thefetus.net. Originally published in The Fetus in. 1994. https://sonoworld.com/Fetus/page.aspx?id=233, 1994.

[2] R. Bhayana, A. Som, M. D. Li et al., "Abdominal imaging findings in COVID-19: preliminary observations," *Radiology*, vol. 297, no. 1, pp. E207–E215, 2020, Epub 2020 May 11. PMID: 32391742, PMCID: PMC7508000.

[3] Y. Liao, B. Wang, J. Wang, J. Shu, W. Zhou, and H. Zhang, "SARS-CoV-2 in the bile of a patient with COVID-19-associated gallbladder disease," *Endoscopy*, vol. 52, no. 12, Article ID 1148, 2020.

[4] K. Morparia, M. J. Park, M. Kalyanaraman, D. McQueen, M. Bergel, and T. Phatak, "Abdominal imaging findings in critically ill children with Multisystem inflammatory syndrome associated with COVID-19," *The Pediatric Infectious Disease Journal*, vol. 40, no. 2, pp. e82–e83, 2021.

[5] F. G. Sileo, L. T. Anna, C. Leone et al., "Pregnant woman infected by Coronavirus Disease (COVID-19) and calcifications of the fetal bowel and gallbladder: a case report," *Minerva Ginecologica*, vol. 23736, pp. 0026–4784, 2020.

[6] J. Juan, M. M. Gil, Z. Rong, Y. Zhang, H. Yang, and L. C. Poon, "Effect of coronavirus disease 2019 (COVID-19) on maternal, perinatal and neonatal outcome: systematic review," *Ultrasound in Obstetrics & Gynecology: The Official Journal of the International Society of Ultrasound in Obstetrics and Gynecology*, vol. 1, pp. 15–27, 2020.

[7] L. Michael, H. Karen, and B. Stephani, "Fetal cholelithiasis," *Journal of Diagnostic Medical Sonography*, vol. 22, no. 6, 2006.

[8] P. Callen, *Ultrasonography in Obstetrics and Gynecology*, W. B. Saunders, Philadelphia, PA, USA, 3rd ed. edition, 1994.

[9] V. Suma, A. Marini, N. Bucci, T. Toffolutti, and E. Talenti, "Fetal gallstones: sonographic and clinical observations," *Ultrasound in Obstetrics and Gynecology*, vol. 12, pp. 439–441, 1998.

[10] P.-Y. Iroh Tam and A. Angelides, "Perinatal detection of gallstones in siblings," *American Journal of Perinatology*, vol. 27, pp. 771–774, 2010.

[11] S. Triunfo, P. Rosati, P. Ferrara, A. Gatto, and g. Scambia, "Fetal Cholelithiasis: a diagnostic update and a literature review," *Clinical Medicine Insights: Case Reports*, vol. 6, pp. 153–158, 2013.

[12] J. Troyano-Luque, A. Padilla-Pérez, I. Martínez-Wallin et al., "Short and long term outcomes associated with fetal cholelithiasis: a report of two cases with antenatal diagnosis and postnatal follow-up," *Case Reports in Obstetrics and Gynecology*, vol. 2014, Article ID 714271, 5 pages, 2014.

[13] Y. Hurni, F. Vigo, B. von Wattenwy, N. Ochsenbein, and C. Canonica, "Fetal cholelithiasis: antenatal diagnosis and neonatal follow-up in a case of twin pregnancy - a case report and review of the literature," *Ultrasound International Open*, vol. 3, no. 1, pp. E8–E12, 2017, A. Smith, B. Jones, G. King, Article title goes here, 1900-2012, Pediatrics, 123, 75–82, 2014. 10.1542/peds.2015-1827.

[14] K. L. Moore, *The Developing Human: Clinically Oriented Embryology*, W. B. Saunders, Philadelphia, PA, USA, 3rd ed. edition, 1982.

[15] K. Hata, S. Aoki, T. Hata, F. Murao, and M. Kitao, "Ultrasonographic identification of the human fetal gallbladder in utero," *Gynecologic and Obstetric Investigation*, vol. 23, pp. 79–83, 1987.

[16] M. H. Moon, J. Y. Cho, J. H. Kim et al., "Utero development of the fetal gall bladder in the Korean population," *Korean Journal of Radiology*, vol. 9, pp. 54–58, 2008.

[17] M. E. Schwab, H. J Braun, V. A. Feldstein, and A. Nijagal, "The natural history of fetal gallstones: a case series and updated literature review," *The Journal of Maternal-Fetal & Neonatal Medicine*, 2020.

[18] N. Munjuluri, N. Elgharaby, D. Acolet, and R. A. Kadir, "Fetal gallstones," *Fetal Diagnosis and Therapy*, vol. 20, pp. 241–243, 2005.

[19] M. Gertner and D. L. Farmer, "Laparoscopic cholecystectomy in a 16-day-old infant with chronic cholelithiasis," *Journal of Pediatric Surgery*, vol. 39, pp. 17–19, 2004.

[20] T. Kiserud, K. Gjelland, H. Bognø, M. Waardal, H. Reigstad, and K. Rosendahl, "Echogenic material in the fetal gallbladder and fetal disease," *Ultrasound in Obstetrics and Gynecology*, vol. 10, pp. 103–106, 1997.

30

An Isolated Hypogonadotropic Hypogonadism due to a L102P Inactivating Mutation of KISS1R/GPR54 in a Large Family

Ahmad J. Alzahrani ⓘ,[1] Azzam Ahmad,[2] Tariq Alhazmi,[1] and Lujin Ahmad[2]

[1]Pediatric Endocrine Department, (A.J.A, T.A), Maternity Children Hospital, Makkah, Saudi Arabia
[2]Umm Al-Qura University, Medical College, (A.A, L.A), Makkah, Saudi Arabia

Correspondence should be addressed to Ahmad J. Alzahrani; zz11ww@yahoo.com

Academic Editor: Vjekoslav Krzelj

KISS1R (GPR54) mutations have been reported in several patients with congenital normosmic idiopathic hypogonadotropic hypogonadism (nIHH). We aim to describe in detail nIHH patients with KISS1R (GPR54) mutations belonging to one related extended family and to review the literature. A homozygous mutation (T305C) leading to a leucine substitution with proline (L102P) was found in three affected kindred (2 males and 1 female) from a consanguineous Saudi Arabian family. This residue is localized within the first exoloop of the receptor, affects a highly conserved amino acid, perturbs the conformation of the transmembrane segment, and impairs its function. In the affected female, a combined gonadotropin administration restored regular period and ovulation and she conceived with a healthy baby boy after 4 years of marriage. We showed that a loss-of-function mutation (p.Tyr305C) in the KISS1R gene can cause (L102P) KISS1 receptor dysfunction and familial nIHH, revealing the crucial role of this amino acid in KISS1R function. The observed restoration of periods and later on pregnancy by an exogenous gonadotropin administration further support, in humans, that the KISS1R mutation has no other harmful effects on the patients apart from the gonadotropin secretion impairment.

1. Introduction

Hereditary isolated hypogonadotropic hypogonadism (IHH) is an uncommon disorder in pediatric and adult population; genetic causes of IHH are increasingly recognized due to the increasing number of genetic testing.

Genetic IHH is classified into two types, depending on the presence or absence of smell defect: Kallmann syndrome when associated with anosmia and normosmic IHH when normal smell is preserved.

Neuroendocrine control of the reproductive axis in humans rests with a group of neurons called GnRH (gonadotropin-releasing hormone) neurons, approximately 1500 in number and dispersed in the hypothalamus. GnRH neurons are originating from the nasal placode during embryogenesis. The hypothalamus synthesizes and releases a neurohormone, GnRH, which then travels via hypothalamic-hypophyseal portal circulation to reach the anterior pituitary, where it binds to the GnRH receptor to stimulate the synthesis and secretion of gonadotropins [1].

IHH is a heterogeneous disorder affecting one in 5000 males, with a three- to fivefold of males over females. Mutations in *KISS1/KISSR, TAC3/TACR3, GNRH1/GNRHR, LEP/LEPR, HESX1, FSHB,* and *LHB* are present in patients with normosmic IHH [2–4].

Several reports have showed the high potency of kisspeptin in regulating LH and FSH secretion in animals and humans [5, 6]. In 2003, two groups independently identified KISS1R as a gatekeeper of puberty: Seminara et al. [1] and de Roux et al. [7].

Inactivating mutations in KISS1R is transmitted as a recessive trait and accounts for 2–4% cases of nIHH. The

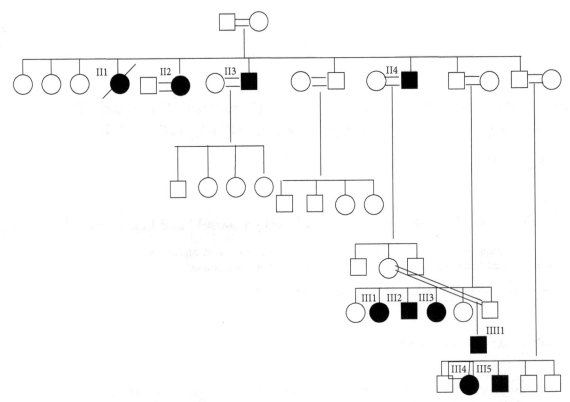

FIGURE 1: Family pedigree of the reported family: black forms indicate affected members. Circles represent female family members and squares indicate male family members. Roman numerals indicate generations and Arabic numbers indicate individuals in each generation. NL: normal.

KISS1R gene is located in locus 19p.13.3. It is also known as the *GPR54* gene, and encodes a G-protein-coupled receptor or receptor for kisspeptins. The GPR54/KISS1R protein is a transmembrane receptor made up of 398 amino acids. It translates signals from the cell surface as part of the signaling pathway for the release of GnRH. The binding of kisspeptin to these receptors in the hypothalamus stimulates the release of GnRH, which in turn stimulates gonadotropin release [8–10].

In this report, we will try to put more light in this group of patients and to show if there is any genotype-phenotype correlation by reporting an extended family of Saudi Arabian origin with KISS1R loss-of-function mutation.

2. Case Report

A large Saudi Arabian family with extensive intermarriage among them sought advice in different medical centers for delayed puberty and infertility. Nine of them had features of idiopathic hypogonadotropic hypogonadism (IHH).

Patients (Figure 1 (III2, III3, and IIII1)) were diagnosed and followed up at our hospital during childhood and adulthood.

Patient III3 was referred to gynecological service to continue her management after she got married. At each visit, growth measurements were recorded: height in cm and weight in kg were plotted in the CDC (Center for Diseases Control and Prevention) growth chart and the pubertal stage was assessed according to Tanner staging. Bone age (BA) was estimated according to the Greulich and Pyle method.

Anterior pituitary hormone activity was evaluated by measuring the basal level of luteinizing hormone (LH), follicular-stimulating hormone (FSH), thyroid-stimulating hormone (TSH), free T4, free T3, and prolactin as well as gonadal steroid (testosterone or estrogen assay using commercial polyclonal RIA).

After informed consent was obtained, genomic DNA was extracted from white blood cells of the three patients and parents of III2 and III3 by using the standard technique.

KISS1R coding exons 1, 2, 3, 4, and 5 and intron-exon junctions were amplified by PCR (polymerase chain reaction) and sequenced, and *GNRHR* (*gonadotropin-releasing hormone receptor*) and other rare sequence variants were also analyzed as previously described [1].

Affected patients were all from consanguineous parents; there were nine affected members in this extended family (Figure 1) with different phenotypes and three of them were attending regularly to our endocrine department.

The first one (Figure 1 (III2)) was a 26-year-old male presented to the clinic with absent puberty, phallus 6 cm, testicular size 5 cc, height 173 cm, weight 65 kg, normal smell, no deafness, no skeletal defects, and no other physical abnormalities.

Laboratory workup showed low serum gonadotropins: LH 0.6 mIU/ml, FSH 3.4 mIU/ml, testosterone 0.1 ng/dl, prolactin 11 ng/ml, and normal TSH, FT3, and FT4. Repeated hormonal assay was almost similar.

Brain magnetic resonance imaging MRI showed empty sella and normal brain structure; otherwise, BA was delayed.

The patient was treated with injectable depot testosterone, gradually increasing the dose from 100 mg to 250 mg with monthly injection.

The patient had adequate pubertal development: P4, phallus 10 cm, and small testes, so the treatment was changed to human chorionic gonadotropin (hCG) (5000 IU twice weekly), and s.c. FSH injection (75 IU twice weekly) was added to enhance testicular growth and spermatogenesis; the testicular size during the last visit was 12 ml, and the patient did not appear for follow-up thereafter.

The second patient (Figure 1 (III3)) was a 17-year-old sister of the first patient who presented to our clinic with absent puberty, primary amenorrhea, normal growth parameters (height 153 cm and weight 49 kg), normal physical examination findings, normal smell, and no skeletal defects. Her hormonal assay was as follows: LH 0.9 mIU/ml, FSH 5.7 mIU/ml, estrogen 5 pg/ml, prolactin 14 ng/ml, and normal thyroid function; repeated assay was almost the same.

Brain MRI showed normal brain structure and BA was delayed.

She was treated with estrogen pills followed by oral combined estrogen/progesterone pills and after she got married she was started on human chorionic gonadotropin (hCG) together with FSH injection as the pulsatile GNRH was not available; fortunately, she got pregnant with a healthy normal boy.

The third patient (Figure 1 (IIII1)) was a 4-year-old boy, a nephew for the previous two cases, who presented with micropenis, stretched length from the pubic ramus to the top of the glans 2.2 cm, testicular volume 2.5 cc, normal physical examination findings, and normal growth parameters. Hormonal assay showed LH 0.1, FSH 0.8, and testosterone 0.2 ng/dl. Thyroid function and prolactin level were normal; the patient received a small dose of depot testosterone (50 mg IM once) and showed significant improvement in phallus size.

On reviewing the family history, it showed the following affected members (Table 1):

(1) Affected aunt (II1) of the first case died at 25 years and was having no breast development, primary amenorrhea, and was married for 4 years with no pregnancy

(2) A 55-year-old aunt (II2) had small breast, primary amenorrhea, married for 30 years, and no children even after pregnancy augmentation

(3) A 45-year-old uncle (II3) with cryptorchidism which was treated and he is married with 5 children after infertility management

(4) A 35-year-old sister (III1) with no puberty, primary amenorrhea, and married for 18 years with no pregnancy even after augmentation

(5) A 30-year-old cousin (III4), lady, with no puberty, no menses, married for 5 years, and had no pregnancy even after augmentation

(6) A 20-year-old cousin (III5), male, with no puberty, small testes, and small phallus

Sequencing of the five exons of the KISS1R gene revealed homozygous mutation in exon 2 in all affected patients (III2, III3, and IIII1) as well as a heterozygous mutation in the parents of III2 and III3. A substitution of a cytosine for thymidine T305C produced a proline substitution for leucine (L102p), and this residue is localized within the first exoloop of the kisspeptin receptors (Figure 2). No mutation was identified in GNRHR or other rare related genes.

3. Discussion

Hereby, we described a loss-of-function mutation in the homozygous state, previously described by Yardena et al. (p.Tyr305C) in the *KISS1R* (*GPR54*) gene leading to p.Leu102Pro in the KISS1 receptor in a highly consanguineous Saudi Arabian family suffering from congenital nIHH [5]. Nine members of this family seem to be affected by this disease, but a longitudinal follow-up of three affected patients revealed inactivation of the gonadotropin axis associated with underdevelopment of external genitalia and absence of puberty.

Our reported cases differ from the previously reported similar mutation by Yardena et al. [5] in certain features: we have a larger collection (nine cases) in one family, complete absence of pubertal signs, and no cryptorchidism in the male patient (Figure 1 (III2)) with better response to treatment in the phallus size of 10 cm and the testicular growth of 12 ml compared to the previously reported cases [5] with a smaller group (three affected) in either family, partial puberty on presentation, cryptorchidism, and poor response to treatment in the male patients with phallus 7.2 cm and testes 4 ml in size which might be due to the late correction of cryptorchidism.

Functional analyses in a previous study by Yardena et al. revealed that the L102P variant led to an almost complete loss-of-function mutation, resulting in a severe phenotype corresponding to lack of pubertal development with cryptorchidism [5].

These results emphasize the role of the KISS1/KISS1R system in initiation of puberty and maintaining reproductive function through the control of GnRH secretion [10, 11].

The phenotypes of the patients appeared to be less severe in our patients as compared with the other mutations, in whom severe micropenis and cryptorchidism were reported [12], indicating that this type of mutation is less severely manifesting than other mutations.

Treating these patients demonstrated that the delayed puberty could be corrected by gonadotropin administration, which further supports the idea that the loss of KISS1R function in pituitary gonadotropic cells does not have clinically significant consequences in humans other than the gonadotropin deficiency and its consequences on health.

In our female patients, fertility was restored by gonadotropin administration where she had a healthy baby boy without miscarriages, indicating that KISS1R loss of function has no direct effect on gonadal or placental function.

The integrity of other anterior pituitary functions in the patients investigated here also shows that loss of KISS1R only affects the gonadotropic axis.

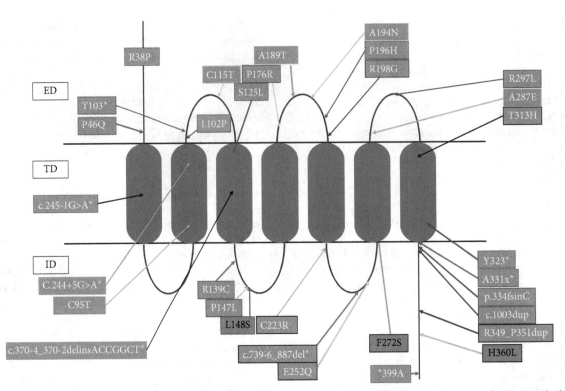

FIGURE 2: Reported mutations and its location in the KISS1 receptor identified in nCHH patients: colored in orange for previously described mutations and in green for our cases. Residues with asterisk indicate nonsense mutations, and residues without asterisk indicate missense mutations. ED: extracellular domain; TD: transmembrane domain; ID: intracellular domain.

TABLE 1: Patients characteristics.

Patient	II1	II2	II3	III1	III2	III3	III4	III5	IIII1
Sex	F	F	M	F	M	F	F	M	M
Age, years	25	55	45	35	26	17	30	20	4
Puberty	No	No	Yes	No	No	No	No	No	Micropenis
Marriage, years	4	30	25	18	2	2	5	0	0
Children	0	0	5	0	0	1	0	0	0
Infertility treatment	Yes	Yes	Yes	Yes	No	Yes	Yes	No	No
LH					Low	Low			Low
FSH					Low	Low			Low
Treatment					Andro., FSH, hCG	hCG			Andro.

F, female; M, male; LH, luteinizing hormone; FSH, follicle-stimulating hormone; hCG, human chorionic gonadotropin; Andro., depot testosterone.

Also in Yardena et al. study, a cell surface-binding analysis revealed normal affinity of the L102P receptor for Kp10 and a small decrease in cell surface expression, which might indicate that this amino acid substitution within the first extracellular loop blocks the normal conformational change of the receptor during activation [5]. This functional analysis shows that a complete defect in the KISS1R receptor signaling results in partial gonadotropic deficiency [5]. The gonadotropic deficiency results in a more quantitative than qualitative defect in the pubertal process, and during 10 min blood sampling, low-amplitude LH pulses can still be detected in patients with KISS1R mutations. Therefore, loss-of-function mutations seem to reduce GNRH without interfering with the intrinsic GNRH pulse generator [2, 13].

One member of this family (Figure 1 (II4)) reported to have anosmia which is not associated with this type of

mutation since it is not reported before to have a smell defect and most likely this is of acquired origin.

Up until mid-2019s, 32 loss-of-function mutations in the KISS1R (GPR54) gene had been described in the literature (Figure 2 and Table 2). These mutations were found to have variable clinical manifestations, varied from incomplete puberty and infertility to severe hypogonadism with microphallus and cryptorchidism in males.

In conclusion, we have identified a novel loss-of-function mutation in the KISS1R (GPR54) gene in three members of highly consanguineous families of Saudi Arabian origin associated with nIHH. This study emphasizes the important role of the KISS1/KISS1R system in maintaining gonadotropin secretion. However, little is known about hypogonadotropic hypogonadism phenotype-genotype relations in patients harboring these mutations. The current report adds to the spectrum of loss-of-function mutations in

TABLE 2: Reported mutations in the KISS1R gene.

DNA mutation	Protein mutation	Functional analysis	Ethnic origin	Ref.
IVS2-4_-2del GCA ins ACCGGCT	Four different abnormal proteins	ND	Brazilian	[14]
c.305C>T	L102P	ND	Saudi Arabian	Present study
c.305C>T	L102P	IP accumulation; residual activity	Arabs	[5, 12]
c.345C>G	p.C115T	No response in luciferase	Caucasian	[12]
c.443T>C	p.L148S	IP accumulation; decreased activity	Saudi Arabian	[1]
155-bp deletion	p.247X	ND	Caucasian	[7]
c.754G>C	p.E252Q	IP accumulation	Brazilian	[14]
c.T815>C	p.F272S	IP accumulation; residual activity	Arabs	[15]
c.1001–1002insC	p.334fsinC.	ND	German	[16]
c.1079A>T	p.H360L	ND	Caucasian	[17]
c.1157G>C	p.R386P	Reduction in the rate of desensitization	Brazilian	[18]
c.667T>C	p.C223R	Ca^{2+} mobilization; low activity	Jamaican-Turkish	[19]
c.891G>T	p.R297L	Ca^{2+} mobilization; low activity	Jamaican-Turkish	[19]
c.991C>T	p.R331X	IP accumulation	Black	[1]
c.1195T>A	p.X399A	IP accumulation; low activity	Black	[1]
c.244 + 5G>A	p.?	ND	Caucasian	[12]
c.285C>G	p.Cys95Trp	No response in luciferase assays	Caucasian	[12]
c.309C>A	p.Tyr103*	No response in luciferase assays	Caucasian	[12]
c.527C>G	p.Pro176Arg	No response in luciferase assays	Caucasian	[12]
c.860C>A	p.Ala287Glu	Shifted response in luciferase assays	Caucasian	[12]
c.113G>C	p.Arg38Pro	ND	Caucasian	[12]
c.137C>A	p.Pro46Gin	ND	Caucasian	[12]
c.374C>T	p.Ser125Leu	ND	Caucasian	[12]
c.592C>G	p.Arg198Gly	ND	Caucasian	[12]
c.969C>A/c.170T>C	p.Y323X/p.L57P	ND	Turkish	[20]
c.440C>T	p.P147L	Impaired receptor function	Japanese	[21]
c.937T>C	p.Tyr313His	ND	Portuguese	[22]
c.305T>C/c.1195T>A	p.L102P/Stop399A	No response in luciferase assays	French	[22]
c.1195T>C	p.X399R	ND	Tunisian	[23]
	R139C	Abolished membrane expression	Turkish	[24]

ND, not done; Ref, references.

the KISS1R gene that results in loss of receptor function. Further identification of KISS1R mutations is needed to define the precise genotype-phenotype relationship.

References

[1] S. B. Seminara, S. Messager, E. E. Chatzidaki et al., "The GPR54 Gene as a regulator of puberty," *New England Journal of Medicine*, vol. 349, no. 17, pp. 1614–1627, 2003.

[2] E. Gianetti and S. Seminara, "Kisspeptin and KISS1R: a critical pathway in the reproductive system," *Reproduction*, vol. 136, no. 3, pp. 295–301, 2008.

[3] L. G. L. Amato, L. R. Montenegro, A. M. Lerario et al., "New genetic findings in a large cohort of congenital hypogonadotropic hypogonadism," *European Journal of Endocrinology*, vol. 181, no. 2, pp. 103–119, 2019.

[4] B. Bhagavath, R. H. Podolsky, M. Ozata et al., "Clinical and molecular characterization of a large sample of patients with hypogonadotropic hypogonadism," *Fertility and Sterility*, vol. 85, no. 3, pp. 706–713, 2006.

[5] T.-R. Yardena, C.-D. Monique, I. André, A. Chantal, A. Osnat, and N. de Roux, "Neuroendocrine phenotype analysis in five patients with isolated hypogonadotropic hypogonadism due to a L102P inactivating mutation of GPR54," *The Journal of Clinical Endocrinology & Metabolism*, vol. 92, no. 3, pp. 1137–1144, 2007.

[6] C. M. Trevisan, E. Montagna, R. de Oliveira et al., "Kisspeptin/GPR54 system: what do we know about its role in human reproduction?," *Cellular Physiology and Biochemistry*, vol. 49, no. 4, pp. 1259–1276, 2018.

[7] N. de Roux, E. Genin, J.-C. Carel, F. Matsuda, J.-L. Chaussain, and E. Milgrom, "Hypogonadotropic hypogonadism due to loss of function of the KiSS1-derived peptide receptor GPR54," *Proceedings of the National Academy of Sciences*, vol. 100, no. 19, pp. 10972–10976, 2003.

[8] N. Chelaghma, S. O. Oyibo, and J. Rajkanna, "Normosmic idiopathic hypogonadotrophic hypogonadism due to a rare KISS1R gene mutation," *Endocrinology, Diabetes & Metabolism Case Reports*, vol. 2018, no. 1, 2018.

[9] U. Boehm, P.-M. Bouloux, M. T. Dattani et al., "European consensus statement on congenital hypogonadotropic hypogonadism-pathogenesis, diagnosis and treatment," *Nature Reviews Endocrinology*, vol. 11, no. 9, pp. 547–564, 2015.

[10] L. G. Silveira, A. C. Latronico, and S. B. Seminara, "Kisspeptin and clinical disorders," *Advances in Experimental Medicine and Biology*, vol. 784, pp. 187–199, 2013.

[11] F. Wahab, R. Quinton, and S. B. Seminara, "The kisspeptin signaling pathway and its role in human isolated GnRH deficiency," *Molecular and Cellular Endocrinology*, vol. 346, no. 1-2, pp. 29–36, 2011.

[12] B. Francou, C. Paul, L. Amazit et al., "Prevalence of KISS1 receptormutations in a series of 603 patients with normosmic congenital hypogonadotrophic hypogonadism and characterization of novel mutations: a single-centre study," *Human Reproduction*, vol. 31, no. 6, pp. 1363–1374, 2016.

[13] J. C. Pallais, Y. Bo-Abbas, N. Pitteloud, W. F. Crowley, and S. B. Seminara, "Neuroendocrine, gonadal, placental, and obstetric phenotypes in patients with IHH and mutations in the G-protein coupled receptor, GPR54," *Molecular and Cellular Endocrinology*, vol. 254-255, pp. 70–77, 2006.

[14] M. G. Teles, E. B. Trarbach, S. D. Noel et al., "A novel homozygous splice acceptor site mutation of KISS1R in two siblings with normosmic isolated hypogonadotropic hypogonadism," *European Journal of Endocrinology*, vol. 163, no. 1, pp. 29–34, 2010.

[15] R. Nimri, Y. Lebenthal, L. Lazar et al., "A novel loss-of-function mutation in GPR54/KISS1R leads to hypogonadotropic hypogonadism in a highly consanguineous family," *The Journal of Clinical Endocrinology & Metabolism*, vol. 96, no. 3, pp. E536–E545, 2011.

[16] F. Lanfranco, J. Gromoll, S. von Eckardstein, E. M. Herding, E. Nieschlag, and M. Simoni, "Role of sequence variations of the GnRH receptor and G protein-coupled receptor 54 gene in male idiopathic hypogonadotropic hypogonadism," *European Journal of Endocrinology*, vol. 153, no. 6, pp. 845–852, 2005.

[17] F. Cerrato, J. Shagoury, M. Kralickova et al., "Coding sequence analysis of GNRHR and GPR54 in patients with congenital and adult-onset forms of hypogonadotropic hypogonadism," *European Journal of Endocrinology*, vol. 155, no. 1, pp. 3–10, 2006.

[18] M. G. Teles, S. D. C. Bianco, V. N. Brito et al., "AGPR54-Activating mutation in a patient with central precocious puberty," *New England Journal of Medicine*, vol. 358, no. 7, pp. 709–715, 2008.

[19] R. K. Semple, J. C. Achermann, J. Ellery et al., "Two novel missense mutations in G protein-coupled receptor 54 in a patient with hypogonadotropic hypogonadism," *The Journal of Clinical Endocrinology & Metabolism*, vol. 90, no. 3, pp. 1849–1855, 2005.

[20] O. Nalbantoglu, G. Arslan, O. Koprulu, F. Hazan, S. Gursoy, and B. Ozkan, "Three siblings with idiopathic hypogonadotropic hypogonadism in a nonconsanguineous family: a novel KISS1R/GPR54 loss-of-function mutation," *Journal of Clinical Research in Pediatric Endocrinology*, 2019.

[21] K. Shimizu, T. Yonekawa, M. Yoshida et al., "Conformational change in the ligand-binding pocket via a KISS1R mutation P147L leads to isolated gonadotropin-releasing hormone deficiency," *Journal of the Endocrine Society*, vol. 1, no. 10, pp. 1259–1271, 2017.

[22] F. Brioude, J. Bouligand, B. Francou et al., "Two families with normosmic congenital hypogonadotropic hypogonadism and biallelic mutations in KISS1R KISS1 receptor: clinical evaluation and molecular characterization of a novel mutation," *PLoS One*, vol. 8, no. 1, Article ID e53896, 2013.

[23] M. Moalla, F. Hadj Kacem, A. F. Al-Mutery et al., "Nonstop mutation in the Kisspeptin 1 receptor KISS1R gene causes normosmic congenital hypogonadotropic hypogonadism," *Journal of Assisted Reproduction and Genetics*, vol. 36, no. 6, pp. 1273–1280, 2019.

[24] A. K. Topaloglu, Z.-L. Lu, I. S. Farooqi et al., "Molecular genetic analysis of normosmic hypogonadotropic hypogonadism in a Turkish population: identification and detailed functional characterization of a novel mutation in the gonadotropin-releasing hormone receptor gene," *Neuroendocrinology*, vol. 84, no. 5, pp. 301–308, 2006.

31

Long-Term Remission of a Spinal Atypical Teratoid Rhabdoid Tumor in Response to Intensive Multimodal Therapy

Fahd Refai,[1] Haneen Al-Maghrabi⬤,[2] Hassan Al Trabolsi,[3] and Jaudah Al-Maghrabi⬤[1,2]

[1]*Department of Pathology, Faculty of Medicine, King Abdulaziz University, Jeddah, Saudi Arabia*
[2]*Department of Pathology, King Faisal Specialist Hospital and Research Centre, Jeddah, Saudi Arabia*
[3]*Oncology Department, King Faisal Specialist Hospital and Research Centre, Jeddah, Saudi Arabia*

Correspondence should be addressed to Jaudah Al-Maghrabi; jalmaghrabi@hotmail.com

Academic Editor: Stacey Tay

Atypical teratoid rhabdoid tumors (ATRTs) are rare and aggressive central nervous system tumors that infrequently arise in spinal locations in young children. Provided clinical and diagnostic suspicion is high, the histopathological diagnosis is relatively straightforward to secure by testing for the characteristic loss of the tumor suppressor protein *SMARCB1/INI1*. Here, we describe a case of thoracic spinal ATRT in a three-year-old boy that showed characteristic aggressive progression until managed with intensive multimodal therapy to achieve durable long-term remission. In doing so, we review the histopathological features, management, and current advances in molecular biology that hold promise for personalized ATRT therapy.

1. Introduction

Atypical teratoid rhabdoid tumors (ATRTs) are rare, aggressive, central nervous system (CNS) tumors that usually arise in the brain in young children but can arise at other sites including the spinal cord [1]. ATRTs need to be considered in the differential diagnosis of small round blue cells and poorly differentiated tumors occurring at peripheral sites, especially when biopsy material is limited, since the tumors are frequently heterogeneous and characteristic rhabdoid cells may be sparsely distributed. However, provided that diagnostic suspicion is high, the diagnosis of ATRT is aided by characteristic and almost pathognomonic molecular features. Here, we describe the rare case of a spinal ATRT occurring in a young boy to illustrate not only the histopathological and molecular features but also the aggressive but rescuable clinical course of ATRT with intensive multimodal management.

2. Case Presentation

A three-and-a-half-year-old boy presented to King Faisal Specialist Hospital & Research Centre, Jeddah, Kingdom of Saudi Arabia, in July 2015 with a ten-day history of back pain and progressive weakness of the lower extremities and an inability to walk. A computerized tomography (CT) scan performed at that time revealed a right suprarenal hypodense mass measuring $2.8 \times 3 \times 4.6$ cm and extending to the spinal canal (T9–T12) to cause spinal cord compression (Figure 1(a)). He underwent urgent laminectomy and decompression followed by debulking one month later, which improved his neurological symptoms. Histopathological examination at that time revealed a highly cellular tumor composed of cells with large nuclei, prominent nucleoli, and a variable amount of cytoplasm. Some of the cells had clear, nearly vacuolated cytoplasm (Figure 1(b)), and scattered cells contained more abundant, eosinophilic cytoplasm, but there were no classic rhabdoid cells with accumulation of intermediate filaments (Figure 1(c)). Immunohistochemistry for antibodies targeting vimentin, smooth muscle actin alpha (SMA) (Figure 1(d)), and p63 was positive, and there was focal positivity for Bcl-2 and focal weak positivity for CD99, CD10, CK8/18, calponin, and epithelial membrane antigen (EMA) (Figure 1(e)). Tumor cells were negative for other immune cell, neural, epithelial cell, germ cell, and smooth muscle cell markers. However, there was loss of

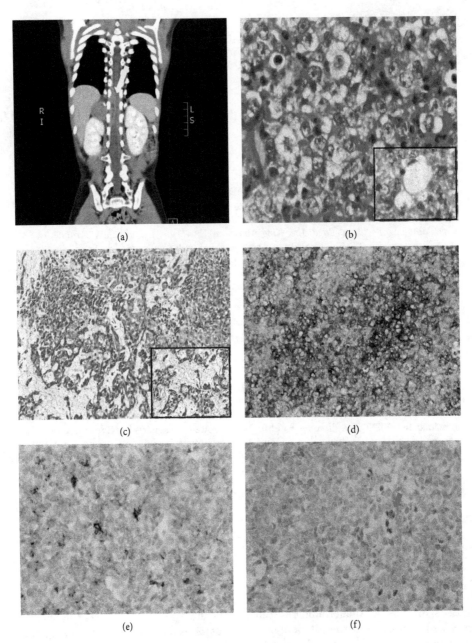

FIGURE 1: (a) Initial CT scan which shows 2.8 cm right suprarenal hypodense mass, extending to the spinal canal (T9–T12) and cause spinal cord compression (yellow arrow). (b) Histology of the tumor is composed of large pleomorphic cells with prominent nucleoli and clear nearly vacuolated cytoplasm (inset); background of scattered acute inflammatory cells are seen (Hematoxylin and eosin (H&E) stain; 40x). (c) Tumor cells containing more abundant eosinophilic cytoplasm, with focal myxoid changes (inset) (Hematoxylin and eosin (H&E) stain; 10x). (d) Tumor cells are diffusely positive for SMA (20x). (e) Focal tumor reactivity for EMA is seen (20x). (f) Complete loss of tumor cells' immunoreactivity for *SMARCB1/INI1*, with maintained internal control in lymphocytes between tumor cells (red arrow) (20x).

tumor cell immunoreactivity for *SMARCB1/INI1* (Figure 1(f)), and Ki-67 was positive in >50% of tumor cells. Fluorescence *in situ* hybridization for EWS/FLI-1 (Ewing sarcoma/PNET) and SYT/SSX (poorly differentiated synovial carcinoma) were all negative. A diagnosis of a malignant poorly differentiated round cell neoplasm was made, and the specific differential diagnosis including atypical teratoid rhabdoid tumor (ATRT) and myoepithelial carcinoma was also made. The case was referred for an external specialist opinion at Boston Children's Hospital, who agreed with the

histopathological assessment that both the morphology and the immunophenotype were consistent with ATRT, the polyphenotypic appearance of the tumor (especially EMA and smooth muscle actin positivity), and the definite loss of *SMARCB1/INI1* expression supporting the diagnosis.

Initial tumor regrowth after surgery was rapid, so the patient received 10 sessions of spinal radiotherapy and dexamethasone IV on a tapering dose in Saudi Arabia. He then went to the USA in September 2015, where he received 29 Gy radiotherapy plus dexamethasone and eight cycles of alternating vincristine, doxorubicin, cyclophosphamide, ifosfamide, cisplatin, and etoposide. He completed chemotherapy in April 2016. While surgical intervention was preferred for local control, this was not possible due to the tumor extent proximity to the spinal cord, so he underwent further 4500 cGy radiotherapy in 25 fractions to the paraspinal area in February and March 2016. A positron emission tomography (PET) scan performed after completion of therapy in 2016 was negative. A follow-up CT scan of the abdomen and pelvis in April 2017 revealed the development of a new soft tissue deposit at the inner aspect of the right 11th rib suggestive of recurrent disease. He had a further course of radiotherapy and chemotherapy which resolved the recurrence, and regular pediatric oncology follow-up with imaging identified no new recurrences over the following eighteen months.

3. Discussion

Atypical teratoid rhabdoid tumor (ATRT) is a rare and aggressive CNS tumor. ATRTs most frequently arise in the posterior cranial fossa (especially at the cerebello-pontine angle) of young children and infants aged under three, with a slight male predominance [1]. However, ATRTs can also rarely arise in spinal locations, as seen here, and also the kidneys and other peripheral, intrabdominal, and retroperitoneal sites [1]. Although in close proximity to the kidney, there was no renal parenchymal involvement of the ATRT described here, so we consider this to be an example of a spinal ATRT, of which about 40 are described in the literature [1–3]. Originally called malignant rhabdoid tumors and described as aggressive variants of Wilms' tumors with rhabdomyosarcomatous features, Rorke et al. [4] fully defined the entity in 1996 before its entry into the World Health Organization (WHO) classification in 2000 [5]. Prior to this, ATRTs were commonly misdiagnosed as medulloblastomas or primitive neuroectodermal tumors (PNETs), because of not only the similar histopathological appearances but also the similar imaging and gross pathological features [5]. The histological features are often mixed. It is not unusual for ATRTs to show minimal rhabdoid features and a predominant undifferentiated blue cell appearance, as seen in this case. Approximately, 30% of tumors contain malignant mesenchymal elements and 25% glandular or squamous epithelial components, although these were not seen here. Accordingly, the immunoreactivity is similarly varied and depends on the tumor composition, but this case showed the fairly typical pattern of vimentin, EMA, and SMA positivity, a high Ki-67 proliferation index, and negativity for desmin and germ cell markers. Critically, this case exhibited loss of SMARCB1/INI1 immunoreactivity, which corresponds to either homozygous deletions or mutations in SMARCB1/INI1, a tumor suppressor gene located on chromosome 22 (22q11.2) [6]. SMARCB1/INI1 is a core subunit of the epigenetic ATP-dependent SWI/SNF chromatin remodeling complex, which is essential for survival and dysregulation of which impacts several important oncogenic pathways involved in proliferation and apoptosis including the p16-RB, WNT, sonic hedgehog, and polycomb

pathways [7]. SMARCB1/INI1 is therefore a *bone fide* tumor suppressor gene and likely driver mutation in ATRTs. SMARCB1/INI1 is mutated in over 90% of ATRTs (with those tumors preserving SMARCB1/INI1, showing loss of the related SWI/SNF complex protein SMARCA4/BRG1) and is only rarely described in other CNS tumors, although is frequently lost in epithelioid sarcoma, pancreatic undifferentiated rhabdoid carcinoma, and epithelioid schwannoma [8], making it an extremely helpful ancillary test in these pediatric brain tumor cases [7]. Indeed, prior to the development of the antibody targeting SMARCB1/INI1, misdiagnosis was especially common if the characteristic rhabdoid cells were not present in the biopsy specimen [9]. Although usually sporadic, germline SMARCB1/INI1 mutations have been described in as many as 35% of cases that give rise to more extensive disease in very young patients [8]. Given that SMARCB1/INI1 is germline lethal, these germline mutations tend to arise *de novo* and hereditary cases are extremely rare [10].

The prognosis of ATRT has generally been regarded as appalling; historically, the majority of patients died within a year of diagnosis [1]. Indeed, our case highlights the rapidly progressive natural disease course in the absence of aggressive multimodal therapy, with the tumor rapidly regrowing after initial debulking. Given the rarity of the tumor and relatively few prospective trials, there has yet to be a consensus on the optimal management of ATRT. Different multimodal strategies combining surgery, radiotherapy, and chemotherapy (conventional and high dose, systemic and intrathecal, and with or without stem cell support) have been used with variable success, and one-year progression-free and overall survival rates have now improved to >50% [11–13]. Nevertheless, five-year survival rates remain only ~30% in pooled analyses [13]. There is now good evidence that while ATRTs are chemosensitive, in order to overcome the early emergence of resistance (usually in the first 24 weeks of diagnosis), the chemotherapy regimen must be intensive and use multiple agents in a dose-dense regimen after surgery and in combination with radiotherapy. Here, we employed a modification of the Medical University of Vienna protocol, which in a retrospective analysis achieved a 100% 5-year overall survival rate and 88.9% event-free survival rate [14]. Although our patient is now approaching four years since the diagnosis, there are no reliable prognostic markers for ATRT, and he will require continuing and close follow-up. With respect to prognosis, recent molecular profiling efforts are starting to define ATRT heterogeneity, with ASCL1 arising risk factors with clinicopathological characteristics and outcomes (supratentorial, improved overall survival) [15]. Of note, ASCL1+ tumors had superior radiation-free survival in this analysis, raising the prospect of a predictive biomarker that might help personalize therapy and spare some patients unnecessary therapies and consequent side effects.

In summary, the characteristic SMARCB1/INI1 mutations seen in ATRT have facilitated its histopathological diagnosis. However, the wider clinical and molecular heterogeneity of ATRT remains unresolved, and further efforts are required to develop prognostic and predictive biomarkers to personalize therapy for these young children. While there has been significant progress in the multimodal management of ATRT, there remains a need for co-ordinated, international, multicenter efforts to standardize management in the context of prospective clinical trials with associated molecular analyses.

Consent

Verbal and written informed consents were obtained from the patients for their anonymized information to be published in this article.

References

[1] M. C. Frühwald, J. A. Biegel, F. Bourdeaut, C. W. M. Roberts, and S. N. Chi, "Atypical teratoid/rhabdoid tumors-current concepts, advances in biology, and potential future therapies," *Neuro-Oncology*, vol. 18, no. 6, pp. 764–778, 2016.

[2] M. Babgi, A. Samkari, A. Al-Mehdar, and S. Abdullah, "Atypical teratoid/rhabdoid tumor of the spinal cord in a child: case report and comprehensive review of the literature," *Pediatric Neurosurgery*, vol. 53, no. 4, pp. 254–262, 2018.

[3] M. F. Chao, Y.-F. Su, T.-S. Jaw, S.-S. Chiou, and C.-H. Lin, "Atypical teratoid/rhabdoid tumor of lumbar spine in a toddler child," *Spinal Cord Series and Cases*, vol. 3, no. 1, Article ID 16026, 2017.

[4] L. B. Rorke, R. J. Packer, and J. A. Biegel, "Central nervous system atypical teratoid/rhabdoid tumors of infancy and childhood: definition of an entity," *Journal of Neurosurgery*, vol. 85, no. 1, pp. 56–65, 1996.

[5] P. Kleihues, D. N. Louis, B. W. Scheithauer et al., "The WHO classification of tumors of the nervous system," *Journal of Neuropathology & Experimental Neurology*, vol. 61, no. 3, pp. 215–225, 2002.

[6] J. A. Biegel, J. Y. Zhou, L. B. Rorke, C. Stenstrom, L. M. Wainwright, and B. Fogelgren, "Germ-line and acquired mutations of INI1 in atypical teratoid and rhabdoid tumors," *Cancer Research*, vol. 59, no. 1, pp. 74–79, 1999.

[7] K. Kohashi and Y. Oda, "Oncogenic roles of SMARCB1/INI1 and its deficient tumors," *Cancer Science*, vol. 108, no. 4, pp. 547–552, 2017.

[8] U. Kordes, S. Gesk, M. C. Frühwald et al., "Clinical and molecular features in patients with atypical teratoid rhabdoid tumor or malignant rhabdoid tumor," *Genes, Chromosomes and Cancer*, vol. 49, no. 2, pp. 176–181, 2010.

[9] C. Haberler, U. Laggner, I. Slavc et al., "Immunohistochemical analysis of INI1 protein in malignant pediatric CNS tumors: lack of INI1 in atypical teratoid/rhabdoid tumors and in a fraction of primitive neuroectodermal tumors without rhabdoid phenotype," *The American Journal of Surgical Pathology*, vol. 30, no. 11, pp. 1462–1468, 2006.

[10] A. C. J. Ammerlaan, A. Ararou, M. P. W. A. Houben et al., "Long-term survival and transmission of INI1-mutation via nonpenetrant males in a family with rhabdoid tumour predisposition syndrome," *British Journal of Cancer*, vol. 98, no. 2, pp. 474–479, 2008.

[11] S. N. Chi, M. A. Zimmerman, X. Yao et al., "Intensive multimodality treatment for children with newly diagnosed CNS atypical teratoid rhabdoid tumor," *Journal of Clinical Oncology*, vol. 27, no. 3, pp. 385–389, 2009.

[12] M. A. Zimmerman, L. C. Goumnerova, M. Proctor et al., "Continuous remission of newly diagnosed and relapsed central nervous system atypical teratoid/rhabdoid tumor," *Journal of Neuro-Oncology*, vol. 72, no. 1, pp. 77–84, 2005.

[13] X. J. Ma, D. Li, L. Wang et al., "Overall survival of primary intracranial atypical teratoid rhabdoid tumor following multimodal treatment: a pooled analysis of individual patient data," *Neurosurgical Review*, pp. 1–12, 2018.

[14] I. Slavc, M. Chocholous, U. Leiss et al., "Atypical teratoid rhabdoid tumor: improved long-term survival with an intensive multimodal therapy and delayed radiotherapy. The Medical University of Vienna Experience 1992–2012," *Cancer Medicine*, vol. 3, no. 1, pp. 91–100, 2014.

[15] J. Torchia, D. Picard, L. Lafay-Cousin et al., "Molecular subgroups of atypical teratoid rhabdoid tumours in children: an integrated genomic and clinicopathological analysis," *The Lancet Oncology*, vol. 16, no. 5, pp. 569–582, 2015.

32

Disseminated Blastomycosis Presenting as Oligoarthritis, Pneumonia and Skin Disease in an Immunocompetent Child

Emily Schildt[ID][1] **and Robyn Bockrath**[ID][2]

[1]*Ann & Robert H. Lurie Children's Hospital of Chicago, Chicago, IL, USA*
[2]*Northwestern University Feinberg School of Medicine, Chicago, IL, USA*

Correspondence should be addressed to Emily Schildt; eschildt@luriechildrens.org

Academic Editor: Sathyaprasad Burjonrappa

Blastomyces species (spp) can cause clinical disease affecting nearly every organ system, including the skeletal system. However, isolated joint involvement without concurrent osteomyelitis is rare, especially in children. We present a pediatric case from a tertiary care center in urban Chicago of disseminated blastomycosis caused by *Blastomyces dermatitidis* presenting as oligoarthritis (in the absence of osteomyelitis), pneumonia, and skin involvement, with clinical improvement on IV amphotericin and oral azole treatment.

1. Introduction

Blastomycosis is a rare endemic fungal infection, primarily found in the eastern half of the United States and Canada [1], caused by the dimorphic fungus *Blastomyces* spp. It predominantly affects adults, with only 5–10% of cases occurring in the pediatric population [2, 3]. Blastomycosis typically causes pulmonary disease first, but disseminated extrapulmonary infection can affect nearly every organ [4]. Studies have shown 21–46% of children with blastomycosis develop extrapulmonary symptoms, most classically involving the skin and skeletal systems [2, 3]. Bony involvement typically manifests as osteomyelitis [5, 6]; arthritis is much less commonly associated with *Blastomyces* spp and is thought to occur from direct extension from bone to nearby joints, resulting in septic arthritis [7].

There have been a few case reports and studies describing septic arthritis caused by blastomycosis in adults [8–15]. However, to our knowledge, this is the first reported pediatric case of disseminated blastomycosis presenting as oligoarthritis (without concurrent osteomyelitis) in association with pneumonia and skin disease in an immunocompetent child.

2. Case Presentation

A previously healthy 14-year-old boy was admitted to a hospital in urban Chicago for 24 hours of monitoring due to cough, tachypnea, and intermittent hypoxemia. He had a lobar infiltrate on chest X-ray and was diagnosed with presumed atypical pneumonia and discharged home to complete a 7-day course of amoxicillin and a 5-day course of azithromycin. However, he continued to experience cough and intermittent shortness of breath, even after completion of antibiotic courses.

One week after discharge, he developed stiffness, pain, and swelling of his left knee with difficulty ambulating. He was seen in the Emergency Department after symptoms had been present for approximately 6 days, at which time he had a bedside arthrocentesis performed by orthopedic surgery for presumed septic arthritis of the left knee. Synovial fluid analysis was significant for >200,000 red blood cells/μL and >4,000 white blood cells/μL with neutrophilic predominance, and serum studies revealed leukocytosis and elevated inflammatory markers. Magnetic resonance imaging (MRI) of the left knee was obtained without evidence of osteomyelitis. He was started on empiric antibiotics and admitted to the general pediatrics service. History was pertinent for no

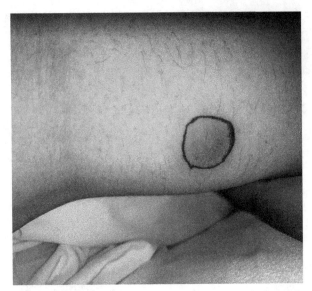

FIGURE 1: Violaceous skin nodule on posterior right lower leg, outlined with surgical marker to track size.

recent travel outside of Chicago, no camping or hiking, and no tick bites.

After admission, the patient developed daily fevers, despite having been reportedly afebrile at home. Bacterial blood cultures were obtained. He was taken to the operating room (OR) for a washout of his knee two days after admission due to persistent fevers, knee swelling, and elevated inflammatory markers. At that time, bacterial, viral, and fungal workup was sent from the synovial fluid. He had no growth from bacterial blood cultures or synovial fluid cultures. Fungal blood culture was not sent, but urine and serum *Histoplasma* and *Blastomyces* spp antibody and antigen testing was obtained.

Urine and serum *Histoplasma* and *Blastomyces* spp antigens resulted as positive, fungal culture from the synovial fluid grew *Blastomyces dermatitidis*, and 18S ribosomal DNA (rDNA) sequencing from the synovial fluid confirmed the presence of *Blastomyces* spp with no evidence of *Histoplasma*. This is indicative of likely cross-reactivity leading to false positive *Histoplasma* result from serum and urine antigen testing. All other studies including potassium hydroxide (KOH) prep, mycobacterium culture, and 16S rDNA sequencing from the synovial fluid were negative.

Of note, this patient's serum *Blastomyces* spp antibody resulted as negative, although in discussion with our infectious disease specialist and review of the literature, lack of antibody positivity is relatively common during acute infection [2].

While awaiting the results of fungal testing, the patient had been continued on empiric antibiotics and was persistently febrile with no improvement in the fever curve. Once the diagnosis was made, he was switched from antibiotics to IV amphotericin for 10 days. He was then transitioned to itraconazole due to acute kidney injury (AKI) attributed to amphotericin. After starting appropriate antifungal therapy, he had gradual improvement in fever curve, knee swelling, and inflammatory markers.

Clinical course was complicated by worsened hypoxemic respiratory distress in the setting of AKI and fluid overload, requiring brief pediatric intensive care unit (PICU) transfer for closer monitoring. Additionally during hospitalization, a 2 cm, raised, violaceous skin nodule on the right leg was identified, thought to be consistent with a blastomycosis skin lesion (Figure 1). No biopsy was performed given its clinical consistency with the patient's diagnosis.

At the time of publication, he is doing well on itraconazole with close outpatient follow-up in the infectious disease clinic and is regaining ambulation and movement of his affected knee with physical therapy.

3. Discussion

In this patient, the combination of recent pneumonia and new onset joint swelling was unusual and prompted a more extensive evaluation to diagnostically connect pulmonary and articular involvement. His inconclusive imaging and laboratory evaluation as well as lack of clinical improvement on antibiotics while awaiting culture and fungal testing results was also concerning and pointed away from a classic bacterial septic arthritis. The development of a nodular skin lesion further raised suspicion for a systemic fungal etiology. Of note, 18S and 16S rDNA gene sequencing studies were sent as part of our workup to evaluate more closely for fungal and bacterial identification, respectively, as our culture came from a patient pretreated with antibiotic therapy.

Blastomycosis is more common in immunocompromised patients, with one review of adult patients showing that only 12% of patients with blastomycosis were immunocompetent [16]. Interestingly, while studies have shown that immunocompromised patients are at higher risk for severe disease, they have similar rates of dissemination as immunocompetent patients [16, 17].

There are only a few isolated reported cases of septic arthritis as the presenting symptom of blastomycosis in children [18, 19], but this is typically in the setting of concurrent osteomyelitis due to the proposed mechanism of joint involvement being secondary to direct bony spread from an affected limb [7]. One case series described 7 children with disseminated blastomycosis causing osteomyelitis with extension to the joint [20], but none of these children had isolated arthritis. Therefore, our patient's presentation of oligoarthritis without osteomyelitis is very unusual and has not been reported in the literature surrounding blastomycosis in children.

Treatment guidelines for blastomycosis in children generally recommend amphotericin B for one to two weeks, following by 6–12 months of itraconazole therapy, with 12 months recommended for patients with osteoarticular disease like the patient we have described. Itraconazole dosing is then adjusted based on serum trough measurements to ensure adequate drug levels. Patients with central nervous system involvement may require longer courses of amphotericin B, followed by treatment with an azole for at least 12 months [21].

Although fungal infections are generally rare in the pediatric population, especially in immunocompetent children, it is important to have a high level of suspicion for the evaluation of fungal etiologies such as *Blastomyces* spp when practicing in an endemic area (such as the case for our patient, who lives in a state adjacent to the Great Lakes which has a relatively high incidence of *Blastomyces* spp [21]) or treating patients who have traveled to an area with fungal pathogens. Blastomycosis can be associated with significant morbidity and mortality, particularly when the diagnosis is delayed [2], highlighting the importance of maintaining a broad differential diagnosis, particularly when a patient does not demonstrate clinical improvement with appropriate antibiotic therapy or when multiple organ systems are involved.

Acknowledgments

The authors acknowledge Dr. Tina Tan and Dr. Alexander Newman for their infectious diseases consultation and expertise

References

[1] https://www.cdc.gov/fungal/diseases/blastomycosis/causes.html.

[2] E. J. Anderson, P. B. Ahn, R. Yogev, P. Jaggi, D. B. Shippee, and S. T. Shulman, "Blastomycosis in children: a study of 14 cases," *Journal of the Pediatric Infectious Diseases Society*, vol. 2, no. 4, pp. 386–390, 2013.

[3] H. M. Frost, J. Anderson, L. Ivacic, and J. Meece, "Blastomycosis in children: an analysis of clinical, epidemiologic, and genetic features," *Journal of the Pediatric Infectious Diseases Society*, vol. 6, no. 1, pp. 49–56, 2017.

[4] C. G. Castillo, C. A. Kauffman, and M. H. Miceli, "Blastomycosis," *Infectious Disease Clinics of North America*, vol. 30, no. 1, pp. 247–264.

[5] R. Jain, K. Singh, I. Lamzabi, A. Harbhajanka, P. Gattuso, and V. B. Reddy, "Blastomycosis of bone," *American Journal of Clinical Pathology*, vol. 142, no. 5, pp. 609–616, 2014.

[6] M. Codifava, A. Guerra, G. Rossi, P. Paolucci, and L. Iughetti, "Unusual osseous presentation of blastomycosis in an immigrant child: a challenge for European pediatricians," *Italian Journal of Pediatrics*, vol. 38, no. 1, p. 69, 2012.

[7] J. A. McBride, G. M. Gauthier, and B. S. Klein, "Clinical manifestations and treatment of blastomycosis," *Clinics in Chest Medicine*, vol. 38, no. 3, pp. 435–449, 2017.

[8] T. Vindenes, B. J. Gardiner, N. Nierenberg, and G. Volpe, "Pneumonia, septic arthritis, and brain abscesses in a construction worker," *Clinical Infectious Diseases*, vol. 60, no. 11, pp. 1722-1723, 2015.

[9] J. Yocum and D. Seligson, "Blastomycosis of the knee and skull after arthroscopy," *The American Journal of Sports Medicine*, vol. 19, no. 6, pp. 670–672, 1991.

[10] M. E. Robert and C. A. Kauffman, "Blastomycosis presenting as polyarticular septic arthritis," *Journal of Rheumatology*, vol. 15, no. 9, pp. 1438–1442, 1988.

[11] R. P. Maioriello and C. F. Merwin, "North American blastomycosis presenting as an acute panniculitis and arthritis," *Archives of Dermatology*, vol. 102, no. 1, pp. 92–96, 1970.

[12] A. L. George Jr., J. T. Hays, and B. S. Graham, "Blastomycosis presenting as monarticular arthritis," *The Role of Synovial Fluid Cytology. Arthritis & Rheumatism*, vol. 28, no. 5, pp. 516–521, 1985.

[13] A. Abril, M. D. Campbell, V. R. Cotten Jr., J. M. Steckleberg,

R. A. El-Azhary, and J. D. O'Duffy, "Polyarticular blastomycotic arthritis," *Journal of Rheumatology*, vol. 25, no. 5, pp. 1019–1021, 1998.

[14] M. Oppenheimer, J. M. Embil, B. Black et al., "Blastomycosis of bones and joints," *Southern Medical Journal*, vol. 100, no. 6, pp. 570–578, 2007.

[15] F. F. Fountain, "Acute blastomycotic arthritis," *Archives of Internal Medicine*, vol. 132, no. 5, pp. 684–688, 1973.

[16] J. A. McBride, K. S. Alana, E. Matkovic, T. B. Aimee, S. N. Gibbons-Burgener, and G. M. Gauthier, "Clinical manifestations and outcomes in immunocompetent and immunocompromised patients with blastomycosis," *Clinical Infectious Diseases*, vol. 72, no. 9, pp. 1594–1602, 2020.

[17] C. Perez, "Blastomycosis in immunocompetent and immunocompromised populations: a single center retrospective analysis between 2002 and 2014," *Open Forum Infectious Diseases*, vol. 3, no. suppl_1, 2016.

[18] A. J. Head, L. K. Myers, J. D. Thompson, S. C. Buckingham, and R. B. Skinner Jr., "Disseminated blastomycosis presenting as oligoarticular septic arthritis in a 12-year-old girl," *Arthritis & Rheumatism*, vol. 53, no. 1, pp. 138–141, 2005.

[19] P. B. MacDonald, G. B. Black, and R. MacKenzie, "Orthopaedic manifestations of blastomycosis," *The Journal of Bone and Joint Surgery*, vol. 72, no. 6, pp. 860–864, 1990.

[20] R. R. Johnson and S. S. Vora, "Blastomycotic multifocal arthritis and osteomyelitis in the urban setting," *Journal of Rheumatology*, vol. 40, no. 9, pp. 1627–1629, 2013.

[21] American Academy of Pediatrics, "Blastomycosis," in *Red Book: 2018 Report of the Committee on Infectious Diseases*, D. W. Kimberlin, M. T. Brady, M. A. Jackson, and S. S. Long, Eds., pp. 249–251, American Academy of Pediatrics, Itasca, IL, USA, 2018.

33

Neonatal Chylothoraces: A 10-Year Experience in a Tertiary Neonatal Referral Centre

Marie K. White [ID],[1] **Ravindra Bhat,**[1,2] **and Anne Greenough** [ID][1,2,3,4]

[1]*Neonatal Intensive Care Centre, Kings College Hospital NHS Foundation Trust, Denmark Hill, London SE5 9RS, UK*
[2]*Department of Women and Children's Health, School of Life Course Sciences, Faculty of Life Sciences and Medicine, King's College London, London SE5 9RS, UK*
[3]*Asthma UK Centre for Allergic Mechanisms in Asthma, King's College London, London SE5 9RS, UK*
[4]*NIHR Biomedical Research Centre at Guy's and St. Thomas' NHS Foundation Trust and King's College London, Guy's Hospital, Great Maze Pond, London SE1 9RT, UK*

Correspondence should be addressed to Anne Greenough; anne.greenough@kcl.ac.uk

Academic Editor: Atul Malhotra

Background. Neonatal chylothorax is a rare condition, but has a high mortality. *Study Objectives.* To analyse the outcomes of a series of neonates with chylothorax and review the literature to determine best practice. *Design.* A case series review and a literature review using electronic databases including the key words neonates and chylothorax. *Results.* Six cases of neonatal chylothorax were identified during a ten-year period, two had congenital chylothoraces and four iatrogenic chylothoraces after thoracic surgery or chest instrumentation. The neonates were ventilated for a median of 30 (range 13–125) days with a median maximum daily pleural fluid output of 218 (range 86–310) ml/kg/day. All the neonates were given medium-chain triglyceride (MCT) feeds which stabilised pleural fluid output in four and reduced it in another. Octreotide was used in three neonates, but the dosage used had no significant effect on pleural output. Two neonates required surgical intervention. The literature review demonstrated MCT feeds can reduce or stabilise pleural fluid output, but highlighted variable use of octreotide and inconsistent dosing regimens and outcomes. No consensus regarding indications for surgical intervention was identified. *Summary and Conclusion.* Neonatal chylothorax is uncommon, but affected neonates require high healthcare utilisation.

1. Introduction

Neonatal chylothorax is a rare condition with an incidence of 1 in 5775 [1] to 24000 [2] and has a high mortality rate of up to 64% [2]. Neonatal chylothorax can be congenital or acquired, the latter most commonly occurs after damage to the thoracic duct during surgery [3]. We have reviewed our experience in a tertiary neonatal surgical unit and set this in the context of a literature review to establish if it was possible to determine best practice.

2. Case Series

2.1. Method. A retrospective study was undertaken to determine the outcomes of all neonates with neonatal chylothoraces admitted to a tertiary medical and surgical neonatal intensive care unit in London, UK, from July 2008 to July 2018. Neonates were identified through the hospital clinical coding and an electronic database (BadgerNet). The diagnosis of a neonatal chylothorax was made if the pleural fluid had a cell count of >1000/ml with a lymphocyte predominance and if the triglyceride level was greater than 1.1 mmol/L in a neonate who was being fed [4]. Initial treatment for our cohort included stabilisation, ventilatory support, and replacement of pleural fluid losses. Specific treatment included medium-chain triglyceride (MCT) feeds, and then octreotide if the pleural fluid output continued, followed by surgical intervention if those interventions failed.

A literature review was undertaken using electronic databases including the key words neonates and chylothorax.

TABLE 1: Perinatal and neonatal characteristics, management, and outcomes.

Neonate	Birth weight (g)	Gestation (weeks)	Antenatal	Mode of delivery	Resuscitation	Diagnoses	MCT feeds	Octreotide and dose	Ventilation (days)	Outcome
1	3080	39	Normal	VD	Thick meconium intubated at 10 minutes	Acquired NC, MAS, multiple pneumothoraces	Yes	No	38	Alive
2	2252	33	Hydrops, bilateral effusions, antenatal shunts	VD	Pleural shunts clamped & intubated at birth	Congenital NC	Yes	Yes (2–8 mcg/kg/hr)	31	Alive
3	4078	38	Left pleural effusion & mediastinal shift	CS	Intubated at birth	Congenital NC	Yes	No	28	Alive
4	2790	37	Left CDH	VD	Intubated at birth	Acquired NC, CDH	Yes	Yes** (1–4 mcg/kg/hr)	125	Died
5	2690	38	Polyhydramnios	VD	No resuscitation	Acquired NC, OA, TOF	Yes	Yes** (1–2 mcg/kg/hr)	13	Alive
6	3350	37	Polyhydramnios	VD	No resuscitation	Acquired NC, OA, TOF	Yes*	No	19	Alive

CDH: congenital diaphragmatic hernia; CS: caesarian section; MAS: meconium aspiration syndrome; MCT: medium-chain triglycerides; NC: neonatal chylothorax; OA: oesophageal atresia; TOF tracheoesophageal fistula; VD: vaginal delivery; *neonate had a reduction in pleural output following introduction of MCT feeds; **octreotide was given prior to surgical intervention.

2.2. Results. There were 54,488 births in the study period, and six neonates were diagnosed with chylothorax, giving a local overall incidence of 1 in 9081 births. The six neonates had a median gestation of $37 + 6$ (range $33 + 5$ to $39 + 6$) weeks and a median birth weight of 2935 (range 2252–4078) grams (Table 1). All neonates had a "lymphocytic" effusion, and three had a raised pleural fluid triglyceride of 2.2 (range 1.7–3.2) mmol/L. Two neonates had genetic variants of unknown significance and one, with subtle dysmorphic features, had a benign copy variant of paternal inheritance.

Four neonates required intubation in the delivery suite, and all required an extended period of mechanical ventilation with a median duration of 30 (range 13–125) days (Table 1). Two neonates required high-frequency oscillation ventilation and inhaled nitric oxide. Five neonates were successfully extubated and self-ventilating in air by a median of 37 (range 30–78) days. The neonates required a median of five (range 2–6) chest drains for a median duration of 36 (range 28–99) days. The median maximum total daily pleural fluid output was 218 (range 86–310) ml/kg/day. The majority of pleural drain losses were replaced by human albumin solution (HAS) or occasionally by 0.9% saline or fresh frozen plasma (FFP).

All the neonates required total parental nutrition and were commenced on MCT feeds after diagnosis. Five achieved full MCT feeds at a median of 37 (range 11–44) days of age. One neonate had resolution of the chylothorax following introduction of MCT feeds. In four neonates, MCT feeds were associated with stabilisation of the pleural fluid output. Two neonates were graded back to either a standard neonatal formula or maternal expressed breast milk, and three were discharged on MCT feeds. One neonate had increased pleural fluid output after the introduction of MCT feeds which were subsequently stopped and the neonate remained on total parental nutrition until reorientation of care.

Three neonates were treated with a continuous octreotide intravenous infusion for a median of seven (range 6–16) days with a starting dose of 1-2 micrograms/kg/hr to a maximum of 2-8 micrograms/kg/hr. One neonate developed transient hypothyroidism and, therefore, remained on low-dose octreotide at 2 micrograms/kg/hr, which was stopped after thoracic duct ligation. Octreotide was stopped in the other two neonates as there was no reduction in pleural fluid output. Two neonates with acquired chylothorax required operative intervention. One had a successful thoracic duct ligation and one had bilateral pleurodesis, but this failed to improve the neonate's outcome. Five neonates survived, and the total length of stay until discharge or death was a median of 68 (range 44–127) days.

3. Discussion

Neonatal congenital chylothorax is a rare condition as evidenced by an incidence of 1 in 27,244 in our cohort, which is in keeping with another study (1 in 24,000 [2]). Our mortality (17%) is in accordance with other studies [1, 2, 12]. Up to 50% of neonates with neonatal chylothorax can be associated with genetic syndromes [1, 14]. In our cohort, although two neonates had genetic variants, none were found to have a defined syndrome.

In our cohort, only one neonate had a reduction in pleural fluid output following the introduction of MCT feeds, but in others the output was stabilised. MCT feeds

TABLE 2: Case series of neonatal chylothorax.

Author and year	Number of neonates	Ventilation (days)	Number given MCT feeds	Number treated with octreotide and dose	Octreotide duration (days)	Octreotide efficacy	Pleurodesis or thoracic duct ligation
Altuncu et al. (2007) [5]	3	N/R	$n = 3$	$n = 1$ (1–10 mcg/kg/hr)	28	No response	$n = 1$
Matsukuma et al. (2009) [6]	2	N/R	$n = 2$	$n = 2$ (0.5–10 mcg/kg/hr)	16–20	No response	$n = 2$
Bellini et al. (2012) [7]	30	30	$n = 28$	$n = 6$ (1–10 mcg/kg/hr)	8–38	Decreased chylous production, but not quantified	$n = 1$
Horvers et al. (2012) [8]	7	16	$n = 7$	$n = 7$ (2–12 mcg/hr)	Median 22 (11–46)	Possible response in two neonates	$n = 0$
Shah and Sinn (2012) [9]	6	30	$n = 6$	$n = 6$ (0.5–10 mcg/kg/hr)	Median 20 (4–41)	Resolution in five neonates	$n = 0$
Downie et al. (2013) [1]	10	8	$n = 7$	$n = 3$ (3.5–10 mcg/kg/hr)	N/R	Response in two neonates: not quantified	$n = 0$
Landis et al. (2013) [10]	11	11	N/R	$n = 6$ (1–13 mcg/kg/hr)	N/R	No response	$n = 0$
Bialkowski et al. (2015) [2]	28	23	$n = 25$	$n = 7$ (3–10 mcg/kg/hr)	Median 21 (10–45)	No response	$n = 0$
Hua et al. (2016) [11]	4	1	N/R	$n = 3$ (N/A)	14	No response	$n = 4$
Yin et al. (2017) [12]	14	13	$n = 12$	$n = 3$ (1–6 mcg/kg/hr)	Median 6	Average drain output significantly lower: three days after treatment. Median 62 ml versus 133 ml ($p = 0.002$)	$n = 0$
Shillitoe et al. (2018) [13]	21	N/R	$n = 2$	$n = 1$ (maximum dose 10 mcg/kg/hr)	N/R	On the maximum dose there was a 50% reduction in five days	$n = 0$
Zaki et al. (2018) [14]	9	N/R	$n = 9$	$n = 9$ (1–10 mcg/kg/hr)	5–66	Resolution in three neonates: not quantified	$n = 0$

N/R: not reported.

have been shown to be effective in reducing lymphatic flow in 25% of neonates with surgically related neonatal chylothorax [15]. Indeed, our literature review (Table 2) demonstrated that the majority of neonates who have a neonatal chylothorax receive MCT feeds.

A systematic review in which the efficacy of octreotide, a somatostatin analogue, was assessed did not recommend its use [4]. Our literature review demonstrated since then multiple case series in which octreotide was used have been published with variable dosing regimens, length of treatment, and outcomes and that octreotide was not used in all neonates (Table 2) [1, 2, 7–14]. A recent systematic review [3] found octreotide to be effective in 47% of neonates with neonatal chylothorax. Many of the papers included, however, did not describe what constituted a clinical improvement or the timescale over which any changes occurred. In our cohort, there was no significant improvement in the pleural fluid output in the three neonates treated with octreotide. None of these neonates reached the dose of 10 micrograms/kg/hr which some studies have used. Multiple side effects have been reported in up to 14% neonates treated with octreotide including hyperglycaemia, necrotising enterocolitis, transient mild cholestasis, transient hypothyroidism, pulmonary hypertension, and severe hypotension [3]. In our cohort, one neonate developed transient hypothyroidism.

The literature review (Table 2) demonstrated only a minority of neonates required either pleurodesis or thoracic duct ligation. This is consistent with the findings of our cohort. A review of a case series of neonatal "surgical" chylothoraces mainly following congenital diaphragmatic hernia repair also demonstrated conservative management was successful in the majority [15]. It would be important to develop evidence-based guidelines as to when such interventions should be used.

4. Conclusions

Our results highlight neonatal chylothorax is an uncommon condition, but is associated with high healthcare utilisation. Neonates require stabilisation with ventilation, pleural drainage, and fluid replacement. MCT feeds can reduce and stabilise pleural fluid output. It is important to optimise the dose of octreotide and monitor for side effects. Multicentre trials are required to identify the optimum evidenced-based management for neonatal chylothorax. Although neonatal chylothorax is an uncommon condition, we believe that multicentre trials would be feasible as shown by the randomised trial of respiratory support in neonates with congenital diaphragmatic hernia [16].

Disclosure

The views expressed are those of the authors and not necessarily those of the NHS, the NIHR, or the Department of Health.

Acknowledgments

This research was supported by the National Institute for Health Research (NIHR) Biomedical Research Centre at Guy's and St Thomas' NHS Foundation Trust and King's College London.

References

[1] L. Downie, A. Sasi, and A. Malhotra, "Congenital chylothorax: associations and neonatal outcomes," *Journal of Paediatrics and Child Health*, vol. 50, no. 3, pp. 234–238, 2014.

[2] A. Bialkowski, C. F. Poets, and A. R. Franz, "Congenital chylothorax: a prospective nationwide epidemiological study in Germany," *Archives of Disease in Childhood Fetal Neonatal Edition*, vol. 100, no. 2, pp. F169–F172, 2015.

[3] C. Bellini, R. Cabano, L. C. De Angelis et al., "Octreotide for congenital and acquired chylothorax in newborns: a systematic review," *Journal of Paediatrics and Child Health*, vol. 54, no. 8, pp. 840–847, 2018.

[4] A. Das and P. S. Shah, "Octreotide of the treatment of chylothorax in neonates," *Cochrane Database of Systematic Reviews*, vol. 9, no. 8, article CD006388, 2010.

[5] E. Altuncu, İ. Akman, G. Kıyan et al., "Report of three cases: congenital chylothorax and treatment modalities," *Turkish Journal of Pediatrics*, vol. 49, no. 4, pp. 418–421, 2007.

[6] E. Matsukuma, Y. Aoki, M. Sakai et al., "Treatment with OK-432 for persistent congenital chylothorax in newborn infants resistant to octreotide," *Journal of Pediatric Surgery*, vol. 44, no. 3, pp. E37–E39, 2009.

[7] C. Bellini, Z. Ergaz, M. Radicioni et al., "Congenital fetal and neonatal visceral chylous effusions: neonatal chylothorax and chylous ascites revisited: a multicenter retrospective study," *Lymphology*, vol. 45, no. 3, pp. 91–102, 2012.

[8] M. Horvers, C. F. Mooij, and T. A. J. Antonius, "Is octreotide treatment useful in patients with congenital chylothorax," *Neonatology*, vol. 101, no. 3, pp. 225–231, 2012.

[9] D. Shah and J. K. Sinn, "Octreotide as therapeutic option for congenital idiopathic chylothorax: a case series," *Acta Paediatrica*, vol. 101, no. 4, pp. e151–e155, 2012.

[10] M. W. Landis, D. Butler, F. Y. Lim et al., "Octreotide for chylous effusions in congenital diaphragmatic hernia," *Journal of Pediatric Surgery*, vol. 48, no. 11, pp. 2226–2229, 2013.

[11] Q.-W. Hua, Z.-Y. Lin, X.-T. Hu, and Q.-F. Zhao, "Treatment of persistent congenital chylothorax with intrapleural injection of sapylin in infants," *Pakistan Journal of Medical Science*, vol. 32, no. 5, pp. 1305–1308, 2016.

[12] R. Yin, R. Zhang, J. Wang et al., "Effects of somatostatin/octreotide treatment in neonates with congenital chylothorax," *Medicine*, vol. 96, no. 29, article e7594, 2017.

[13] B. M. J. Shillitoe, J. Berrington, and N. Athiraman, "Congenital pleural effusions: 15 years single-centre experience from North-East England," *Journal of Maternal-Fetal & Neonatal Medicine*, vol. 31, no. 15, pp. 2086–2089, 2018.

[14] S. A. Zaki, M. H. Krishnamurthy, and A. Malhotra, "Octreotide use in neonates: a case series," *Drugs in R&D*, vol. 18, no. 3, pp. 191–198, 2018.

[15] K. M. Costa and A. K. Saxena, "Surgical chylothorax in neonates: management and outcomes," *World Journal of Pediatrics*, vol. 14, no. 2, pp. 110–115, 2018.

[16] K. G. Snoek, I. Capolupo, J. van Rosmalen et al., "Conventional mechanical ventilation versus high-frequency oscillatory ventilation for congenital diaphragmatic hernia," *Annals of Surgery*, vol. 263, no. 5, pp. 867–874, 2016.

34

Late Treatment and Recurrence of Kawasaki Disease in a Moroccan Infant

R. Elqadiry ⓘ, **O. Louachama, N. Rada, G. Draiss, and M. Bouskraoui**

Pediatric A Department, Mother-Child Pole, Mohammed VI University Hospital, Marrakesh, Morocco

Correspondence should be addressed to R. Elqadiry; rabiy.elqadiry@gmail.com

Academic Editor: Yusuke Shiozawa

Introduction. While the diagnosis of typical form of Kawasaki disease (KD) is obvious, this multifaceted disease continues to surprise us. We report the case of a recurrent Kawasaki disease in an infant. *Case.* At the age of 13 months, the infant was diagnosed with complete Kawasaki disease; he presented with prolonged fever, bilateral conjunctivitis, enanthem, exanthema, edema of the lower limb, peeling, and biological inflammatory syndrome. He was treated with intravenous immunoglobulin (IVIG) associated with a high dose of aspirin and then an antiplatelet dose with a good clinical-biological evolution. The echocardiography was normal. Seven months later, the patient was again admitted, in a similar picture: a prolonged fever evolving for 7 days, bilateral conjunctivitis, enanthem, cervical adenopathy of 1.5 cm/1 cm, scarlatiniform erythema, pruriginous of the trunk and limb, and peeling of the toes, with indurated edema of the hands and feet. The rest of the examination was normal except the irritability. The diagnosis of recurrent KD was made according the five criteria of the American Heart Association. The echocardiography was normal again. The infant received IVIG with good outcome. *Conclusion.* Despite its rarity, the possibility of recurrence of KD should be known by clinicians, so as not to delay the specific management of vasculitis whose stakes in terms of prevention of coronary artery lesions are well known. Our case confirms the possibility of this recurrence.

1. Introduction

Kawasaki disease (KD) is an acute multisystemic vasculitis that affects young children and infants with predilection. After its first description in Japan, Kawasaki disease (KD) has been reported worldwide. Its incidence is variable from one country to another, and its severity was attributed from the outset, in the absence of diagnosis and treatment, to cardiovascular complications, mainly coronary.

The recurrence of KD is frequently reported in Japan and the USA, respectively, in 3-4% and 0.8% of cases [1], but it is rarely reported in Morocco.

We report a case of recurrent KD in its complete form and make through this observation a brief review of the literature.

2. Case

We report the case of a 20-month-old infant, whose parents are no consanguineous, the youngest of three siblings. Seven months ago, the diagnosis of complete form of KD was made because he presented with prolonged fever, bilateral conjunctivitis, enanthem, exanthema, edema of the lower limbs, and peelings and a biological inflammatory syndrome. The patient was treated with IVIG and acetylsalicylic acid with good outcome and no coronary abnormalities in echocardiography.

The infant was again admitted, 7 months later, in a similar picture: he had a fever at 39–40°C, persisting and resistant to the antipyretic drugs evolving for seven days, associated with a generalized scarlatiniform rash. The patient was initially treated in ambulatory with 3rd generation cephalosporin and macrolide antibiotics without improvement and then referred to our department for further management.

Physical examination revealed an irritable infant, febrile with temperature at 39°C, icterus, bilateral nonpurulent conjunctivitis, bleeding cheilitis with "strawberry tongue," scarlatiniform erythema, and pruriginous in the trunk and limbs associated with indurated edema of the hands and feet with peelings of the toes (Figure 1). Otherwise, examination of the lymph nodes noted noninflammatory cervical lymphadenopathy measuring 1.5 cm/1 cm.

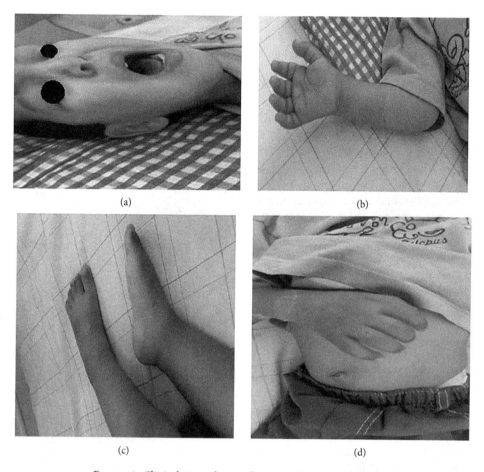

FIGURE 1: Clinical signs that made it possible to confirm KD.

Biological investigations showed an elevated leukocyte count with 20 100/mm^3, with a predominance of neutrophils at 11,000/mm^3 and thrombocytes at 7,61,000/mm^3, elevated CRP at 104 mg/l, elevated SV at 86 mm at the first hour, and moderate elevations in serum transaminases (SGPT at 125 UI/l and SGOT at 80 UI/l). Urinanalysis revealed an aseptic leucocyturia, and the blood cultures were sterile.

The patient was treated with IVIG, 2 g/kg in a single infusion, together with high doses of aspirin (80 mg/kg/d) related by antiplatelet doses (3 mg/kg/d) after resolution of the inflammatory syndrome (in 4 weeks), according to the recommendations of the literature.

The infant has been afebrile after 48 hours of IVIG treatment, and the evolution was favorable, with regression of conjunctivitis and cutaneous signs and progression of CRP from 104 mg/l to 6 mg/l, and echocardiographic control was still normal.

3. Discussion

So many words express the many faces of Kawasaki. Since its first description in Japan, several hypotheses have been advanced, but no etiological factor has been identified.

The diagnosis of this lymphadeno-mucocutaneous syndrome, based on clinical criteria, can only be retained after excluding the other differential diagnosis [2].

Furthermore, the differential diagnosis of KD includes viral infections (measles, adenovirus, rubella, and mononucleosis) that present acute oropharyngitis, fever, and cervical lymphadenopathy, but with fewer systemic inflammatory signs and no involvement of the extremities. Of the same, the systemic juvenile idiopathic arthritis can mimic KD, but the absence of joint involvement after prolonged follow-up has excluded it in our patient. The patient had normal hemodynamic parameters, excluding streptococcal toxic shock. Furthermore, no improvement of symptomatology with 3rd generation cephalosporin and macrolide excludes in our patient the possibility of scarlet fever and rickettsioses [3]. The diagnosis of recurrent KD was then retained and reinforced by the very high inflammatory syndrome. The good response of the two episodes to immunoglobulin infusion also reinforced our diagnosis.

The recurrence of KD is defined by the reappearance of symptoms two months after the first episode [4]. A Japanese study has tried to identify risk factors for this recurrence: age less than 2 years, prolonged fever over 10 days, anemia, high levels of transaminases, and coronary lesion during the first episode [5]. During the first episode, our patient had a prolonged fever because of the infusion delay of 18-day immunoglobulins. Outside of the young age, none of the other criteria were found. However, mucocutaneous jaundice was observed with cytolysis during the second episode.

The cases of KD recurrence are rare in Europe; on the contrary, the relapses were reported in Japan, China, Taiwan, Korea, and the United States at rates of 3%, 3.5%, 1.82%, 1.5%, and 0.8%, respectively. The disease appears to recur more frequently in the first two years after diagnosis, with the highest rates seen in children between 1 and 2 years of age, as in our patient [4].

4. Conclusion

The rarity of recurrence of KD and atypical clinical presentation made diagnosis difficult, but currently, any clinicians should know it. The major challenge of KD is diagnosing and treating it before irreversible coronary damage appears.

The recurrence of KD is possible, so the pediatricians should know it.

References

[1] H.-m. Yang, Z.-D. Du, and P.-p. Fu, "Clinical features of recurrent Kawasaki disease and its risk factors," *European Journal of Pediatrics*, vol. 172, no. 12, pp. 1641–1647, 2013.

[2] N. M. Osman, "Recurrent Kawasaki disease resistant to initial treatment with intravenous immunoglobulin," *Sudanese Journal of Paediatrics*, vol. 12, no. 2, pp. 65–69, 2012.

[3] P. Verma, N. Agarwal, and M. Maheshwari, "Recurrent Kawasaki disease," *Indian Pediatrics*, vol. 52, no. 2, pp. 152–154, 2015.

[4] C. Tissandier, M. Lang, J. R. Lusson, B. Bœuf, E. Merlin, and C. Dauphin, "Kawasaki shock syndrome complicating a recurrence of Kawasaki disease," *Pediatrics*, vol. 134, no. 6, pp. e1695–e1699, 2014.

[5] S. Hirata, Y. Nakamura, and H. Yanagawa, "Incidence rate of recurrent Kawasaki disease and related risk factors: from the results of nationwide surveys of Kawasaki disease in Japan," *Acta Paediatrica*, vol. 90, no. 1, pp. 40–44, 2001.

35

Severe Cardiorespiratory and Neurologic Symptoms in a Neonate due to Mepivacaine Intoxication

Maurike de Groot-van der Mooren ⓘ,[1] **Sabine Quint,**[1] **Ingmar Knobbe,**[2] **Doug Cronie,**[3] **and Mirjam van Weissenbruch**[1]

[1]*Department of Neonatology, Emma Children's Hospital and VU University Medical Center, Boelelaan 1117, Amsterdam 1081 HV, Netherlands*
[2]*Department of Pediatric Cardiology, Emma Children's Hospital and VU University Medical Center, Boelelaan 1117, Amsterdam 1081 HV, Netherlands*
[3]*Department of Obstetrics and Gynaecology, Onze Lieve Vrouwe Gasthuis, Jan Tooropstraat 164, Amsterdam 1061 AE, Netherlands*

Correspondence should be addressed to Maurike de Groot-van der Mooren; md.degroot@amsterdamumc.nl

Academic Editor: Maria Moschovi

Local anesthesia with mepivacaine is used for vaginal deliveries and for minor surgeries of the vagina and perineum as repair of an episiotomy or perineal laceration. Neonatal intoxication caused by local anesthesia with mepivacaine for maternal episiotomy has been rarely reported. We present a case of a term female infant with unexplained cardiorespiratory distress and several neurologic findings, including seizures, one hour after birth. Electrocardiogram showed a second-degree atrioventricular block and a left-bundle branch block. Blood measures in the patient revealed a high mepivacaine level following local anesthesia for maternal episiotomy. Because of the increasing practice of local anesthesia, high awareness for neonatal intoxication and further research in safe elimination therapy in neonates is needed.

1. Introduction

Local anesthetics with mepivacaine are used for vaginal deliveries and for minor surgeries of the vagina and perineum as repair of an episiotomy or perineal laceration [1]. Neonatal complications are uncommon. We here present a newborn with sudden respiratory, neurologic, and cardiac signs, shortly after birth, following maternal episiotomy after perineal nerve block with mepivacaine 100 milligrams (mg) per milliliter (ml) (10 mg/ml, 10 ml) during labor.

2. Case Presentation

A term female infant who was born in a referral hospital was transferred to our neonatal intensive care unit (NICU) after unexpected signs of hypothermia (35. 3°C) and an episode of recurrent apnea, irregular respiration, bradycardia, signs of hypotonia, and suspected convulsions one hour after birth.

In the mother, a healthy 27-year-old primigravida, labor was induced at 38 weeks and 3 days, because of suspicion of intrauterine growth restriction. During 34 weeks, pregnancy abdominal circumference (AC) was at the 37th percentile (p37) and estimated fetal weight (EFW) at the p18. At 35 weeks, pregnancy AC was at the p17 and EFW at the p11. Besides the fetal growth restriction, no other abnormal findings were found during pregnancy. The mother had a remarkable short stature, 149 centimeters (cm), and weighed less than 45 kilograms (kg) but was healthy. Family anamnesis revealed no neurological or cardiac diseases. There was no history of maternal medication use or drugs abuse during pregnancy. There were no risk factors for infection during pregnancy and birth.

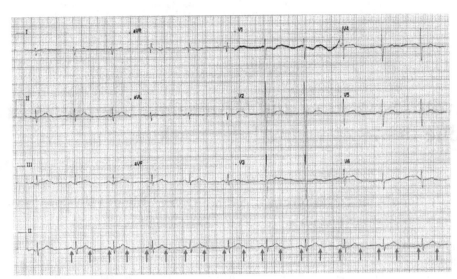

FIGURE 1: ECG during bradycardia showed a second-degree AV block with an atrial frequency of 130/min and a ventricular frequency of 65/min. QRS 76 ms; QTc 590 ms. Red arrows are pointed towards the P-waves, at times hidden in the T-waves. Settings 25 mm/s; 10 mm/mV.

The mother underwent episiotomy after perineal nerve block with 100 mg of mepivacaine (10 ml, 10 mg/ml), about twenty minutes before delivery. External intrapartum fetal monitoring showed no signs of fetal distress. The time interval between delivery and cord clamping was five minutes. Umbilical-cord blood gas analysis was normal.

A girl was born with Apgar scores 9 and 10 after 1 and 5 minutes, respectively. She had a birthweight of 2854 grams (p20), a birth length of 50 cm (p67), and a head circumference of 33 cm (p23), all in normal range. Breastfeeding was initiated immediately. Because of the clinical deterioration one hour after birth, the newborn was first admitted to the neonatology ward of the referral hospital. During the episodes of apneas, fasciculation of the tongue, tremor of the lips, and smacking movements of the mouth were noticed. Extremities were put in flexion, with pointed toes, hands in fists, and pupillary mydriasis fixed to light. Before the apnea, a short crying was observed. In between these seizures, she was hypotonic but normal neonatal reflexes could be provoked. Venous access was difficult to obtain, so an umbilical venous catheter was inserted and phenobarbital 20 mg/kg was given intravenously. One and a half hours after birth, there was a sudden decrease in the heart rate of 80–90 beats/minute. Atropine was given but had no effect on the heart rate. The blood pressure and body temperature were stable and in normal range.

Based on the above findings, she was intubated and thereafter transferred to our NICU. Physical examination showed an encephalopathic, nonresponsive neonate on the ventilator, with bradycardia of 65 beats/minute and well saturated. Neurological examination showed a decorticated posture, hypotonia and pupillary mydriasis fixed to light, without brainstem reflexes.

Laboratory tests showed normal glucose, blood cell count, electrolytes, and kidney function. In addition, bilirubin 64 micromol per liter (μmol/L), creatinine kinase 854 units per liter (U/L), and lactate 1.5 millimol per liter (mmol/L) were normal. ALT was raised (435 U/L), AST and

gamma GT were hemolytic, and ammoniac was slightly elevated to 120 μmol/L, however, normalized to 64 μmol/L 5 hours after birth. A low level of C-reactive protein was found (3 milligrams per liter (mg/L)).

Brain monitoring using 2-channel amplitude-integrated EEG (aEEG) showed a status epilepticus and again she was treated with phenobarbital 10 mg/kg intravenously. The bradycardia recovered after administering phenobarbital suggesting the bradycardia was related to convulsions.

Some hours later and during local transportation to the radiology department to undergo a magnetic resonance imaging (MRI) of the brain, again a bradycardia was present. aEEG at that time could not be registered. Because bradycardia was thought to be a symptom of a convulsion, a third phenobarbital dose was administered intravenously (10 mg/kg). However, it did not show any effect on the heart rhythm. Evaluation of the electrocardiogram (ECG) showed a second-degree atrioventricular (AV) block (Figure 1).

Figure 2 shows the heart rate over time with a sudden decline in the heart rate and sudden recovery from 2 : 1 AV conduction to normal AV conduction. A 21-channel video EEG at that time showed no epileptic activity, suggesting bradycardia was not related to convulsions. A few hours later, bradycardia resolved spontaneously and ECG showed a left bundle branch block (Figure 3).

Empirical antibiotics were started, but cultures of blood and cerebrospinal fluid remained negative. Antibiotics were stopped after 48 hours. Also, liquor polymerase chain reaction (PCR) on neurotropic viruses was negative. Metabolic screening in cerebrospinal fluid and urine was normal. Brain ultrasound and MRI/magnetic resonance spectroscopy (MRS) at days 1 and 2 showed no abnormalities. The infant improved further, and on the second day of life, her physical and neurologic examination restored to normal whereafter she was extubated. The ECG normalized. Seven days later, the neonate was fully recovered and could be discharged from the NICU. In retrospection, an intoxication with a local

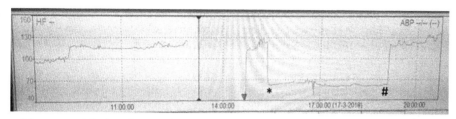

FIGURE 2: Illustration of the curve of the heartbeat with episodes of a sudden bradycardia (*) and spontaneous recovery to normal AV conduction (#). Y-axis: heart rate in beats per minute; X-axis: time in hours.

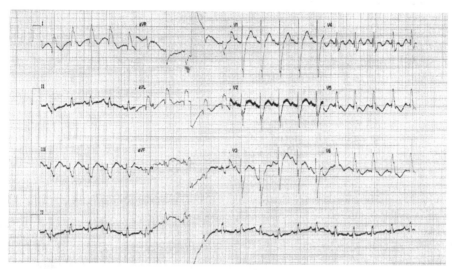

FIGURE 3: ECG on the right showed normal heart frequency (131 beats/minute) with 1 : 1 AV conduction, with a left bundle branch block (QRS 120 ms). Settings 25 mm/s; 10 mm/mV.

anesthetic was suspected. The consulted obstetrician confirmed the use of mepivacaine for a perineal infiltration during delivery. Therefore, blood samples obtained from the first days of life were analyzed. On the first day, the mepivacaine level was 20 mg/L, and on the second day, it was 2 mg/L. There was no injection site visible on the scalp. The mother did not show any signs of intoxication during or after delivery. Following up at 8 months of age, the infant's neurodevelopmental examination was in normal range.

3. Discussion

Apnea, bradycardia, prolonged QRS complexes, cyanosis, hypotonia, pupillary mydriasis fixed to light, and seizures are characteristic features for an intoxication with local anesthetics in neonates. The mother in this case received local anesthesia with mepivacaine for maternal episiotomy. The neonate had typical symptoms of an intoxication, and the blood sample on the first day revealed a mepivacaine level of 20 mg/L. Toxic effects in neonates have been described with levels as low as 3 mg/L. Furthermore, the neonate was fully recovered on the second day, which was coherent with a mepivacaine level of 2 mg/L.

Perinatal infection or metabolic causes were excluded. Although perinatal asphyxia may also explain these symptoms, differences in the early course of patients can differentiate for an intoxication. Hypoxic-ischemic encephalopathy caused by perinatal asphyxia is usually not characterized by high Apgar scores followed by a symptomless period after birth before the onset of hypotonia, tonic seizures, and arrest of spontaneous respiration or with fixed dilated pupils and eyes fixed in the oculocephalic reflex. Furthermore, brain imaging and blood results were not suggestive for asphyxia during pregnancy or labor. The onset of all the signs observed in our case might therefore be caused by intoxication from local anesthesia [2].

Mepivacaine similar to lidocaine is an amide-type local anesthetic agent. It reversibly blocks the sodium channels of nerve fibers, thereby inhibiting the conduction of nerve impulses. As mepivacaine affects the function of skeletal muscles, it reduces conduction of the AV node (second-degree AV block) and conduction over the His bundle causing a left bundle branch block. Without the knowledge of mepivacaine treatment in our case, a second-degree AV block and pseudoblock with QTc around 590 ms were considered. However, in mepivacaine intoxication, AV conduction disturbances are much more likely than prolonged repolarization (pseudoblock). Mepivacaine is known to cross the placental barrier and can affect the fetus. Two possibilities for transmission are described in the literature: first, trans-placental transmission following perineal infiltration for maternal episiotomy [3] and second, accidental injection (in the fetal scalp) during infiltration for paracervical and pudendal blocks during labor [4].

Lidocaine intoxication is better known in neonatal intoxication after local anesthesia [5, 6]. Recently, a case report described a toxic lidocaine level in a cord blood sample, so trans-placental intoxication of lidocaine was verified [7]. In our case, the mepivacaine level was not examined in the cord blood; however, trans-placental intoxication seems to be most likely. The perineal infiltration technique was applied lege artis, keeping the fingers between the needle and the fetal skull. Throughout the procedure, the perineum bulged as the mepivacaine was injected. Because no skull laceration was seen in our case, direct injection in the skull seems highly unlikely but cannot completely ruled out because of a hairy skull. However, the birth attendant confirmed this did not happen.

Pharmacokinetic studies show diverse fetal/maternal lidocaine ratios depending on the route of administration (perineal infiltration, lumbar epidural anesthesia, pudendus block, or paracervical block). Because mepivacaine is like lidocaine, an amide-type local anesthetic agent, the same explanations may be given for the high fetal/maternal ratio after perineal infiltration of mepivacaine as for lidocaine. First, the local anesthesia is injected in a highly vascularized zone. Second, there is anatomic proximity of the perineum to the fetus. Third, mepivacaine is a weak base which will rapidly cross the placenta in the unionized state. Because of fetal acidosis in the second stage of labor, there is an increased conversion to ionized mepivacaine in the fetus; the ratio ionized to unionized mepivacaine rises. This leads to an accumulation of mepivacaine in the fetus. This phenomenon is called "trapping" of the anesthesia in the ionized form. This explains the strong correlation between the fetal/maternal ratio and the length of the second stage of labor and in fetal asphyxia. Additionally, half-life time of mepivacaine is at least three times longer in neonates than in adults, respectively, 9 hours versus 2 to 3 hours. Toxic effects in neonates have been described with levels as low as 3 mg/L [8]. Because local anesthetics accumulate preferentially in acidic media, elimination can be enhanced with gastric lavage (however, the risk for aspiration should be taken into account) and forced diuresis. Elimination by exchange transfusion is possible too. Furthermore, intravenous intralipid administration is described to resolve toxicity in neonates caused by local anesthetic procedures. Intralipid is an emulsion of soybean oil in water, predominantly neutral triglycerides, made isotonic with glycerin. In blood, these fat droplets form a lipid compartment, separate from the plasma aqueous phase, into which a lipophilic substance like mepivacaine might dissolve (lipid sink therapy). A concentration gradient develops between tissue and blood which causes local anesthetics to move from the heart or brain (areas of high concentrations) to the "lipid sink". Because of the increasing practice of local anesthesia, further research in safe elimination therapy as intralipid in neonates is therefore needed [9]. By the time the diagnosis was established in this current case, the patient was already recovered and elimination therapy was not necessary.

Exact morbidity and mortality of infants following intoxication by local anesthetics is not known. Long-term follow-up studies documenting neurologic and developmental outcome are necessary; however, this characteristic syndrome after maternal local anesthetics is rare and may therefore often be unrecognized.

This case presents a term newborn with respiratory, cardiac, and neurologic signs shortly after birth most probably caused by intoxication with mepivacaine following perineal infiltration for maternal episiotomy. Although this is an uncommon complication, we advise that in case of unexplained symptoms, intoxication involving the fetus during labor has always to be taken into account.

Consent

Parents have given their written informed consent to publish this case.

Acknowledgments

The authors thank T. Smits, Hospital Pharmacy Resident at Emma Children's Hospital and VU University Medical Center, Amsterdam UMC, University of Amsterdam, Amsterdam.

References

[1] J. Shah, E. G. Votta-Velis, and A. Borgeat, "New local anesthetics," *Best Practice & Research Clinical Anaesthesiology*, vol. 32, no. 2, pp. 179–185, 2018.

[2] M. S. Pignotti, G. Indolfi, R. Ciuti, and G. Donzelli, "Perinatal asphyxia and inadvertent neonatal intoxication from local anaesthetics given to the mother during labour," *BMJ*, vol. 330, no. 7489, pp. 34-35, 2005.

[3] M. Amato, A. Carasso, and C. Ruckstuhl, "Neonatal mepivacaine poisoning following episiotomy," *Z Geburtshilfe Perinatol*, vol. 187, no. 4, pp. 191–193, 1983.

[4] L. S. Hillman, R. E. Hillman, and W. E. Dodson, "Diagnosis, treatment, and follow-up of neonatal mepivacaine intoxication secondary to paracervical and pudendal blocks during labor," *Journal of Pediatrics*, vol. 95, no. 3, pp. 472–477, 1979.

[5] C. De Praeter, P. Vanhaesebrouck, N. De Praeter, P. Govaert, M. Bogaert, and J. Leroy, "Episiotomy and neonatal lidocaine intoxication," *European Journal of Pediatrics*, vol. 150, no. 9, pp. 685-686, 1991.

[6] W. Y. Kim, J. J. Pomerance, and A. A. Miller, "Lidocaine intoxication in a newborn following local anesthesia for episiotomy," *Pediatrics*, vol. 64, no. 5, pp. 643–645, 1979.

[7] V. Demeulemeester, H. Van Hautem, F. Cools, and J. Lefevere, "Transplacental lidocaine intoxication," *Journal of Neonatal-Perinatal Medicine*, vol. 11, no. 4, pp. 439–441, 2018.

[8] P. D. Walson, M. A. Ott, and D. E. Carter, "Lidocaine and mepivacaine in cord blood," *Pediatr Pharmacol (New York)*, vol. 2, no. 4, pp. 341–348, 1982.

[9] K. Patil, "Use of intralipid for local anesthetic toxicity in neonates," *Pediatric Anesthesia*, vol. 21, no. 12, pp. 1268-1269, 2011.

36

Type IV Laryngotracheoesophageal Cleft Associated with Type III Esophageal Atresia in 1p36 Deletions Containing the RERE Gene: Is There a Causal Role for the Genetic Alteration?

Gloria Pelizzo ⓘ,[1] Aurora Puglisi,[2] Maria Lapi,[2] Maria Piccione,[3] Federico Matina,[4] Martina Busè,[3] Giovanni Battista Mura,[1] Giuseppe Re,[2] and Valeria Calcaterra[5]

[1]Pediatric Surgery Unit, Pediatric Surgery Unit, Children's Hospital "G. Di Cristina", ARNAS "Civico-Di Cristina-Benfratelli", Palermo, Italy
[2]Pediatric Anesthesiology and Intensive Care Unit, Pediatric Anesthesiology and Intensive Care Unit, Children's Hospital "G. Di Cristina", ARNAS "Civico-Di Cristina-Benfratelli", Palermo, Italy
[3]Department of Sciences for Health Promotion and Mother and Child Care "Giuseppe D'Alessandro", University of Palermo, Palermo, Italy
[4]Neonatal Intensive Care Unit, A.O.U.P. "P. Giaccone", Department of Sciences for Health Promotion and Mother and Child Care "G. D'Alessandro", Palermo, Italy
[5]Pediatrics and Adolescentology Unit, Department of Internal Medicine University of Pavia and Fondazione IRCCS Policlinico San Matteo, Pavia, Italy

Correspondence should be addressed to Gloria Pelizzo; gloriapelizzo@gmail.com

Academic Editor: Larry A. Rhodes

The causes of embryological developmental anomalies leading to laryngotracheoesophageal clefts (LTECs) are not known, but are proposed to be multifactorial, including genetic and environmental factors. Haploinsufficiency of the RERE gene might contribute to different phenotypes seen in individuals with 1p36 deletions. We describe a neonate of an obese mother, diagnosed with type IV LTEC and type III esophageal atresia (EA), in which a 1p36 deletion including the RERE gene was detected. On the second day of life, a right thoracotomy and extrapleural esophagus atresia repair were attempted. One week later, a right cervical approach was performed to separate the cervical esophagus from the trachea. Three months later, a thoracic termino-terminal anastomosis of the esophagus was performed. An anterior fundoplication was required at 8 months of age due to severe gastroesophageal reflux and failure to thrive. A causal role of 1p36 deletions including the RERE gene in the malformation is proposed. Moreover, additional parental factors must be considered. Future studies are mandatory to elucidate genomic and epigenomic susceptibility factors that underlie these congenital malformations. A multiteam approach is a crucial factor in the successful management of affected patients.

1. Introduction

Complete laryngotracheoesophageal clefts (LTECs), types III and IV, are rare congenital anomalies that occur when the primitive foregut fails to separate into the tracheobronchial tree and the esophagus [1]. These malformations are the most challenging to diagnose and manage since they are life-threatening conditions [1–6]. LTECs have been associated with many other congenital anomalies, such as defects of the gastrointestinal and genitourinary tracts and cardiovascular anomalies [7]. The causes of embryological developmental anomalies leading to LTECs are not known, but are proposed to be multifactorial, including genetic and environmental factors, such as maternal risks [4–6, 8].

The arginine-glutamic acid dipeptide repeats gene (RERE (MIM: 605226)) is located in the proximal 1p36 critical region [9, 10]. RERE encodes a widely expressed nuclear receptor coregulator [11, 12] that positively regulates retinoic acid signaling in multiple tissues during embryonic development [13–15]. Data from animal models suggest that haploinsufficiency of RERE might contribute to intellectual disability, developmental delay, structural brain anomalies, vision problems, hearing loss, congenital heart defects, cardiomyopathy, and renal anomalies seen in individuals with 1p36 deletions [16]. However, the exact role that RERE deficiency plays in 1p36 deletion syndrome, and more generally in human disease, remains unclear [9].

We describe a neonate diagnosed with type IV LTEC and type III esophageal atresia in which a 1p36 deletion including the RERE gene was detected. The surgical and anesthesiological decision-making and management of the newborn are detailed. The roles of multifactorial factors in the pathogenesis of the malformation are also discussed.

2. Case Presentation

A Caucasian male neonate, weighing 3080 g, was born by cesarean section at the 37th week of pregnancy. Prenatally, at 23 weeks' gestation, microgastria without polyhydramnios was detected and a suspicion of type III esophageal atresia was suggested. Prenatal MRI was not available due to severe maternal obesity. The Apgar scores were 7 and 9 at 1 and 5 minutes, respectively. At birth, clinical examination revealed hypotonia and pathological transmitted sounds from the upper airways without respiratory distress. No dysmorphic features, eye anomalies, vertebral or limb abnormalities, or genitalia malformations were noted.

A posterior-anterior chest radiograph at 3 h of age confirmed the prenatal suspicion of esophageal atresia. At bronchoscopy, type IV LTEC was diagnosed associated with type III esophageal atresia. Illustration of the malformation is shown in Figure 1(a).

On the second day of life, a right thoracotomy and extrapleural esophagus atresia repair were attempted. Following induction, the patient was intubated with a 3.5 mm uncuffed endotracheal tube. The tracheoesophageal fistula was sutured first. Multiple episodes of desaturation were immediately controlled after the dissection of the proximal esophageal pouch from the trachea. The neoesophageal tube was separated from the trachea using running sutures (Figure 1(b)). A nonresorbable biologic-tissue patch was positioned in between the anterior esophageal wall and the trachea in order to consolidate the tracheal pars membranacea. The proximal and distal pouches were stitched to the right thoracic paravertebral region to obtain progressive elongation. Gastrostomy for feeding was also performed.

One week later, a right cervical approach was performed to separate the cervical esophagus from the trachea (Figure 1(c)). After surgery, the child was gradually weaned off a ventilator, and after 13 days, sufficient respiratory autonomy was obtained. Enteral feeding was started. The postoperative course was characterized by *Klebsiella* septicemia, a thromboembolic event and bronchopneumonia *ab ingestis*. Three months later, the thoracic termino-terminal anastomosis of the esophagus was performed (Figure 1(d)). An anterior fundoplication was required at eight months of age due to severe gastroesophageal reflux and failure to thrive.

Genetic testing and genomic DNA sequencing were performed. No evidence of cystic fibrosis or phenylketonuria was detected. CHD7 sequencing and deletion and duplication analysis did not reveal any pathological variants. Array-CGH analysis documented a 1p36.33 deletion of approximately 50 kb (position from 8.779.410 to 8.830.261), containing the RERE gene. Array-CGH analysis in both parents showed that the rearrangement was of paternal origin. The child exhibited the associated anomalies, unilateral hypoplastic and ptotic right kidney. No pathological neurological signs or symptoms were revealed. The proband's father had a normal phenotype but was severely obese.

3. Discussion

To the best of our knowledge, this is the first report on a 1p36 deletion containing the RERE gene in a neonate with type IV LTEC and type III esophageal atresia. Genetic alterations can contribute to the development of these congenital malformations; moreover, the role of environmental factors should not be excluded.

Subjects with terminal and interstitial deletions of chromosome 1p36 have a spectrum of defects that include eye anomalies, postnatal growth deficiency, structural brain anomalies, seizures, cognitive impairment, delayed motor development, behavior problems, hearing loss, cardiovascular malformations, cardiomyopathy, and renal anomalies [9, 16]. The proximal 1p36 genes that contribute to these defects have not been clearly delineated. RERE is located in the proximal region of chromosome 1p36. Due to its role as a nuclear receptor coregulator and the role it plays in retinoic acid signaling, it is considered a candidate gene, which could contribute to the development of several phenotypes seen in individuals with proximal interstitial deletions or large terminal deletions of 1p36 [9].

The function of RERE in development has been explored using mouse models. In these models, RERE plays a critical role in the development and function of multiple organs including the eye, brain, inner ear, heart, and kidney. To date, mutations in RERE have not been implicated as the cause of a specific disease or syndrome in humans; however, in 16% and 13% of the individuals with isolated 1p36 deletions that include RERE, orofacial clefts and genitourinary anomalies have, respectively, been reported [9].

The estimated annual incidence of LTEC is 1/10,000 to 1/20,000 live births, accounting for 0.2% to 1.5% of congenital malformations of the larynx. It is often associated with other congenital abnormalities (16% to 68%), mostly malformations of the digestive tract [7]. Our neonate presented with LTEC associated with esophageal atresia. There are scattered reports of patients with this association, but the actual incidence of this particular association is difficult to

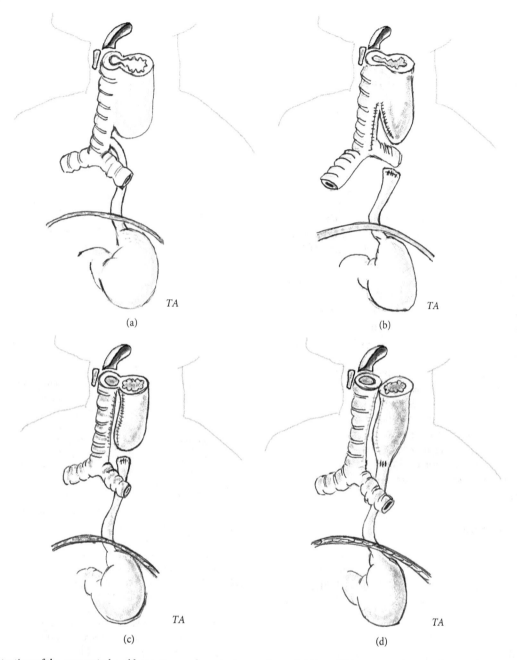

FIGURE 1: Illustration of the congenital malformation and surgical procedures. (a) Type IV laryngotracheoesophageal clefts (LTEC) and type III esophageal atresia. (b) Step 1: suture of the tracheoesophageal fistula, dissection of the proximal esophageal pouch from the trachea, and separation of the neoesophageal tube from the trachea. (c) Step 2: separation of the cervical esophagus from the trachea. (d) Step 3: thoracic termino-terminal anastomosis of the esophagus (drawn by Dr. Salvatore Amoroso).

assess because most of the reports regarding this association are in the form of case reports or limited series [17–21].

It has been hypothesized that LTECs result from the complex interplay of multiple genes and environmental factors. In our patient, in whom LTEC and EA were also associated with a renal anomaly, the paternal origin of the genetic rearrangement was revealed. Even though the father had a normal phenotype, the causal role of RERE in malformations is supported. Indeed, the deletions in RERE may contribute alone or in conjunction with other genetic or environmental factors to the development of the phenotype

seen in affected subjects [10]. The role of maternal obesity as a candidate cofactor is also proposed. The effects of maternal obesity extend to the fetus, with several large population-based analyses demonstrating independent risks of fetal neural tube defects, cardiac malformations, and orofacial clefts. The mechanism for the observed association between obesity and birth defects is not known, but several possible explanations have been proposed [22]. Firstly, obese women have metabolic alterations, such as hyperglycemia/diabetes or elevated insulin or estrogen levels that increase the risk for birth defects. Secondly, women who are obese also might have nutritional deficits, resulting from dieting behaviors or poor-quality diets that increase their risk for congenital anomalies. Additionally, obese women might have an increased requirement for certain nutrients (e.g., folic acid) known to be protective against birth defects. Associations between maternal obesity, epigenetic alterations, and congenital malformations have also been proposed [23, 24]. Finally, also considering the father's severe obesity, the role of the epigenetic paternal profile should not be excluded [25].

The surgical and anesthesiological management of patients affected by LTEC is generally complicated and presents a challenge in the preoperative, perioperative, and postoperative periods [5]. Recent advances in knowledge, diagnosis, and, above all, the treatment of LTEC have led to significant improvements in survival and quality of life for these patients, as obtained in this reported patient. As reported by Chitkara et al., critical factors in the successful management of these patients include a team-oriented approach with experience in airway surgery, safe management of the airway, early and aggressive management of gastric reflux, nutritional sustenance, and early surgical intervention [5].

In summary, we describe a neonate affected by type IV LTEC and type III esophageal atresia, in which a 1p36 deletion containing the RERE gene was detected and a multiteam approach resulted in successful surgical treatment. The causal role of the genetic profile was proposed; moreover, the fetal effects of concurrent parental factors should be considered. Future studies are mandatory to elucidate genomic and epigenomic susceptibility factors, which underlie these congenital malformations.

Acknowledgments

The authors thank Dr. Salvatore Amoroso for the illustration, Dr. Laurene Marguerite Kelly for English revision of the manuscript, and the association "4CHILDREN C&C Onlus" for supporting the research in their Pediatric Surgery Unit.

References

[1] J. Merei and J. Hutson, "Embryogenesis of tracheo esophageal anomalies: a review," *Pediatric Surgery International*, vol. 18, no. 5-6, pp. 319–326, 2002.

[2] K. Mochizuki, M. Shinkai, H. Take et al., "Type IV laryngotracheoesophageal cleft repair by a new combination of lateral thoraco-cervical and laryngoscopic approaches," *Pediatric Surgery International*, vol. 30, no. 9, pp. 941–944, 2014.

[3] A. L. Kawaguchi, P. K. Donahoe, and D. P. Ryan, "Management and long-term follow-up of patients with types III and IV laryngotracheoesophageal clefts," *Journal of Pediatric Surgery*, vol. 40, no. 1, pp. 158–164, 2005.

[4] K. Sonmez, R. Karabulut, Z. Turkyilmaz et al., "Our experience in two cases of type IV laryngotracheoesophageal cleft (LTEC) with a diagnosis of antenatal esophageal atresia," *Pan African Medical Journal*, vol. 26, p. 55, 2017.

[5] A. E. Chitkara, M. Tadros, H. J. Kim, and E. H. Harley, "Complete laryngotracheoesophageal cleft: complicated management issues," *Laryngoscope*, vol. 113, no. 8, pp. 1314–1320, 2003.

[6] K. Geller, Y. Kim, J. Koempel, and K. D. Anderson, "Surgical management of type III and IV laryngotracheoesophageal clefts: the three-layered approach," *International Journal of Pediatric Otorhinolaryngology*, vol. 74, no. 6, pp. 652–657, 2010.

[7] N. Leboulanger and E. N. Garabédian, "Laryngo-tracheo-oesophageal clefts," *Orphanet Journal of Rare Diseases*, vol. 6, no. 1, p. 81, 2011.

[8] F. B. Essien and A. Maderious, "A genetic factor controlling morphogenesis of the laryngotracheo-esophageal complex in the mouse," *Teratology*, vol. 24, no. 2, pp. 235–239, 1981.

[9] B. Fregeau, B. J. Kim, A. Hernández-García et al., "De novo mutations of RERE cause a genetic syndrome with features that overlap those associated with proximal 1p36 deletions," *American Journal of Human Genetics*, vol. 98, no. 5, pp. 963–970, 2016.

[10] B. J. Kim, H. P. Zaveri, O. A. Shchelochkov et al., "An allelic series of mice reveals a role for RERE in the development of multiple organs affected in chromosome 1p36 deletions," *PLoS One*, vol. 8, no. 2, Article ID e57460, 2013.

[11] L. Wang, H. Rajan, J. L. Pitman, M. McKeown, and C. C. Tsai, "Histone deacetylase-associating Atrophin proteins are nuclear receptor corepressors," *Genes and Development*, vol. 5, pp. 525–530, 2005.

[12] J. S. Zoltewicz, N. J. Stewart, R. Leung, and A. S. Peterson, "Atrophin 2 recruits histone deacetylase and is required for the function of multiple signaling centers during mouse embryogenesis," *Development*, vol. 131, no. 1, pp. 3–14, 2004.

[13] S. Kumar and G. Duester, "Retinoic acid controls body axis extension by directly repressing Fgf8 transcription," *Development*, vol. 141, no. 15, pp. 2972–2977, 2014.

[14] G. C. Vilhais-Neto, M. Fournier, J. L. Plassat et al., "The WHHERE coactivator complex is required for retinoic acid-dependent regulation of embryonic symmetry," *Nature Communications*, vol. 8, p. 728, 2017.

[15] G. C. Vilhais-Neto, M. Maruhashi, K. T. Smith et al., "Rere controls retinoic acid signalling and somite bilateral symmetry," *Nature*, vol. 463, no. 7283, pp. 953–957, 2010.

[16] V. K. Jordan, B. Fregeau, X. Ge et al., "Genotype-phenotype correlations in individuals with pathogenic RERE variants," *Human Mutation*, vol. 35, no. 5, pp. 666–675, 2018.

[17] C. Eriksen, D. Zwillenberg, and N. Robinson, "Diagnosis and management of cleft larynx–literature review and case report," *Annals of Otology, Rhinology & Laryngology*, vol. 99, no. 9, pp. 703–708, 1990.

[18] N. Burroughs and L. L. Leape, "Laryngotracheoesophageal cleft: report of a case successfully treated and review of the literature," *Pediatrics*, vol. 53, pp. 516–522, 1974.

[19] K. L. Evans, R. Courteney-Harris, C. M. Bailey, J. N. Evans, and D. S. Parsons, "Management of posterior laryngeal and laryngotracheoesophageal clefts," *Archives of Otolaryngology-Head and Neck Surgery*, vol. 121, no. 12, pp. 1380–1385, 1995.

[20] L. P. Glossop, R. J. Smith, and J. G. Evans, "Posterior laryngeal cleft: an analysis of ten cases," *International Journal of Pediatric Otorhinolaryngology*, vol. 7, no. 2, pp. 133–143, 1984.

[21] S. R. Cohen, "Cleft larynx. A report of seven cases," *Annals of Otology, Rhinology & Laryngology*, vol. 84, no. 6, pp. 747–756, 1975.

[22] M. L. Watkins, S. A. Rasmussen, M. A. Honein, L. D. Botto, and C. A. Moore, "Maternal obesity and risk for birth defects," *Pediatrics*, vol. 111, pp. 1152–1158, 2003.

[23] S. Chandrasekaran and G. Neal-Perry, "Long-term consequences of obesity on female fertility and the health of the offspring," *Current Opinion in Obstetrics and Gynecology*, vol. 29, no. 3, pp. 180–187, 2017.

[24] N. N. Mathur, G. J. Peek, C. M. Bailey, and M. J. Elliott, "Strategies for managing Type IV laryngotracheoesophageal clefts at Great Ormond Street Hospital for Children," *International Journal of Pediatric Otorhinolaryngology*, vol. 70, no. 11, pp. 1901–1910, 2006.

[25] G. Raad, M. Hazzouri, S. Bottini, M. Trabucchi, J. Azoury, and V. Grandjean, "Paternal obesity: how bad is it for sperm quality and progeny health?," *Basic and Clinical Andrology*, vol. 27, p. 20, 2017.

37

Severe Hypernatremia in a Significantly Underweight Female Child

Megan B. Coriell ⑩,[1] Prasanthi Gandham,[1,2] Kupper Wintergerst,[1,2] and Bradly Thrasher[1,2]

[1]*University of Louisville School of Medicine, Louisville, KY, USA*
[2]*Norton Children's Hospital, Louisville, KY, USA*

Correspondence should be addressed to Megan B. Coriell; megan.buttleman@louisville.edu

Academic Editor: Junji Takaya

In this study, we present the case of a 5-year-old female who presented for evaluation of dehydration with labs that revealed significant hypernatremia concerning for diabetes insipidus (DI). Further evaluation revealed that she had underlying chronic malnutrition. Her diagnostic work up for DI produced some evidence consistent with DI while other data indicated otherwise, bringing up the possibility of partial DI. She was ultimately diagnosed with sporadic vasopressin release secondary to her chronic malnutrition. This case illustrates another effect chronic malnutrition can have on pediatric patients along with the importance of a broad differential for patients with severe hypernatremia.

1. Introduction

It is well known that chronic malnutrition in childhood can have both short-term and long-term health consequences. Malnutrition in childhood not only effects physical growth and brain development but has also been shown to delay puberty [1, 2]. However, there is a paucity of data on the possible effects malnutrition can have on vasopressin and the hypothalamic-pituitary-adrenal axis. In this article, we present the case of a 5-year-old female whose initial chief complaint was dehydration. She had significant hyper-natremia concerning for diabetes insipidus (DI) and was found to have underlying chronic malnutrition. This case illustrates another health consequence of chronic malnu-trition along with the importance of a broad differential for patients with severe dehydration and hypernatremia.

2. Case Presentation

A 5-year-old female presented to the emergency department with a three-day history of poor oral intake, mild upper respiratory symptoms, and concerns for dehydration. Her history was notable for premature birth at 29 weeks, neonatal respiratory distress syndrome, and necrotizing enterocolitis. History was limited as patient's father was present during her medical evaluation, and patient was in mother's care prior to arrival. Of note, parents were separated but still shared custody.

Initial evaluation at an outside facility included a comprehensive metabolic panel (CMP), which revealed a sodium of 176 mmol/L. She was given a lactated Ringer's bolus, resulting in a decrease of her sodium to 171 mmol/L. Table 1 provides the initial lab results. Other testing included a rapid strep test, chest X-ray, complete blood count, and influenza and COVID-19 testing, all of which were unre-markable. A urinalysis was notable for specific gravity 1.020, ketones 5 mg/dL, protein 500 mg/dL, nitrite negative, leu-kocyte esterase 100, and white blood cells 10–15 HPF. She was then transferred to Norton Children's Hospital for further management of hypernatremia. During transport, the patient reported hunger and stated that she was not given food at home.

On arrival to our facility, a basic metabolic panel (BMP) was repeated which was notable for sodium 158 mmol/L, potassium 2.7 mmol/L, chloride 119 mmol/L, carbon diox-ide 32 mmol/L, and glucose 108 mg/dL. Random urine

TABLE 1: Initial electrolytes obtained at outside facility.

Lab	Initial CMP	BMP after fluid bolus	Reference ranges (adult ranges)
Sodium (mmol/L)	176 (H)	171 (H)	136–145 mmol/L
Potassium (mmol/L)	3.38 (L)	3.20 (L)	3.5–5 mmol/L
Chloride (mmol/L)	137 (H)	135 (H)	98–107 mmol/L
Carbon dioxide (mmol/L)	26	25	21–31 mmol/L
Glucose (mg/dL)	165 (H)	168 (H)	80–100 mg/dL
BUN (mg/dL)	33 (H)	33 (H)	7–25 mg/dL
Creatine (mg/dL)	0.77	0.79	0.6–1.3 mg/dL
Total protein (g/dL)	7.2		6.4–8.9 g/dL
Albumin (g/dL)	4.60		3.5–5.7 g/dL
Calcium (mg/dL)	9.5	9.3	8.6–10.8 mg/dL
AST (IU/L)	26		13–35 IU/L
ALT (IU/L)	24		7–52 IU/L
Alkaline phosphatase (IU/L)	91		38–104 IU/L
Total bilirubin (mg/dL)	0.5		0.3–1.0 mg/dL

sodium and random urine creatinine were within normal limits. Random urine osmolality was decreased at 99.5 mOsm/kg, and serum osmolality was increased at 330 mOsm/kg. Given these findings, pediatric endocrinology was consulted due to hypernatremia and concern for DI. Additional labs showed a low prealbumin of 8 mg/dL (reference range: 11.0–23.0 mg/dL), normal renin activity of 4.5 ng/mL/hr, low aldosterone of <3.0 ng/dL (reference range 4.0–44.0 ng/dL), and normal AM cortisol of 13.7 ug/dL. She was started on normal saline fluids, given oral potassium-chloride replacement, and admitted to the pediatric ICU for further management.

On day 2 of admission, her sodium level trended down to 155 mmol/L with fluid resuscitation and her appetite improved. However, her urine output (UOP) was significantly elevated at 8.28 mL/kg/hr. Dad denied any history of polyuria or polydipsia. She was toilet trained and had no history of accidents. She had been meeting developmental milestones and doing well in virtual kindergarten.

Her weight on admission was 15.1 kg (1.8th percentile), height was 106 cm (8.9th percentile), and BMI was 13.44 kg/m^2 (4.8th percentile). Of note, at 2 years of age, her height was in the 71st percentile and weight in the 30th percentile. Given these findings along with her significant electrolyte abnormalities on presentation, forensics was consulted due to concerns for chronic malnutrition. Additional work up included thyroid studies, which showed a thyroid stimulating hormone (TSH) of 6.050 IU/mL (reference range: 0.470–4.680 IU/mL) and free thyroxine (T4) of 1.49 ng/dL (reference range: 0.78–2.19 ng/dL). Her celiac panel was negative, and growth factors were normal for age.

Our patient's sodium level improved with IV fluids and oral intake. Her hypokalemia and alkalosis also improved with potassium-chloride replacement. She was noted to have a mild acute kidney injury on admission with an elevated creatinine of 0.77 mg/dL, but her creatinine level normalized quickly with rehydration. Although clinical evidence of dehydration resolved, including physical examination findings and normalization of her heart rate and blood pressure, her sodium level rose to 149–150 mmol/L each time IV fluids were weaned. She also continued to have

polyuria, although this slowly improved throughout admission. Due to the persistent hypernatremia and polyuria, DI continued to be a concern, and a modified water deprivation test was performed. During a traditional water deprivation test, the patient is made NPO, and serial labs are checked every 1-2 hours. These labs include serum sodium, serum osmolality, urine osmolality, and urine specific gravity. If the patient has DI, the urine osmolality and specific gravity will remain low despite a high serum osmolality and hypernatremia [3]. In our patient's case, she was made NPO at midnight, and fasting AM labs were obtained. Initial labs were concerning for DI with a low urine osmolality in the setting of a high serum sodium and serum osmolality. Desmopressin (DDAVP) was ordered to determine if administration would lead to concentration of urine. This would differentiate central from nephrogenic DI. However, before DDAVP could be given, father allowed the patient to drink. Of note, her UOP had decreased significantly, and so the decision was made to monitor. Another water deprivation test was performed overnight, and results were not consistent with DI. The lab results from her water deprivation tests are given in Table 2.

While these mixed results were not consistent with a frank diagnosis of complete vasopressin deficiency, the possibility of a partial DI diagnosis was considered. A pituitary MRI with and without contrast was obtained to look for abnormalities that may explain her findings. This showed a normal pituitary gland with decreased bright spot on T1 weighted imaging, likely within range of normal. This decrease in the bright spot has been reported in patients with DI but is also a normal variant found in 10% of the general population [4].

At discharge, our patient's sodium level had remained within normal range for several days off IV fluids and despite fasting for prolonged periods of time. Her weight increased from 15.1 kg to 16.3 kg during admission. She was discharged in the care of her father per child protective services with a plan for close follow-up.

She was seen by pediatric endocrinology two weeks after hospital discharge, and her father reported no signs of excessive urination or excessive thirst. Her weight was up to

Table 2: Water deprivation test results.

Lab	Test 1				Test 2	
	11/11/20 at 2157	11/12/20 at 0544	11/12/20 at 0845	11/12/20 at 1150	11/13/20 at 0629	11/13/20 at 1135
Serum sodium (mmol/L)	145	147 (H)	139	140	139	140
Serum osmolality (mOsm/kg)	305 (H)	311(H)	296	305	298	300
Urine sodium (mmol/L)	27	34	186	189	40	
Urine osmolality (mOsm/kg)	101.5 (L)	221 (L)	504	518.5	253.5 (L)	255.5 (L)
Specific gravity		1.006	1.012	1.011	1.008	1.010

17.3 kg from 16.3 kg at discharge. A BMP, thyroid function studies, and repeat growth factors were all within normal limits. At her endocrinology follow-up three months later, a repeat CMP was still normal, and she had no symptoms of polyuria or polydipsia. She continued to have appropriate weight gain. Based on her course, findings, and resolution of symptoms with adequate weight gain, she was diagnosed with hypernatremia and dehydration related to sporadic vasopressin release secondary to her malnutrition.

3. Discussion

The differential for severe hypernatremia in this clinical vignette included DI, hypernatremic dehydration, salt intoxication, primary hyperaldosteronism, and Gitelman/Bartter syndrome. The diagnostic criteria for DI includes polydipsia and polyuria in the setting of hypernatremia, serum osmolality >300 mOsm/kg, urine osmolality <300 mOsm/kg, and urine specific gravity <1.010 [4, 5]. Polyuria is defined as > 100–110 mL/kg/day in children ≤2 years of age and >50 mL/kg/day in older children [5]. DI was high on the differential given our patient's low urine osmolality and low urine specific gravity in the setting of a high serum osmolality and hypernatremia. She also had significant polyuria during the first 24 hours of admission with a UOP of 8.28 mL/kg/hr. However, there was no history of polyuria prior to admission. Later during admission, labs were no longer consistent with DI. This brought up the possibility of partial DI. Patients with partial DI have a partial deficiency of or partial response to vasopressin. They can typically somewhat concentrate their urine, with urine osmolality between 300 and 800 mOsm/kg following a water deprivation test. They typically have a <50% increase in urine osmolality after administration of DDAVP as compared to a >50% increase in urine osmolality in patients with complete DI [3, 5, 6].

Hypernatremic dehydration was also high on the differential given her significant dehydration and concerns for malnutrition on presentation. Hypernatremic dehydration occurs when water loss is more than solute loss and serum sodium is > 150 mmol/L [7]. The history of very poor oral intake for 2-3 days in the setting of a possible illness further supports this diagnosis. If this was our patient's diagnosis, we would anticipate her UOP to slowly return to baseline as her hydration status improved.

Salt intoxication usually involves a random urine sodium of >25 mmol/L and a fraction of excreted sodium (FENa) of >2%. Patients also typically have altered mental status (AMS) due to the acute change in their serum sodium level [8]. This diagnosis was less likely in our patient given her initial random urine sodium of 23 mmol/L, FENa of 2%, and no episodes of AMS before or during admission.

Primary hyperaldosteronism presents with hypernatremia and hypokalemia. This is a very rare condition, and patients typically have hypertension and mild volume expansion. Our patient had no hypertensive episodes and was dehydrated, as opposed to volume expanded, on presentation. Her renin and aldosterone were both appropriately suppressed in the setting of hypernatremia and hypokalemia, ruling out primary hyperaldosteronism.

Our patient's history of poor growth over the past several months was concerning for long standing malnutrition. Her thyroid studies showed a slightly elevated TSH and a normal free T4. The patient was clinically euthyroid. These lab findings were most likely due to her acute presentation. Her short stature was likely secondary to chronic malnutrition as growth factors were normal for age.

After narrowing down our differential, we found that no diagnosis completely fit our patient's case. We then turned to the literature to look for similar cases. Review of the literature revealed case reports of abnormal arginine vasopressin (AVP) axis function in patients with anorexia nervosa (AN). It is hypothesized that refeeding patients with severe malnutrition secondary to AN led to the development of DI [9]. These patients' AVP axes recovered over time, usually over the course of two weeks to several months [9, 10]. Several studies have shown alterations of osmoregulation in patients with AN, which is thought to be associated with severity of and duration of AN [11]. Additionally, it has been noted that these patients tend to have sporadic release of vasopressin [10]. Sporadic release of vasopressin could lead to a combination of both normal labs and labs consistent with DI. It is possible that our patient was experiencing a similar phenomenon occurring secondary to her chronic malnutrition. Our patient experienced complete resolution of her symptoms and lab abnormalities with appropriate nutrition and weight gain.

4. Conclusion

This case illustrates that severe electrolyte abnormalities can be seen in the setting of severe/prolonged malnutrition, and thus malnutrition should be considered in these cases. As demonstrated in patients with AN, severe/prolonged malnutrition can cause sporadic vasopressin release, leading to labs consistent with partial DI. In cases of sporadic vasopressin release secondary to malnutrition, adequate healthy weight gain will result in normalization of vasopressin function and, ultimately, resolution of symptoms.

Data Availability

This is a case report of a single patient; to protect privacy and respect confidentiality, none of the raw data have been made available in any public repository. The original reports, laboratory studies, imaging studies, and outpatient clinic records are retained as per normal procedure within the medical records of our institution.

References

[1] M. R. Corkins, "Why is diagnosing pediatric malnutrition important?" *Nutrition in Clinical Practice*, vol. 32, no. 1, pp. 15–18, 2017.

[2] M. J. Vazquez, I. Velasco, and M. Tena-Sempere, "Novel mechanisms for the metabolic control of puberty: implications for pubertal alterations in early-onset obesity and malnutrition," *Journal of Endocrinology*, vol. 242, no. 2, pp. R51–R65, 2019.

[3] G. Priya, S. Kalra, A. Dasgupta, and E. Grewal, "Diabetes insipidus: a pragmatic approach to management," *Cureus*, vol. 13, no. 1, Article ID e12498, 2021.

[4] A. Weiner and P. Vuguin, "Diabetes insipidus," *Pediatrics in Review*, vol. 41, no. 2, pp. 96–99, 2020.

[5] M. Christ-Crain, D. G. Bichet, W. K. Fenske et al., "Diabetes insipidus," *Nature Reviews Disease Primers*, vol. 5, no. 1, p. 54, 2019.

[6] T. Cheetham and P. H. Baylis, "Diabetes insipidus in children," *Pediatric Drugs*, vol. 4, no. 12, pp. 785–796, 2002.

[7] K. S. Powers, "Dehydration: isonatremic, hyponatremic, and hypernatremic recognition and management," *Pediatrics in Review*, vol. 36, no. 7, pp. 274–285, 2015.

[8] E. Blohm, A. Goldberg, A. Salerno, C. Jenny, E. Boyer, and K. Babu, "Recognition and management of pediatric salt toxicity," *Pediatric Emergency Care*, vol. 34, no. 11, pp. 820–824, 2018.

[9] E. L. Rosen, A. Thambundit, P. S. Mehler, and S. D. Mittelman, "Central diabetes insipidus associated with refeeding in anorexia nervosa: a case report," *International Journal of Eating Disorders*, vol. 52, no. 6, pp. 752–756, 2019.

[10] P. W. Gold, W. Kaye, G. L. Robertson, and M. Ebert, "Abnormalities in plasma and cerebrospinal-fluid arginine vasopressin in patients with anorexia nervosa," *New England Journal of Medicine*, vol. 308, no. 19, pp. 1117–1123, 1983.

[11] F. Evrard, M. Pinto da Cunha, M. Lambert, and O. Devuyst, "Impaired osmoregulation in anorexia nervosa: a case-control study," *Nephrology Dialysis Transplantation*, vol. 19, no. 12, pp. 3034–3039, 2004.

38

Pantoea agglomerans Infections in Children: Report of Two Cases

Shraddha Siwakoti ⓘ,[1] Rinku Sah,[1] Rupa Singh Rajbhandari,[2] and Basudha Khanal[1]

[1]Department of Microbiology, B.P. Koirala Institute of Health Sciences, Dharan, Nepal
[2]Department of Pediatrics, B.P. Koirala Institute of Health Sciences, Dharan, Nepal

Correspondence should be addressed to Shraddha Siwakoti; shraddha.siwakoti@bpkihs.edu

Academic Editor: Larry A. Rhodes

Introduction. *Pantoea agglomerans*, primarily an environmental and agricultural organism has been reported as both commensal and pathogen of humans. We present two case reports of *P. agglomerans* infections in children that involved the meninges and bloodstream. *Case Presentations.* A 6-month-old female baby, diagnosed as congenital hydrocephalus secondary to aqueduct stenosis with ventriculoperitoneal shunt in situ, operated 14 days back was brought to the pediatric emergency with a two-day history of high fever associated with vomiting, irritability, excessive crying, and decreased feeding. Postoperative meningitis was confirmed as cerebrospinal fluid culture revealed *P. agglomerans*. She responded well with a 14-day intravenous (IV) course of ceftriaxone. Also, we report a case of a 3-year-old male child referred to our center with a provisional diagnosis of UTI with chickenpox for further evaluation. During his 24-hour stay at the local hospital, he had received oral antibiotics and urinary catherization. Urine culture of catheter clamp urine was sterile. *P. agglomerans* was grown in blood culture. He was treated successfully with IV ceftriaxone and amikacin. *Conclusion.* *P. agglomerans* can cause postsurgical meningitis and bloodstream infection in children. The clinical course of infection was mild and timely administration of proper antibiotic resulted in a favorable outcome.

1. Introduction

Pantoea agglomerans is a gram-negative aerobic bacillus that belongs to the family Enterobacteriaceae. It is primarily an environmental and agricultural organism that inhabits plants, soil, and water. This bacterium has been reported as both commensal and pathogen of animals and humans [1]. Human infections may be associated with trauma caused by penetration of vegetative material and also with secondary bacteremia or nosocomial infections that are related to medical equipment such as intravenous catheters or contaminated intravenous fluids and parenteral nutrition [2–4]. Spontaneously occurring bacteremia and meningitis caused by this pathogen have rarely been reported, especially in children. Here, we present two case reports of *P. agglomerans* infections in children that involved the meninges and bloodstream.

2. Case Report 1: Meningitis

This case was a six-month-old female infant, diagnosed as congenital hydrocephalus secondary to aqueduct stenosis with VP shunt in situ. Fourteen days earlier, the child had undergone ventriculoperitoneal (VP) shunt surgery. The patient presented to the pediatric emergency with a two-day history of high fever associated with vomiting (2 episodes), irritability, excessive crying, and decreased feeding. On examination, her heart rate was 136/min, respiratory rate was 60/min, and temperature was 37.7°C. Central nervous system examination showcased normal cry, hypertonia, decreased power, and exaggerated reflexes on both upper and lower limbs. Pupils were bilaterally equal and reacting to the light. Examination results of the respiratory system, cardiovascular system, and abdomen were within normal limits. The child was treated empirically with IV vancomycin and ceftriaxone after collecting the CSF sample by lumbar puncture. CSF analysis showed an elevated white blood cell count of 400×10^6/L (95% polymorphs and 5% lymphocytes), raised protein level of 141 mg/dl, and decreased glucose level of 40 mg/dl (blood glucose level: 70 mg/dl). Gram stain of direct CSF smear showed few pus cells and few gram negative bacilli. CSF culture on chocolate and 5% sheep blood agar showed yellow pigmented, smooth surface colonies (Figure 1) and Mac Conkey's agar grew a nonlactose fermenting bacillus after 48-hours of aerobic incubation at 35°C. Based on biochemical reactions (Table 1), the colony was identified as *Pantoea agglomerans*. Antimicrobial susceptibility by Kirby–Bauer disc diffusion method showed the isolate to be resistant to ampicillin and sensitive to amikacin, ceftriaxone, ciprofloxacin, cotrimoxazole, and meropenem. After receiving the CSF culture report, vancomycin was discontinued, and IV ceftriaxone was continued for 2 weeks. The child's condition improved, and she was discharged after 15 days of hospital stay.

3. Case Report 2: Blood Stream Infection

A 3-year-old male child from the eastern part of Nepal was referred to our tertiary center after 24 hours admission at a local hospital with a provisional diagnosis of UTI with chickenpox for further evaluation. The child had a four-day history of abdominal pain, pain and difficulty with urination, urinary retention, and fever (up to 39°C). Urinary catheterization was done, and oral antibiotic was administered at the local hospital. The patient had also experienced rashes for 3 days, which started from lower limb and was later generalized. The patient had a recent history of UTI one month back. On the current admission, examination revealed temperature to be 37°C and skin showed multiple, erythematous rashes with dew drop appearance. Routine urine microscopic examination revealed the presence of 2 to 3 pus cells per high power field. Urine culture of catheter clamp urine did not yield a growth. Abdominal ultrasound showed mild hydronephrosis bilaterally and dense internal echoes within the urinary bladder lumen. A voiding cystourethrogram showed typical findings of a posterior urethral valve (PUV) with grade III vesicoureteral reflux. Blood culture grew *Pantoea agglomerans* sensitive to ampicillin, amikacin, ceftriaxone, ciprofloxacin, cotrimoxazole, and meropenem. Other laboratory parameters were within normal range. The child was empirically treated with IV ceftriaxone and amikacin which was continued for 7 days after getting the antibiotic sensitivity report. The child was successfully treated and discharged on the 8th day of hospital stay. He is currently being followed up at pediatric outpatient department and managed conservatively for PUV.

4. Discussion

Human infections caused by *P. agglomerans* are most often associated with wound infection with plant material or hospital acquired due to contamination of medical equipment and fluids. The most common infections caused by this

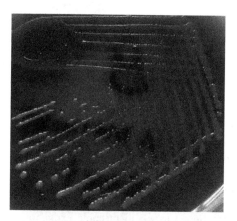

FIGURE 1: Growth of *Pantoea agglomerans* in blood agar.

TABLE 1: Biochemical tests to differentiate *P. agglomerans*.

Biochemicals	Interpretation
Catalase	Produced
Oxidase	Not produced
Citrate (Simmons)	Utilized
Urease, hydrogen sulfide, indole	Not produced
Motility	Motile
Nitrate	Reduced to nitrite
Glucose, xylose, arabinose, maltose, trehalose, rhamnose, mannitol	Fermented
Lactose, sucrose, sorbitol	Not fermented
Oxidative fermentative (OF)	Fermentative
Methyl red, Voges–Proskauer	Positive
Lysine, ornithine, arginine	Not decarboxylated

pathogen in children are blood stream infection, abscess, osteomyelitis, septic arthritis, and urinary tract infection. And, the source of these infections as described in literature is due to thorn pricks, infected parenteral fluids, and indwelling catheters [4]. *Pantoea* spp. seems to be a relatively uncommon cause of meningitis. In our case, the absence of any bacteria other than *P. agglomerans* on the CSF culture confirmed that this pathogen was responsible for the postoperative meningitis. Similarly, Wang and Fraser have isolated *P. agglomerans* from the brain abscess that developed after infarction and hemicraniectomy [5]. A case report of *Pantoea calida* causing postsurgical meningitis in a 52-year-old female has been reported by Fritz et al. [6]. Our isolation of *P. agglomerans* from a similar case indicates that *Pantoea* spp. must be considered as an opportunistic Enterobacteriaceae pathogen responsible for postsurgical meningitis. This *P. agglomerans* isolate displayed *in vitro* sensitivity to all the commonly used antibiotics, and accordingly, the child recovered with proper antibiotic treatment. A similar finding of antimicrobial sensitivity pattern was reported by Fritz et al. of their *P. calida* isolate from postsurgical meningitis where the patient had full recovery after 14 days of treatment with meropenem [6]. This depicts that meningitis caused by *Pantoea* spp. can have a mild clinical course, and administration of an effective antibiotic can cure the infection.

In our second case report, *P. agglomerans* was isolated from blood culture from a child. There can be two possible causes for this blood stream infection. It is conceivable that this bacteremia could be secondary to the UTI episode. The child had clinical features of UTI and was diagnosed with PUV, an important risk factor for UTI. Microbiology testing revealed a sterile urine culture which can be explained by the recent antibiotic administration at the local hospital. Instead, this bacteremia could be an event of primary blood stream infection; by definition not secondary to localized foci, as the exact source of bacteremia could not be established. Moreover, there was no identifiable exogenous source of infection. Most of the cases of *P. agglomerans* bacteremia in the literature have been documented in association with the contamination of intravenous fluid, total parenteral nutrition, and blood products [2, 3]. Conversely, the spontaneously occurring bacteremia has rarely been reported, especially for children. A study by Cruz et al. reported 23 culture-documented *P. agglomerans* infections in children with 21 central venous line- (CVL-) related bacteremic episodes and 2 nonCVL-associated spontaneous bacteremic episodes over 6 years [4]. Likewise 5 cases of sporadic *P. agglomerans* septicemia in preterm neonates with full recovery of all cases due to proper antibiotic therapy have been reported [7]. A case report of bloodstream infection caused by *Pantoea* spp. in a vaginally delivered 4-day-old baby from India had a favorable outcome after antibiotic therapy [8]. The outcome in our case was also benign after antibiotic treatment which may be partly due to early diagnosis and the adequacy of the antibiotics. Moreover, we believe that this favorable outcome of our child was probably because of infection caused by relatively less virulent strain. In contrary, there are several previously reported cases in the literature that had a fatal outcome [3, 4, 7]. Bergman et al. reported mortality of 3 cases of sporadic septicemia out of 125 infections with *P. agglomerans* among 6,383 newborns hospitalized in an intensive care unit [9]. This lethal outcome may be due to decline of patient's immunity caused by underlying disease, prematurity, and/or hospital procedures.

To the best of our knowledge, these are the first case reports of *P. agglomerans* causing infections in children from Nepal. Being an uncommon agent of human infection, *P. agglomerans* may be underreported or reported as any other member of Enterobacteriaceae in the routine settings. Due to the ubiquitous presence of *P. agglomerans* in nature, strict compliance to infection control practices would prevent the infection with this agent.

5. Conclusion

P. agglomerans can be the opportunistic agent for postsurgical meningitis and pathogen for bloodstream infection in children. The clinical course of infection caused by this bacterium can be mild, probably due to infection caused by relatively less virulent strain and can be treated with proper antibiotic therapy.

Consent

Written informed consent was obtained from the patient's legal guardian for publication of these case reports.

References

[1] F. Gavini, J. Mergaert, A. Beji et al., "Transfer of *Enterobacter agglomerans* (Beijerinck 1888) Ewing and Fife 1972 to *Pantoea* gen. nov. as *Pantoea agglomerans* comb. nov. and description of *Pantoea dispersa* sp. nov.," *International Journal of Systematic Bacteriology*, vol. 39, no. 3, pp. 337–345, 1989.

[2] N. S. Matsaniotis, V. P. Syriopoulou, M. C. Theodoridou, K. G. Tzanetou, and G. I. Mostrou, "*Enterobacter* sepsis in infants and children due to contaminated intravenous fluids," *Infection Control*, vol. 5, no. 10, pp. 471–477, 1984.

[3] H. Habsah, M. Zeehaida, H. Van Rostenberghe et al., "An outbreak of *Pantoea* spp. in a neonatal intensive care unit secondary to contaminated parenteral nutrition," *Journal of Hospital Infection*, vol. 61, no. 3, pp. 213–218, 2005.

[4] A. T. Cruz, A. C. Cazacu, and C. H. Allen, "*Pantoea agglomerans*, a plant pathogen causing human disease," *Journal of Clinical Microbiology*, vol. 45, no. 6, pp. 1989–1992, 2007.

[5] J. Wang and J. F. Fraser, "An intracranial petri dish? formation of abscess in prior large stroke after decompressive hemicraniectomy," *World Neurosurgery*, vol. 84, no. 5, pp. 1495. e5–1495.e9, 2015.

[6] S. Fritz, N. Cassir, R. Noudel, S. De La Rosa, P.-H. Roche, and M. Drancourtt, "Postsurgical *Pantoea calida* meningitis: a case report," *Journal of Medical Case Reports*, vol. 8, no. 1, p. 195, 2014.

[7] N. Y. Aly, H. N. Salmeen, R. A. Lila, and P. A. Nagaraja, "*Pantoea agglomerans* bloodstream infection in preterm neonates," *Medical Principles and Practice*, vol. 17, no. 6, pp. 500–503, 2008.

[8] S. Tiwari and S. S. Beriha, "*Pantoea* species causing early onset neonatal sepsis: a case report," *Journal of Medical Case Reports*, vol. 9, no. 1, p. 188, 2015.

[9] K. A. Bergman, J. P. Arends, and E. H. Schölvinck, "*Pantoea agglomerans* septicemia in three newborn infants," *Pediatric Infectious Disease Journal*, vol. 26, no. 5, pp. 453–454, 2007.

39

Severe Generalized Epidermolysis Bullosa Simplex in Two Hong Kong Children due to *De Novo* Variants in *KRT14* and *KRT5*

Shuk Ching Chong ⓘ,[1,2] Kam Lun Hon ⓘ,[1] Fernando Scaglia ⓘ,[2,3,4] Chung Mo Chow ⓘ,[1] Yu Ming Fu ⓘ,[5] Tor Wo Chiu ⓘ,[6] and Alexander K. C. Leung ⓘ[7]

[1]Department of Paediatrics, The Chinese University of Hong Kong, Prince of Wales Hospital, Shatin, Hong Kong
[2]The Chinese University of Hong Kong, Baylor College of Medicine Joint Center for Medical Genetics, Prince of Wales Hospital, Shatin, Hong Kong
[3]Department of Molecular and Human Genetics, Baylor College of Medicine, Houston, Texas, USA
[4]Texas Children's Hospital, Houston, Texas, USA
[5]Department of Paediatrics and Adolescent Medicine, Princess Margaret Hospital, Kwai Chung, Hong Kong
[6]Division of Plastic Reconstructive and Aesthetic Surgery, The Chinese University of Hong Kong, Prince of Wales Hospital, Shatin, Hong Kong
[7]Department of Pediatrics, The University of Calgary and the Alberta Children's Hospital, Calgary, Alberta, Canada

Correspondence should be addressed to Kam Lun Hon; ehon@hotmail.com

Academic Editor: Yann-Jinn Lee

We report two Hong Kong children with severe generalized epidermolysis bullosa simplex (EBS), the most severe form of EBS, without a family history of EBS. EBS is a rare genodermatosis usually inherited in an autosomal dominant fashion although rare autosomal recessive cases have been reported. Genetic studies in these patients showed that the first case was due to a novel *de novo* heterozygous variant, c.377T>G (NM_000526.5 (c.377T>G, p.Leu126Arg)) in the *KRT14* gene and the second case was due to a rare *de novo* heterozygous variant c.527A>G (NM_000424.4, c.527A>G, p.Asn176Ser) in the *KRT5* gene. To our knowledge, the c.377T>G variant in the *KRT14* gene has not been previously reported, and the c.527A>G variant in the *KRT5* gene is a rare cause of severe generalized EBS. In severe generalized EBS, infants exhibit severe symptoms at the onset; however, they tend to improve with time. A precise genetic diagnosis in these two cases aided in counseling the families concerning the prognosis in their affected children and the recurrence risk for future pregnancies.

1. Introduction

Epidermolysis bullosa (EB) is a heterogeneous group of rare inherited connective tissue disorders characterized by marked fragility of epithelial tissues with prototypic blistering, erosions, and nonhealing ulcers following minimal rubbing or frictional trauma [1–10]. EB is classified into four major categories, each with many subtypes based on the precise location at which separation or blistering occurs, namely, epidermolysis bullosa simplex (EBS; intraepidermal skin separation), epidermolysis bullosa junctional (EBJ; skin separation in lamina lucida or central basement membrane zone (BMZ)), dystrophic epidermolysis bullosa or epidermolysis bullosa dystrophica (EBD; sublamina densa BMZ separation), and Kindler syndrome (multiple cleavage planes) [2–4, 6, 8, 11–14]. The fundamental pathology of EB lies on the increase in collagenase activity, leading to collagen degeneration and hence splitting of various epidermal layers or at the transition between epidermis and dermis [5, 15]. EBS is the most common type of EB, accounting for 75 to 85% of cases of EB in the Western world [16]. EBS is usually caused by pathogenic variants in the keratin genes (*KRT5* and *KRT14*) with resultant formation of a cleavage plane at the level of the basal keratinocytes [17]. Localized

EBS (formerly known as Weber–Cockayne EBS), usually associated with little or no extracutaneous involvement, is the mildest and most common form of EBS. Nail dystrophy is rare and generally mild. Severe generalized EBS (formerly known as Dowling–Meara EBS) is the most severe form of EBS and presents with widespread friction-induced blistering at birth. Involvement of the oral mucosa and nail dystrophy are common. Generalized intermediate EBS (formerly known as Koebner EBS) may present at birth with blistering and possibly with milder clinical courses [18–21].

A retrospective review of EB cases diagnosed and evaluated at the Department of Pediatrics at Prince of Wales Hospital in Hong Kong was conducted [22]. There were only two cases of congenital EBS diagnosed over the past 20 years (1999 to 2019). Their demographic details, clinical presentation, histopathology findings, and genetics findings were reviewed. Genetic testing included a next generation sequencing (NGS) EB panel and Sanger sequencing technologies to cover the full coding regions and ~10 bp of noncoding DNA flanking region of each exon of the genes related to EB. Genomic DNA was extracted from the patient and parents' blood specimens. For NGS, patients' DNA was captured, and then sequenced using Illumina's Reversible Dye Terminator (RDT) platform. Sanger sequencing was used for parental sample testing. Ethics approval was obtained from the NTEC-Chinese University of Hong Kong Ethics Committee to review these cases, and consent was obtained from both families.

In this report, we describe two Hong Kong children with severe generalized EBS. The first case was due to a novel *de novo* heterozygous c.377T>G (NM_000526.5 (c.377T>G, p.Leu126Arg)) variant in the *KRT14* gene, and the second case was due to a rare *de novo* heterozygous c.527A>G (NM_000424.4, c.527A>G, p.Asn176Ser) variant in the *KRT5* gene. To our knowledge, the c.377T>G variant in the *KRT14* gene has not been reported previously, and the c.527A>G variant in the *KRT5* gene is a rare cause of generalized severe EBS.

2. Case Series

2.1. Case 1. A female neonate was born to non-consanguineous Southern Chinese parents at term following an uncomplicated pregnancy and normal spontaneous vaginal delivery. Her birth weight was 2.455 kg. She was noted to have extensive bullous lesions over the whole body and blisters in the buccal mucosa at birth. Dystrophic nail changes in the fingers and toes were also noted. There was no family history of bullous disease. A skin biopsy was performed. Attachment of the basement membrane to the blister roof could not be clearly determined by light microscopy. Electron microscopy revealed EBS characterized by a diffuse cytolysis in basal cells with intraepidermal cleavage.

NGS detected a novel *de novo* heterozygous c.377T>G variant in the *KRT14* gene that predicted to result in the amino acid substitution p.Leu126Arg (NM_000526.5 (c.377T>G, p.Leu126Arg)). No copy number variants were found in *KRT14*. She also had a novel *ITGB4* variant

(NM_000213.5 (c.3554A>G, p.Asn1185Ser)). Clinically, this patient did not have pyloric atresia. The asymptomatic father did not carry the same variants on *ITGB4* nor *KRT14* gene. Both her asymptomatic mother and elder brother carried the same *ITGB4* variant. This patient had recurrent crops of generalized bullous formation and significant failure to thrive. She had poor weight gain and frequent infections during the first few months of life. The condition of this patient was still very severe at follow-up at 9 months of age.

2.2. Case 2. A female neonate was born at term following an uncomplicated pregnancy and normal vaginal delivery with a birth weight of 2.3 kg. Parents were healthy non-consanguineous Southern Chinese. She had extensive bullae over the whole body from the skull to the soles at birth. There were blisters present in the oral mucous membranes. Dystrophic nail changes in the fingers and toes were also noted (Figure 1). There was no family history of bullous disease. Genetic testing confirmed a *de novo* heterozygous variant in *KRT5*, c.527A>G (NM_000424.4, c.527A>G, p.Asn176Ser). No copy number variants were found in *KRT5*. The patient had poor weight gain and recurrent bacterial infections which required treatment with antibiotics. New bullae continued to develop all over her body over the first few months of life (Figure 2). The function of her joints was not affected. With the molecular diagnosis, no skin biopsy was obtained from this patient. She was treated with special enriched milk to increase the caloric intake and supplemented with trace elements. The skin and nails were still severely affected in the first year of life, and the child received intensive care for the first 9 months of life.

3. Discussion

Severe generalized EBS is devastating both to patients and their families. Obstetricians and pediatricians must be familiar with the mode of inheritance, age-related morbidity, and mortality associated with this rare but severe disease in order to provide timely counseling on the natural history of the disease, recurrence risk, and reproductive options to the families. Histopathology and molecular studies play an important role in prognostication and counseling. NGS detected that the first patient had a *de novo* heterozygous novel c.377T>G variant in the *KRT14* gene (NM_000526.5 (c.377T>G, p.Leu126Arg)), which was predicted to result in the amino acid substitution p.Leu126Arg. This *KRT14* variant has not been reported in the literature and is not found in ExAC or 1000 genomes. The *in silico* prediction for this variant by SIFT and Polyphen-2 is damaging, and the amino acid residue is highly conserved across species. This variant is also predicted to be deleterious when analyzed by the Mutation Taster software (http://www.mutationtaster.org/). No copy number variants were found in the *KRT14* gene. She also had an *ITGB4* variant (NM_000213.5 (c.3554A>G, p.Asn1185Ser)), which has not been reported in the literature to date, and it was predicted to be of uncertain clinical significance according to American College of Medical Genetics and Genomics (ACMG) guidelines.

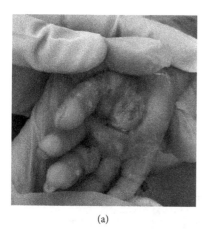
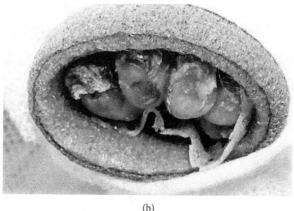

(a)   (b)

FIGURE 1: (a) Severely dystrophic fingernails of right hand and (b) toenails of the left foot wrapped in multiple layers of protective dressings.

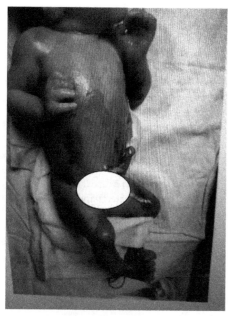

FIGURE 2: Severe generalized EBS with denuded skin following rupture of bullae involving the face, torso, and the limbs.

ITGB4 encodes for the hemidesmosomal protein integrin *β*4. Pathogenic variants in *ITGB4* may cause the rare subtype of EB with pyloric atresia (EB-PA). This patient did not exhibit pyloric atresia. Both her asymptomatic mother and elder brother carried the same *ITGB4* variant. These findings help narrow down the variant in *KRT14* variant as responsible for her EBS. Genetic information of the first case was especially relevant for counseling because two EB gene variants were present, one responsible for EBS while the other was deemed not relevant in this case. Precise genetic diagnosis is highly relevant for counseling in EBS, especially in a patient without a skin biopsy as is illustrated in the second case or if the skin biopsy result is ambiguous or inconclusive. *KRT5* c.527A>G (p.Asn176Ser) is a rare variant in individuals with sporadic EBS [23]. The prognosis of *KRT5* variants has been reported among Chinese and other Asian patients [23].

EBS is almost always inherited in an autosomal dominant fashion, although rare autosomal recessive forms have been reported [24]. *De novo* pathogenic variants in *KRT14* and *KRT5* genes account for the occurrence of severe generalized EBS in these two patients in the absence of a family history of EBS. One limitation of this study is that no screening was performed in these two cases for possible somatic or germline mosaicism in their parents. However, although somatic and germline mosaicism have been found to be the underlying cause in some seemingly sporadic cases thought to be caused by *de novo* pathogenic variants [25], another study has reported a high rate of 37% for *de novo* pathogenic variants in *KRT14* and *KRT5* [26]. The cause for the high percentage of *de novo* variants is not entirely clear, but highly mutable CpG dinucleotides have been found in some codons more frequently affected by these *de novo* variants in multiple families [26].

The genetics of EBS have been reported in Korean, Japanese, and Chinese patients, but not in patients from Hong Kong (Table 1) [18, 20, 28, 29]. The current report expands the molecular spectrum of EBS. Knowledge of the exact genetics of EBS helped in counseling the families regarding the prognosis of their affected children and recurrence risk for future pregnancies.

Unlike EBD and EBJ, EBS is usually a milder disease and not associated with high mortality [30]. Our two patients had severe generalized EBS based on the onset of the disease at birth, disseminated friction or trauma-induced blistering, involvement of oral mucosa, and presence of nail dystrophy. Despite these findings, symptoms observed in severe generalized EBS tend to improve with time [30]. The main causes of early morbidity and mortality in severe generalized EB are septicemia, malnutrition, and electrolyte disturbances [1–4]. Hence, skin care and nutrition support must be meticulous [31]. Malnutrition can be attributed to recurrent mucosal lesions, feeding difficulties, high energy consumption from accelerated skin turnover, transcutaneous loss of nutrients, and catabolic state from recurrent infections [22, 31]. It is therefore important to involve dietitians to prepare easy-to-consume recipes, identify high-caloric and protein-fortified foods and beverages to replace

TABLE 1: Genetics of Congenital EBS in selected Asian reports.

Ethnicity	Genetics [27]	Year of publication (reference number)
Southern Chinese (Hong Kong) $n = 2$	KRT14 (NM_000526.4 (c.377T>G, p.Leu126Arg)) KRT5 (NM_000424.3 (c.527A>G, p.Asn176Ser))	Present series
Japanese, $n = 16$	KRT 5 KRT14	2013 [18]
Chinese, $n = 1$	KRT5	2016 [20]
Korean, $n = 15$	KRT5 (p.Val143Phe, p.Arg265Pro, p.Cys479X, p.Asn177del, and p.Glu477Lys) KRT14 (p.Arg125Leu, p.Leu401Pro, and p.Arg125His)	2010 [28]
Chinese, $n = 2$ pedigrees	KRT5 (a heterozygous T>A transition at nucleotide 1730, changing phenylalanine (Phe) to tyrosine (Tyr) at position 577) KRT5 (two recurrent mutations c.1649delG (p.Gly550AlafsX77) and c.508G>(p.Glu170Lys in Chinese patients with mottled pigmentation EBS and localized EBS, respectively)	2009 [29]

protein lost in draining blisters, suggest vitamin and mineral nutritional supplements, and recommend dietary adjustments to prevent gastrointestinal problems, such as constipation, diarrhea, or painful defecation [4, 11, 12]. During hospitalization, the importance of adequate nutritional intake should be reinforced. When indicated, the option of gastrostomy should be discussed with the patient and his/her family for those patients who remain cachectic despite conservative measures.

4. Conclusion

Herein, we report two children with severe generalized EBS in Hong Kong. Severe generalized EBS is an inherited blistering skin disease associated with significant morbidity and mortality, and the prognosis is better with the autosomal dominant inherited or *de novo* EBS cases than in those with the rare autosomal recessive inherited EBS. The first case was due to a novel *de novo* heterozygous variant c.377T>G in *KRT14*, and the second case was due to a rare *de novo* heterozygous variant with c.527A>G in the *KRT5* gene. These molecular findings corroborate the elevated rate of seemingly *de novo* variants in *KRT5* and *KRT14* found in previous studies. Exact genetic diagnosis of severe generalized EBS aided in counseling the families concerning the prognosis of this disease in their affected children and the recurrence risk for future pregnancies. It would be most useful to establish a registry for EB in Hong Kong to evaluate the natural history of these disorders in order to facilitate patient management via a multidisciplinary team approach and facilitate novel therapeutic approaches such as gene therapy trials in the upcoming future.

References

[1] K. L. Hon, P. C. L. Choi, A. Burd, and N. M. Luk, "Epidermolysis bullosa dystrophica in a Chinese neonate," *Hong Kong Journal of Paediatrics*, vol. 12, no. 2, 2007.

[2] A. C. Fu, K. L. Hon, and P. C. Choi, "A neonate with generalised bullae and pyloric atresia," *Hong Kong Medical Journal*, vol. 19, no. 19, pp. 188–192, 2013.

[3] K. L. E. Hon, A. Burd, P. C. L. Choi, and N. M. T. Luk, "Epidermolysis bullosa in three Chinese neonates," *Journal of Dermatological Treatment*, vol. 18, no. 5, pp. 306–311, 2007.

[4] J.-D. Fine, R. A. J. Eady, E. A. Bauer et al., "The classification of inherited epidermolysis bullosa (EB): report of the third international consensus meeting on diagnosis and classification of EB," *Journal of the American Academy of Dermatology*, vol. 58, no. 6, pp. 931–950, 2008.

[5] S. C. Chong, K. L. Hon, L. Yuen, C. L. Choi, W. G. G. Ng, and T. Chiu, "Neonatal epidermolysis bullosa: lessons to learn about genetic counselling," *Journal of Dermatological Treatment*, vol. 29, pp. 1–14, 2018.

[6] L. R. A. Intong and D. F. Murrell, "Inherited epidermolysis bullosa: new diagnostic criteria and classification," *Clinics in Dermatology*, vol. 30, no. 1, pp. 70–77, 2012.

[7] C. H. Hsieh, C. J. Huang, and G. T. Lin, "Death from colonic disease in epidermolysis bullosa dystrophica," *BMC Dermatology*, vol. 6, no. 2, p. 2, 2006.

[8] G. A. Ergun, A. N. Lin, A. J. Dannenberg, and D. M. Carter, "Gastrointestinal manifestations of epidermolysis bullosa a study of 101 patients," *Medicine*, vol. 71, no. 3, pp. 121–127, 1992.

[9] R. A. J. Eady, "Epidermolysis bullosa: scientific advances and therapeutic challenges," *The Journal of Dermatology*, vol. 28, no. 11, pp. 638–640, 2001.

[10] C. Prodinger, J. Reichelt, J. W. Bauer, and M. Laimer, "Epidermolysis bullosa: advances in research and treatment," *Experimental Dermatology*, vol. 28, no. 10, pp. 1176–1189, 2019.

[11] J.-D. Fine, J. McGrath, and R. A. J. Eady, "Inherited epidermolysis bullosa comes into the new millenium: a revised classification system based on current knowledge of pathogenetic mechanisms and the clinical, laboratory, and epidemiologic findings of large, well-defined patient cohorts," *Journal of the American Academy of Dermatology*, vol. 43, no. 1, pp. 135–137, 2000.

[12] J.-D. Fine, R. A. J. Eady, E. A. Bauer et al., "Revised classification system for inherited epidermolysis bullosa," *Journal of the American Academy of Dermatology*, vol. 42, no. 6, pp. 1051–1066, 2000.

[13] E. B. Lane, E. L. Rugg, H. Navsaria et al., "A mutation in the conserved helix termination peptide of keratin 5 in hereditary skin blistering," *Nature*, vol. 356, no. 6366, pp. 244–246, 1992.

[14] J. Uitto, "Epidermolysis bullosa: diagnostic guidelines in the laboratory setting," *British Journal of Dermatology*, vol. 182, pp. 526-527, 2020.

[15] A. Nakano, S.-C. Chao, L. Pulkkinen et al., "Laminin 5 mutations in junctional epidermolysis bullosa: molecular basis of Herlitz vs non-Herlitz phenotypes," *Human Genetics*, vol. 110, no. 1, pp. 41-51, 2002.

[16] J. A. Sa'd, M. Indelman, E. Pfendner et al., "Molecular epidemiology of hereditary epidermolysis bullosa in a middle eastern population," *Journal of Investigative Dermatology*, vol. 126, no. 4, pp. 777-781, 2006.

[17] S. E. Sheppard, L. E. Anderson, C. Sibbald et al., "Generalized, severe epidermolysis bullosa simplex caused by a Keratin 5 p.E477K mutation," *Pediatric Dermatology*, vol. 36, no. 6, pp. 1007-1009, 2019.

[18] S. Minakawa, H. Nakano, K. Nakajima et al., "Mutational analysis on 16 Japanese population cases with epidermolysis bullosa simplex," *Journal of Dermatological Science*, vol. 72, no. 3, pp. 330-332, 2013.

[19] H. M. Horn and M. J. Tidman, "The clinical spectrum of epidermolysis bullosa simplex," *British Journal of Dermatology*, vol. 142, no. 3, pp. 468-472, 2000.

[20] J. Zhang, M. Yan, J. Liang, M. Li, and Z. Yao, "A novel KRT5 mutation associated with generalized severe epidermolysis bullosa simplex in a 2-year-old Chinese boy," *Experimental and Therapeutic Medicine*, vol. 12, no. 5, pp. 2823-2826, 2016.

[21] Y. C. Kho, L. M. Rhodes, S. J. Robertson et al., "Epidemiology of epidermolysis bullosa in the antipodes: the Australasian Epidermolysis Bullosa Registry with a focus on Herlitz junctional epidermolysis bullosa," *Archives of Dermatology*, vol. 146, no. 6, pp. 635-640, 2010.

[22] K. L. Hon, J. J. Li, B. L. Cheng et al., "Age and etiology of childhood epidermolysis bullosa mortality," *Journal of Dermatological Treatment*, vol. 26, no. 2, pp. 1-5, 2014.

[23] K. Stephens, P. Ehrlich, M. Weaver, R. Le, A. Spencer, and V. P. Sybert, "Primers for exon-specific amplification of the KRT5 gene: identification of novel and recurrent mutations in epidermolysis bullosa simplex patients," *Journal of Investigative Dermatology*, vol. 108, no. 3, pp. 349-353, 1997.

[24] P. Khani, F. Ghazi, A. Zekri et al., "Keratins and epidermolysis bullosa simplex," *Journal of Cellular Physiology*, vol. 234, no. 1, pp. 289-297, 2018.

[25] M. Nagao-Watanabe, T. Fukao, E. Matsui et al., "Identification of somatic and germline mosaicism for a keratin 5 mutation in epidermolysis bullosa simplex in a family of which the proband was previously regarded as a sporadic case," *Clinical Genetics*, vol. 66, no. 3, pp. 236-238, 2004 Sep.

[26] M. C. Bolling, H. H. Lemmink, G. H. L. Jansen, and M. F. Jonkman, "Mutations in KRT5 and KRT14 cause epidermolysis bullosa simplex in 75% of the patients," *British Journal of Dermatology*, vol. 164, no. 3, pp. 637-644, 2011.

[27] J. T. den Dunnen, R. Dalgleish, D. R. Maglott et al., "HGVS recommendations for the description of sequence variants: 2016 update," *Human Mutation*, vol. 37, no. 6, pp. 564-569, 2016.

[28] T. W. Kang, J. S. Lee, S. E. Kim, S. W. Oh, and S. C. Kim, "Novel and recurrent mutations in Keratin 5 and 14 in Korean patients with Epidermolysis bullosa simplex," *Journal of Dermatological Science*, vol. 57, no. 2, pp. 90-94, 2010.

[29] H. Y. Tang, W. D. Du, Y. Cui et al., "One novel and two recurrent mutations in the keratin 5 gene identified in Chinese patients with epidermolysis bullosa simplex," *Clinical and Experimental Dermatology*, vol. 34, no. 8, pp. e957-e961, 2009.

[30] E. Kim, A. Harris, L. Bingham, W. Yan, J. Su, and D. Murrell, "A review of 52 pedigrees with epidermolysis bullosa simplex identifying ten novel mutations in KRT5 and KRT14 in Australia," *Acta Dermato Venereologica*, vol. 97, no. 9, pp. 1114-1119, 2017.

[31] S. Allman, L. Haynes, P. MacKinnon, and D. J. Atherton, "Nutrition in dystrophic epidermolysis bullosa," *Pediatric Dermatology*, vol. 9, no. 3, pp. 231-238, 1992.

40

Torticollis as Presentation for Atypical Kawasaki Disease Complicated by Giant Coronary Artery Aneurysms

Tracey Dyer ⓘ, Paul Dancey ⓘ, John Martin, and Suryakant Shah

Department of Pediatrics, Memorial University, 300 Prince Phillip Drive, St. John's, NL, Canada A1B 3V6

Correspondence should be addressed to Tracey Dyer; a35tmd@mun.ca

Academic Editor: Junji Takaya

Kawasaki disease (KD) is an acute systemic vasculitis of childhood. The diagnosis can be made in a patient who presents with a prolonged high fever and meeting at least four of five criteria including polymorphous rash, mucosal changes, extremity changes (including swelling and/or palmar and plantar erythema), bilateral nonsuppurative conjunctivitis, and unilateral cervical lymphadenopathy. Atypical KD refers to patients who have not met the full criteria and in whom atypical features may be present. We discuss a case of a 6-year-old male who presented to the Emergency Department with torticollis. A series of investigations for elevated inflammatory markers revealed dilated coronary artery aneurysms on echocardiogram, and thus he was diagnosed with atypical KD. His only other criteria were bilateral nonsuppurative conjunctivitis and a prior brief febrile illness. He was treated with high-dose intravenous immune globulin (IVIG) and low-dose aspirin. Low-molecular-weight heparin and atenolol were added due to the presence of giant aneurysms.

1. Introduction

Kawasaki disease (KD) is an acute systemic vasculitis of childhood diagnosed by high fever for 5 days accompanied by at least four of the following symptoms: polymorphous rash, mucosal changes (including dry, cracked lips and strawberry tongue), extremity changes (including palmar and/or plantar erythema, swelling, and desquamation), bilateral nonsuppurative conjunctivitis, and cervical lymphadenopathy [1]. It is the second most common vasculitis of childhood with a peak age of 2-3 years and rarely seen above the age of 7 years. KD is now the most common cause of acquired heart disease in children in developed countries [2]. Atypical KD refers to patients who have not met the full criteria and in whom atypical features may be present [3]. Risk factors for development of coronary artery aneurysms with KD include prolonged fever, prolonged elevation of inflammatory markers, age younger than 1 year or older than 6 years at onset, and male gender [1]. KD is treated with aspirin and intravenous immune globulin (IVIG) which reduces the incidence of coronary artery involvement from approximately 25% to less than 4% [4].

2. Case Presentation

A previously healthy 6-year-old boy presented to a pediatric hospital with a 3-week history of torticollis. He had symptoms of an upper respiratory tract infection four weeks prior and had 2 days of documented fever at home during that time. He had been treated with a 7-day course of amoxicillin by the primary care physician for suspected streptococcal pharyngitis. Four days into the course of antibiotics, he woke up from sleep with pain on the left side of his neck. Despite taking ibuprofen and acetaminophen, he presented to the Emergency Department 3 weeks later due to persisting torticollis. Pain was worse with movement. There was no history of head/neck trauma. At the time of presentation, the infectious symptoms had resolved. Some fatigue was noted but he remained generally active, continuing to play hockey. There was no history of rash, peripheral joint pain, or weight loss. Past medical history and family history were unremarkable.

On examination, the patient was afebrile with normal blood pressure for age and a maximum heart rate of 110 beats per minute. The patient's head was tilted to the right with chin rotation to the left. No lymphadenopathy or masses were noted on palpation of the neck. There was no tenderness to palpation of bilateral sternocleidomastoid muscles. There was a limited range of motion in all planes of rotation of the neck secondary to pain, particularly in lateral flexion. Bilateral injected conjunctivas were present. The oropharynx was normal with no erythema or mucus membrane changes. Cardiovascular exam revealed normal peripheral pulses, a quiet precordium with normal heart sounds, and no murmur. Respiratory exam was normal. The abdomen was soft with no distension, tenderness, or hepatosplenomegaly. There were no bruits heard on auscultation of major vessel regions. There were no rashes or desquamation of the skin. Neurological exam was normal.

At the time of presentation, laboratory investigations revealed an elevated white blood cell count of 17.4×10^9/L with a neutrophil count of 14.1×10^9/L. Hemoglobin was normal for age at 110 g/L. Inflammatory markers were elevated including platelet count of 860×10^9/L and CRP of 38.5 mg/L. Renal function (BUN and creatinine) and liver function (ALP and ALT) were normal for age. Because of the unexplained elevated white blood cell count and evidence of inflammation, a chest X-ray was performed which revealed normal lung fields but an enlarged cardiac silhouette. X-ray of the cervical spine was normal with no atlantoaxial rotary subluxation demonstrated. Ultrasound of the neck revealed mild thickening of the left sternocleidomastoid muscle and no lymphadenopathy. Abdominal ultrasound with Doppler was normal.

Additional investigations included a normal throat swab for group A streptococci and a negative anti-streptolysin O antibody titer. High-sensitivity troponin was elevated to 176 ng/L. Creatinine kinase was normal. ANCA was normal. Electrocardiogram showed normal sinus rhythms without evidence of chamber hypertrophy. The patient underwent an echocardiogram to further characterize the enlarged cardiac silhouette identified on the chest X-ray. This revealed massive ectasia and aneurysmal dilatation of the right coronary artery, left main artery, left anterior descending artery, and circumflex arteries, as seen in Figure 1. Left ventricular function was normal. The aortic arch was normal as were the proximal neck vessels.

Because of the dilated coronary aneurysms, the patient was diagnosed with KD. Despite lack of fever, given the evidence of ongoing inflammation and initial presence of bilateral nonsuppurative conjunctivitis, in addition to the coronary artery changes, the patient was treated with high-dose IVIG (2 g/kg) and started on daily low-dose aspirin. Low-molecular-weight heparin was started as antithrombotic therapy and once stabilized, daily atenolol was initiated. Activity was restricted as much as possible.

Inflammatory markers were followed. Platelets revealed a peak of 952×10^9/L and CRP a peak of 54.6 mg/L. After treatment, both platelet and CRP levels normalized.

The patient's neck pain and the limited range of movement resolved immediately after treatment, as did the

bilateral conjunctivitis. The patient was stable and appeared well at time of discharge. His aspirin, low-molecular-weight heparin, and atenolol were continued. The CT angiogram performed after discharge revealed massively dilated and aneurysmal coronary arteries, as shown in Figure 2.

In follow-up cardiology and rheumatology clinics, he has been doing well with no further neck pain or stiffness. He did not develop desquamation during follow-up, and the repeat echocardiogram one month after discharge was unchanged. He will continue long-term anticoagulation therapy with low-dose heparin with a target level greater than 0.5 IU/ml. He will also continue low dose aspirin and atenolol. His family was advised to have the annual influenza vaccine.

3. Discussion

Our patient was diagnosed with KD after dilated coronary artery aneurysms were found on the echocardiogram. He had a history of fever for two days that occurred three weeks prior to presentation, and no further fevers were documented or recognized by his parents. The only criteria of KD met on history and examination at presentation was bilateral nonsuppurative conjunctivitis. Blood work did reveal evidence of ongoing inflammation. Risk factors for KD with coronary involvement were male gender and a delayed presentation prior to diagnosis. It is possible that he had fever longer than the reported two days as the parents had not measured it regularly at home. Presumably, the inflammatory markers had been elevated for up to three weeks prior to diagnosis; however, no blood work had been performed during the initial febrile period.

Although unusual, there have been several reports in the literature of KD presenting as torticollis or neck tilt. Different pathophysiologies have been described including KD associated with Grisel's syndrome, a rare, nontraumatic atlantoaxial subluxation [5]; KD with retropharyngeal edema and arthritis of the small joints in the head and neck region [6]; and KD with severe cervical spine and bilateral temporomandibular joint arthritis [7]. Our patient did not have any other signs of arthritis, and there was no cervical lymphadenopathy to explain the torticollis. During the admission, an X-ray of the cervical spine and ultrasound of the neck did not reveal any underlying pathology. The torticollis resolved after treatment with IVIG and aspirin and did not recur.

Despite giant coronary aneurysms, our patient has remained well since discharge from hospital and is closely followed by Cardiology and Rheumatology. He has had no further neck pain or stiffness and has not developed any further symptoms including desquamation or arthritis. Repeat echocardiograms have remained stable. He will require long-term anticoagulation therapy.

Our patient was brought to medical attention due to his torticollis. While the exact reason for the torticollis is unclear, we feel it is important to raise the awareness of this rare

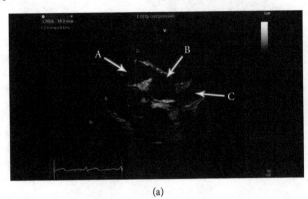
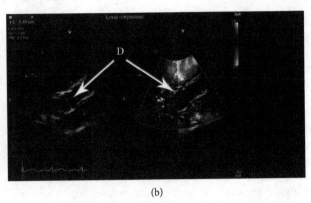

(a)

(b)

Figure 1: Echocardiogram: (a) Massive ectasia and aneurysmal dilatation of the right coronary artery (16 mm × 17 mm) (A), aorta (B), and left coronary artery (C). (b) Massive ectasia and aneurysmal dilatation of left main artery (13 mm × 13 mm) (D).

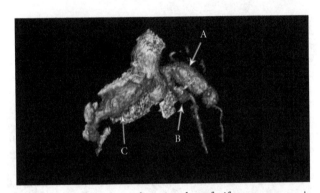

Figure 2: CT angiogram: there is a long fusiform aneurysm involving the proximal LAD measuring approximately 12 mm × 12 mm and extending over a length of 2.3 cm (A). The left circumflex is aneurysmal proximally measuring approximately 5 mm × 5.5 mm (B). There is a long fusiform aneurysm of right coronary artery measuring 16 mm × 16 mm and extending over a length of at least 3.2 cm (C).

Consent

Written consent was obtained.

References

[1] W. E. Nelson, K. J. Marcdante, and R. M. Kliegman, *Nelson Essentials of Pediatrics*, Elsevier Saunders, Philadelphia, PA, USA, 2015.

[2] B. W. Mccrindle, A. H. Rowley, J. W. Newburger et al., "Diagnosis, treatment, and long-term management of Kawasaki disease: a scientific statement for health professionals from the american heart association," *Circulation*, vol. 135, no. 17, pp. e927–e999, 2017.

[3] R. E. Petty, R. M. Laxer, C. B. Lindsley, and L. Wedderburn, *Textbook of Pediatric Rheumatology*, Elsevier, New York, NY, USA, 2016.

[4] J. W. Newburger, M. Takahashi, A. S. Beiser et al., "A single intravenous infusion of gamma globulin as compared with four infusions in the treatment of acute Kawasaki syndrome," *New England Journal of Medicine*, vol. 324, no. 23, pp. 1633–1639, 1991.

[5] F. Nozaki, T. Kusunoki, Y. Tomoda et al., "Grisel syndrome as a complication of Kawasaki disease: a case report and review of the literature," *European Journal of Pediatrics*, vol. 172, no. 1, pp. 119–121, 2012.

[6] L. Puhakka, R. Saat, T. Klockars, L. Kajosaari, E. Salo, and T. Nieminen, "Retropharyngeal involvement in Kawasaki disease—a report of four patients with retropharyngeal edema verified by magnetic resonance imaging," *International Journal of Pediatric Otorhinolaryngology*, vol. 78, no. 10, pp. 1774–1778, 2014.

[7] M. Jen, L. A. Brucia, A. N. Pollock, and J. M. Burnham, "Cervical spine and temporomandibular joint arthritis in a child with Kawasaki disease," *Pediatrics*, vol. 118, no. 5, pp. e1569–e1571, 2006.

41

Tubular Dysfunction and Ruptured Ureter in a Child with Menkes Syndrome

Wun Fung Hui ⓘ,[1] Kam Lun Hon ⓘ,[1] Alexander K. C. Leung ⓘ,[2] Kristine Kit Yi Pang,[3] and Michael Wai Yip Leung[3]

[1]*Department of Paediatrics and Adolescent Medicine, The Hong Kong Children's Hospital, Kowloon, Hong Kong*
[2]*Department of Paediatrics, The University of Calgary and Pediatric Consultant at The Alberta Children's Hospital, T2M 0H5, Calgary, Alberta, Canada*
[3]*Department of Surgery, The Hong Kong Children's Hospital, Kowloon, Hong Kong*

Correspondence should be addressed to Kam Lun Hon; ehon@hotmail.com

Pannee Visrutaratna

Children with Menkes disease may develop various urological and renal problems that evolve as the disease progresses. A 4-year-old boy with Menkes disease had multiple bladder diverticula and a history of recurrent urinary tract infection caused by urea-splitting organisms. The child developed urosepsis and right pyelonephritis. Subsequent investigations revealed multiple right renal stones and a ruptured right ureter. The child also developed hypokalemia, hypophosphatemia, and normal anion gap metabolic acidosis that required electrolyte and potassium citrate supplement. Further assessment revealed renal tubular dysfunction. Our case suggests that regular imaging surveillance, monitoring of renal function and electrolyte profile, and tubular function assessment should be considered in children with Menkes disease.

1. Introduction

Menkes syndrome, also known as Menkes kinky hair syndrome, is a rare X-linked recessive disease caused by mutation of the *ATP7A* gene. The gene encodes a transmembrane copper-transporting P-type ATPase; mutation of the gene may lead to impaired copper metabolism. Most patients have severe developmental delay, seizures, failure to thrive, and connective tissue abnormality resulting in blood vessel tortuosity and the characteristic kinky hair [1]. Besides, urological abnormalities and related complications such as recurrent urinary tract infection may also be encountered [2, 3]. We report a 4-year-old boy with Menkes disease who presented with urosepsis, and subsequent workup identified a ruptured right ureter resulting from a ureteric stone. The child was also found to have multiple bladder diverticula and tubular dysfunction; the latter led to multiple electrolyte disturbances. Our case illustrated that uncommon urological and renal complications may develop in children with Menkes disease.

2. Case History

A 4-year-old boy with Menkes disease was admitted for increased abdominal distension and discomfort for two days associated with reduced oral intake. There was no vomiting, and his urine output and urine appearance were normal. He also developed fever and dyspnea for one day.

During infancy, the child was suspected to have Menkes disease due to fair skin, sparse, kinky, unruly, and steely gray-colored hair, failure to thrive, seizures, and developmental delay. The diagnosis was confirmed at 5 months of age by genetic analysis which showed a *de novo* pathogenic mutation of the *ATP7A* gene. He had been given copper-histidine injection since 8 months of age. He had a gastrostomy with fundoplication performed at 2 years of age and had intractable chronic diarrhea. The child had several episodes of urinary tract infections (UTIs) caused by *Klebsiella* and *Proteus* species since one year of age. An ultrasound of the urinary system at 14 months of age revealed normal kidneys, diffuse urinary bladder wall thickening, and bladder diverticula. There was no ureterocele. The child was found to have a neurogenic bladder with poor bladder emptying, requiring regular intermittent catheterization of the bladder since 19 months of age. The frequency of UTI significantly reduced thereafter, and he was given trimethoprim prophylaxis till 29 months of age. The initial micturating cystourethrogram (MCUG) and DMSA appointments were defaulted. Urodynamic study was unfortunately not performed, and there was no regular imaging surveillance of the urinary system.

Physical examination on admission showed stable vital signs, and his temperature was 36.2°C. The hydration status was satisfactory. The abdomen was distended, and there was generalized tenderness. Investigations showed hemoglobin 8.5 g/dL, white blood cell count 8.97×10^9/L, and platelet count 179×10^9/L. The child was found to have stage 1 acute kidney injury with urea and creatinine levels raised to 11 mmol/L and 47 umol/L, respectively (baseline creatinine level: 25 umol/L). The electrolyte profile showed serum sodium 137 mmol/L, potassium 3.4 mmol/L, chloride 106 mmol/L, calcium 2.74 mmol/L, and phosphate 0.89 mmol/L. There was also normal anion gap metabolic acidosis with venous blood gas showing pH of 7.31, bicarbonate of 14.5 mmol/L, base excess of −10.2 mmol/L, and a calculated anion gap of 16.5 mmol/L. The C-reactive protein was also raised to 212 mg/L. The child was empirically started on intravenous Augmentin after sepsis workup.

An urgent CT abdomen and pelvis showed diminished right kidney parenchymal enhancement, multiple right kidney and pelvis stones up to 1.5 cm in size, and a right mid-ureteric stone of 0.5 cm with proximal hydroureteronephrosis. A focal wall defect was noted at the posterior aspect of the proximal ureter with contrast extravasation resulting in contrast accumulation around the ureter and in the retroperitoneal space suggestive of a ruptured proximal ureter with urinary leakage (Figure 1). There were multiple bladder diverticula and bladder stones.

The child evolved to develop thrombocytopenia and mildly deranged clotting profile suggestive of disseminated intravascular coagulation. The clinical diagnosis was pyelonephritis and urosepsis complicated with multiple renal stones and ureteric rupture, together with a normal anion gap metabolic acidosis. An emergency operation was then arranged. Intraoperative cystoscopy found stone debris with turbid urine inside the bladder. Multiple bladder diverticula were identified with the left ureteral orifice buried inside a diverticulum, and the right ureteral orifice was not identified. A right percutaneous nephrostomy was performed. The child was then transferred to pediatric intensive care unit for further management.

The urinary drainage was satisfactory after the operation. The blood culture isolated non-typhoidal *Salmonella* Group B. Urinary culture from both the percutaneous nephrostomy, and bladder catheterization identified multiple bacterial species including *Proteus mirabilis*, *Klebsiella pneumoniae*, *Escherichia coli*, *Salmonella* Group B, *Morganella morganii*, and *Streptococcus anginosus*. The antibiotics were later switched to meropenem according to the sensitivity profile.

The patient developed hypokalemia and hypophosphatemia with diuresis requiring electrolyte replacement. The metabolic acidosis also persisted. The acute kidney injury resolved with creatinine returning to baseline levels. Further metabolic and renal tubular function workup was then performed for the renal stone and multiple electrolyte disturbances, and the results revealed tubular dysfunction (Table 1). Because of the active urosepsis, an ammonium chloride loading test was not performed.

He was initially given bicarbonate infusion followed by oral potassium citrate supplement to keep the urine pH > 7.0 and serum bicarbonate level >20 mmol/L. Phosphate supplement was also required to maintain a normal serum phosphate level. Adequate fluid was administered, and a total course of 4-week antibiotics was given. After a thorough discussion, parents agreed for further definitive treatment regarding the urological problem. Right pyeloplasty was then performed 6 weeks later by dividing the ureter proximally at the ureteropelvic junction and distally below the ureteric stricture followed by a ureteropelvic anastomosis, and the stones over the right renal pelvis were also removed. The ureteric stricture that was secondary to ureteric rupture was surrounded by thick fibrotic tissue and attached firmly to the retroperitoneal space. A J-J stent was inserted into the right ureter. Analysis of the right ureteric stone showed 98% carbonate apatite and 2% calcium oxalate monohydrate.

3. Discussion

Children with Menkes disease may develop various urological abnormalities, and bladder diverticulum is the most frequently reported one, with a reported prevalence ranging from 36.8% to 57.1% [2, 3]. Lysyl oxidase is a copper-dependent and elastic-fiber-associated coenzyme responsible for lysine-derived cross-linking of collagen and elastin in connective tissue. The function of lysyl oxidase is defective in patients with Menkes syndrome, which leads to connective tissue abnormality including the formation of multiple bladder diverticula [3, 4]. This may lead to neurogenic bladder with urinary stasis, incomplete bladder emptying, and recurrent UTI as illustrated in our patient, which are risk factors for development of pyelonephritis and chronic kidney disease.

Our patient had a ruptured ureter, which is a rare complication of ureteric stone. It may potentially lead to urinoma, retroperitoneal abscess, and urosepsis [5]. Most of the reported cases are associated with ureteric stones [6, 7], and rarely bladder outlet obstruction [8] or connective tissue abnormality [9]. All these risk factors were present in our patient. Hence, the ureteric rupture in our patient could possibly be explained by the formation of urinary tract stones due to recurrent UTI by urea-splitting organisms, together with other predisposing urological or systemic factors.

Given the high incidence of urological abnormalities with their complications in children with Menkes disease, renal system imaging surveillance such as regular ultrasound of the urinary system should be considered to identify and

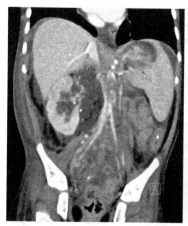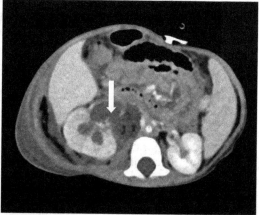

FIGURE 1: CT image showing rupture of the right ureter. A focal wall defect was noted at the posterior aspect of the right proximal ureter, just distal to the right ureteropelvic junction (arrow) with adjacent fluid surrounding the ureter.

TABLE 1: Urinary indices of tubular function assessment.

Urinary indices	Value
Urine pH	6.5
Urine anion gap	10
Urine beta-2-microglobulin (ug/ml) (normal: <0.2 ug/ml)	65.1
Aminoaciduria (%)*	100%
Urine potassium-creatine ratio (mmol/mmol Cr)	18.0
Transtubular potassium gradient	8.0
24-hour urinary calcium (mmol/kg/day) (renal wasting: >0.1 mmol/kg/day)	0.15
Tubular maximum phosphate reabsorption (renal wasting: <1.15)	0.38
Tubular reabsorption of phosphate (%) (renal wasting: <85%)	24.4%
24-hour urinary magnesium (mmol/day) (renal wasting: >1 mmol/day)	0.28
24-hour urinary uric acid (mmol/day) (normal: 1.2–5.9)	1.0

*Expressed as percentage of types of amino acids with measured values exceeding the upper limit of normal range. Tubular dysfunction was suggested by the presence of β-2-microglobulinuria, generalized aminoaciduria, and urinary electrolyte wasting. The chronic diarrhea in our patient confounded the interpretation of urine anion gap.

monitor the progression of any urological abnormalities and to detect stone formation. More invasive investigations such as MCUG or cystoscopy may be considered on an individual basis. There is currently no consensus on how to investigate and manage the urological abnormalities among children with Menkes disease. A thorough discussion among the medical team and parents should be encouraged as Menkes disease is considered a life-limiting condition and parents may opt not to perform invasive investigations as in our present case.

Our patient also had tubular dysfunction with pattern of both proximal and distal tubular involvement. Traditionally, urine anion gap is used to differentiate between patients with proximal or distal renal tubular acidosis. However, our patient's chronic diarrhea confounded the results of urinary anion gap, making it difficult for interpretation. In the present case, tubular dysfunction was suggested by the presence of β-2-microglobulinuria, generalized aminoaciduria, and urinary electrolyte wasting. Tubular dysfunction in Menkes disease is not well studied compared to Wilson's disease, another disorder of copper metabolism. Previous reports showed conflicting results regarding the tubular

function assessment in patients with Menkes disease [10, 11]. Urinary β-2-microglobulin level has been used as a marker for copper-histidine therapy-associated proximal tubular dysfunction among children with Menkes disease [12]. Although copper deposition has been demonstrated in the proximal renal tubules among patients with Menkes disease receiving copper-histidine treatment [13], there were also reports describing tubular dysfunction in children not given copper-histidine therapy [10]. Ozawa et al. reported the results of serial renal function assessment on three patients with Menkes disease that were given copper-histidine therapy, and one of them showed an elevated pretreatment urinary β-2-microglobulin level [10]. Interestingly, the urinary β-2-microglobulin level increased in all three of them as the patient grew older. It is still not certain whether tubular dysfunction is purely a clinical manifestation of children with Menkes disease or a consequence of copper-histidine therapy. Currently, there are no longitudinal data on the evolution of tubular dysfunction among children with Menkes disease and its relation to the administration of copper-histidine therapy. However, the results of our patient suggest that regular monitoring of renal function and electrolyte profile with tubular function assessment may be required in children diagnosed with Menkes disease, especially for those who have been given copper-histidine therapy.

4. Conclusion

Menkes disease is a multisystem disorder caused by defective copper metabolism. Urological abnormality is not uncommon, which may lead to rare complications such as a ruptured ureter. In addition, tubular dysfunction may also be encountered leading to electrolyte and acid-base disturbances. Hence, regular imaging surveillance of the urinary system, monitoring of renal function and electrolyte profile, and renal tubular function assessment may be needed in these patients.

References

[1] L. B. Møller, M. Mogensen, and N. Horn, "Molecular diagnosis of Menkes disease: genotype-phenotype correlation," *Biochimie*, vol. 10, pp. 1273–1277, 2009.

[2] M. Y. Kim, J. H. Kim, M. H. Cho et al., "Urological problems in patients with Menkes disease," *Journal of Korean Medical Science*, vol. 34, no. 1, p. e4, 2018.

[3] M. Zaffanello, C. Maffeis, V. Fanos, M. Franchini, and G. Zamboni, "Urological complications and copper replacement therapy in childhood Menkes syndrome," *Acta Paediatrica*, vol. 95, no. 7, pp. 785–790, 2006.

[4] P. M. Royce and B. Steinmann, "Markedly reduced activity of lysyl oxidase in skin and aorta from a patient with Menkes' disease showing unusually severe connective tissue Manifestations1," *Pediatric Research*, vol. 28, no. 2, pp. 137–141, 1990.

[5] A. Eken, T. Akbas, and T. Arpaci, "Residency programs in colon and rectal surgery," *Diseases of the Colon & Rectum*, vol. 58, no. 2, pp. e29–e31, 2015.

[6] S. Koga, Y. Arakaki, M. Matsuoka, and C. Ohyama, "Spontaneous peripelvic extravasation of urine," *International Urology and Nephrology*, vol. 24, no. 5, pp. 465–469, 1992.

[7] K. Stravodimos, I. Adamakis, G. Koutalellis et al., "Spontaneous perforation of the ureter: clinical presentation and endourologic management," *Journal of Endourology*, vol. 22, no. 3, pp. 479–484, 2008.

[8] H. Akpinar, A. R. Kural, İ. Tüfek et al., "Spontaneous ureteral rupture: is immediate surgical intervention always necessary? Presentation of four cases and review of the literature," *Journal of Endourology*, vol. 16, no. 3, pp. 179–183, 2002.

[9] S. Reva and Y. Tolkach, "Spontaneous pelvic rupture as a result of renal colic in a patient with klinefelter syndrome," *Case reports in urology*, vol. 2013, p. 374973, 2013.

[10] H. Ozawa, H. Kodama, H. Kawaguchi, T. Mochizuki, M. Kobayashi, and T. Igarashi, "Renal function in patients with Menkes disease," *European Journal of Pediatrics*, vol. 162, no. 1, pp. 51-52, 2003 Jan.

[11] H. Kodama, I. Okabe, A. Kihara, Y. Mori, and M. Okaniwa, "Renal tubular function of patients with classical Menkes disease," *Journal of Inherited Metabolic Disease*, vol. 15, no. 1, pp. 157-158, 1992.

[12] S. G. Kaler, C. S. Holmes, D. S. Goldstein et al., "Neonatal diagnosis and treatment of Menkes disease," *New England Journal of Medicine*, vol. 358, no. 6, pp. 605–614, 2008.

[13] M. Kinebuchi, A. Matsuura, T. Kiyono, Y. Nomura, and S. Kimura, "Diagnostic copper imaging of Menkes disease by synchrotron radiation-generated X-ray fluorescence analysis," *Scientific Reports*, vol. 6, no. 1, Article ID 33247, 2016.

42

Pseudohypertriglyceridemia: A Novel Case with Important Clinical Implications

Ankur Rughani (ID),[1] **Kenneth Blick,**[2] **Hui Pang,**[3] **Monica Marin,**[1] **Jonathan Meyer,**[1] **and Jeanie B. Tryggestad**[1]

[1]*Department of Pediatrics, Section of Diabetes and Endocrinology, University of Oklahoma Health Sciences Center, Oklahoma City, Okla, USA*
[2]*Department of Pathology, University of Oklahoma Health Sciences Center, Oklahoma City, Okla, USA*
[3]*Department of Pediatrics, Section of Genetics, University of Oklahoma Health Sciences Center, Oklahoma City, Okla, USA*

Correspondence should be addressed to Ankur Rughani; ankur-rughani@ouhsc.edu

Academic Editor: Gulay Karagüzel

Pseudohypertriglyceridemia is an overestimation of serum triglyceride levels that may incorrectly lead to a diagnosis of hypertriglyceridemia. Glycerol kinase deficiency is a condition in which glycerol cannot be phosphorylated to glycerol-3-phosphate, resulting in elevated levels of serum glycerol. Laboratory assays that measure triglycerides indirectly may be affected by elevated glyerol levels and incorrectly report serum tryglyceride levels. We present a case of a novel missense mutation in the *GK* gene leading to isolated glycerol kinase deficiency and pseudohypertriglyceridemia in a male infant of a mother with gestational diabetes. This paper reviews glycerol kinase deficiency, describes the challenges in diagnosing pseudohypertriglyceridemia, and provides suggestions on improving diagnostic accuracy. Additionally, a potential maternal-fetal interaction between gestational diabetes and glycerol kinase deficiency is discussed.

1. Introduction

Pseudohypertriglyceridemia is an overestimation of serum triglyceride levels due to laboratory assays that measure free glycerol concentrations instead of triglycerides directly [1]. Specifically, laboratory assays commonly used today rely on microbial lipase enzymes to hydrolyze triglycerides into free fatty acids and glycerol, followed by enzymatic quantitation and therefore measure monoglycerides, diglycerides, triglycerides, and free glycerol [2]. Chemical methods used in the past to measure triglycerides directly by separating phospholipids from glycerol are too labor-intensive for automated commercial laboratories [3]. Consequently, conditions presenting with elevated levels of endogenous or exogenous free glycerol, such as glycerol kinase deficiency, result in an overestimation of serum triglycerides. While triglycerides are an important marker of metabolism, cardiovascular, and pancreatic health, overestimation of the triglyceride levels can lead to inappropriate and futile medical therapy which unnecessarily attempts

to lower triglyceride levels in efforts to reduce the risk of cardiometabolic disease [4].

Glycerol kinase deficiency (GKD) is a rare X-linked recessive condition due to a mutation in the *GK* gene, which is found on the short (*p*) arm of chromosome X at position 21.2 [5]. The mutation leads to a condition in which glycerol cannot be phosphorylated to glycerol-3-phosphate and, therefore, cannot be used as a substrate in gluconeogenesis [6]. Glycerol blanking has occasionally been used to control the overestimation of triglycerides, but this method is not always available [7].

2. Case Presentation

The subject was a term male infant born to a previously healthy mother with gestational diabetes mellitus (GDM) requiring insulin (type A2). He was admitted to the NICU for hypoxic ischemic encephalopathy secondary to meconium aspiration. He was born at the 41st week of gestation by emergency Caesarean section for non-reassuring fetal heart pattern after failed induction. APGAR scores after birth were 2 at 1 minute of life, 6 at 5 minutes of life, and 7 at 10 minutes of life. The infant was intubated at 10 minutes of life due to severe respiratory distress as a result of severe pulmonary hypertension and underwent therapeutic hypothermia for 3 days. On physical examination, the infant's birth weight was 5430 grams (WHO Z-score +3.6, large for gestational age), and he did not have any dysmorphic features, midline defects, or organomegaly. His neurologic exam was remarkable for mild hypotonia and several beat clonus at the ankles. The infant received total parenteral nutrition for 17 days, including intralipids for the first 7 days. Routine laboratory tests incidentally noted elevated triglycerides (961 mg/dL) on day of life 7, after which intralipids were discontinued. His lipid panel was otherwise unremarkable given his age: total cholesterol was 69 mg/dL, non-HDL cholesterol was 44 mg/dL, and HDL cholesterol was 28 mg/dL. The rest of his workup, including electrolytes, glucose, liver function, thyroid function, and essential fatty acids, were within normal limits for age. The newborn screens at 24 hours and 2 weeks of life were normal. Posthypothermia MRI of the brain was unremarkable. Ophthalmic exam was significant for bilateral foveal hemorrhages but negative for lipemia retinalis. No fat necrosis was identified. The infant received a gastrostomy tube due to poor oral intake. There was no known family history of dyslipidemia.

The infant was transitioned from parenteral to enteral nutrition with high medium-chain triglycerides (MCT) formula. He was initially on casein-based formula with 55% MCT and then placed on casein-based formula with 84% MCT. However, serum triglycerides remained relatively unchanged despite changes in formula, persisting between 900 mg/dL and 1280 mg/dL. Sequencing of genes associated with chylomicronemia (APPL1, BLK, CEL, GCK, HNF1A, HNF1B, HNF4A, INS, KCNJ11, KLF11, NEUROD1, PAX4, PDX1, APOA5, APOC2, GPIHBP1, LMF1, and LPL) showed no variants. A chromosomal microarray was also unremarkable with no regions of homozygosity. Whole exome sequencing revealed a missense variant c.763 G > A (p.Gly255Arg) in the GK gene (NM_000167.5) consistent with isolated GKD, resulting in pseudohypertriglyceridemia. This variant in exon 9 leads to the replacement of the amino acid glycine at position 255 with arginine in a region that is highly conserved across 13 species. In silico analysis tools predict this variant to be damaging to the glycerol kinase function or structure [8–10]. Segregation analysis was not performed per family preference. Corrected triglycerides, after blanking, were subsequently measured and found to be 82 mg/dL, and serum glycerol was 101 mg/dL (reference range 5–20 mg/dL [11]), confirming pseudohypertriglyceridemia. Glycerol kinase enzyme activity has not been assessed.

3. Discussion

The etiology of hypertriglyceridemia in children includes (i) familial hypertriglyceridemia, an autosomal dominant condition that results from hepatic secretion of large VLDL

particles that are triglyceride-rich; (ii) familial chylomicronemia syndrome, which is caused by defective lipoprotein lipase activity; (iii) fat necrosis, which may occur in infants undergoing therapeutic hypothermia; and (iv) iatrogenic causes such as the administration of intralipids [12, 13]. When the history and biochemical findings are not consistent with any of these etiologies in a patient with elevated triglycerides, pseudohypertriglyceridemia secondary to glycerol kinase deficiency should be considered [1].

GKD, first described in 1978, is an X-linked recessive disorder due to a variant in the GK gene on Xp21 in which glycerol—a product of lipolysis—cannot be phosphorylated to glycerol-3-phosphate; therefore, it can neither be used as a substrate in gluconeogenesis nor be esterified to free fatty acids [14, 15]. Biochemically, this results in elevated serum and urine glycerol levels [14]. There are currently three accepted forms of GKD corresponding with their symptoms: complex, isolated symptomatic, and isolated benign [6, 14]. Complex GKD involves two additional genes that are contiguous with GK, namely, DAX1 and DMD. The deletion of DAX1 leads to primary adrenal insufficiency secondary to congenital adrenal hypoplasia manifested by signs of glucocorticoid and mineralocorticoid deficiencies such as hypoglycemia, hyperpigmentation, and electrolyte disturbances during adrenal crises and in periods of stress and illness; the involvement of the DMD gene, known to cause Duchenne muscular dystrophy, leads to progressive muscular disease [14, 16]. Additionally, patients with complex GKD present with triangular facies with an "hourglass" midface appearance, mental retardation, emesis, and metabolic acidosis [16].

In contrast to complex GKD, isolated GKD may be either symptomatic or asymptomatic; however, the phenotype may change over time, suggesting no strict genotype-phenotype correlation [17]. The symptomatic form, also referred to as the juvenile form, presents with intermittent emesis, ketosis and acidosis, lethargy, hypoglycemia, unconsciousness, and seizures in early childhood, but symptoms appear to improve with time [17]. The variation of symptoms between childhood and adulthood has been attributed to a relative glucose deficit in children in which hepatic glucose output is unable to meet the metabolic demands during periods of prolonged starvation or catabolism [17]. Management of isolated GKD, therefore, is focused on avoiding prolonged fasting and on treatment with dextrose-containing fluids in hospitalized patients who are unable to tolerate oral intake. Long term, elevated glycerol levels do not appear to have a clinically significant negative impact on cardiovascular health, though they may contribute to insulin resistance making monitoring for hyperglycemia and type 2 diabetes mellitus an important goal of surveillance [4].

This case has several implications. The missense mutation in the GK gene, c.763 G > A (p.Gly255Arg), leading to isolated glycerol kinase deficiency is a novel variant not previously reported to cause disease. Furthermore, our case illustrates the clinical challenges of diagnosing pseudohypertriglyceridemia. Glycerol blanking differentiates pseudohypertriglyceridemia from true hypertriglyceridemia but is not widely available. The consequences of unidentified pseudohypertriglyceridemia include overtreatment and pursuing additional, often expensive, specialized testing, including genetic sequencing, unnecessarily. Given the uncertain prevalence of isolated GKD and its asymptomatic nature, it is likely underdiagnosed and often incidentally discovered, leading to needless medical therapy, potentially unnecessary testing of family members, as well as increased patient anxiety. To avoid these problems, one should consider requesting the laboratory either blank for glycerol or otherwise correct for hyperglycerolemia in cases of hypertriglyceridemia without other lipid abnormalities or in asymptomatic cases. Alternatively, laboratories should consider reflexing to glycerol blanking in cases of hypertriglyceridemia in which the total cholesterol levels are unusually normal, e.g., by estimation using the Friedewald equation [18]. The addition of the *GK* gene to commercially available chylomicronemia or hypertriglyceridemia gene sequencing panels may also aid in making the appropriate diagnosis sooner rather than later. In this case, for instance, the diagnosis of GKD would have been made a lot sooner, and with less expense had the *GK* gene been included in the chylomicronemia gene panel. Instead, whole exome sequencing was pursued at added expense and resource utilization after the chylomicronemia panel was unrevealing.

It is noteworthy that the proband's mother was diagnosed with GDM requiring insulin. It has previously been noted that *GK* likely plays an important role in insulin signaling, insulin resistance, and type 2 diabetes mellitus [19]. Furthermore, a maternal-fetal association has previously been reported between GDM in a mother who was a GKD carrier and her male fetus with isolated GKD [20]. A similar maternal-fetal genotype interaction has been reported between maternal fatty liver disease and fetuses with 3-hydroxyacyl-CoA dehydrogenase deficiency [21]. Although the maternal genotype here is unknown, the intriguing finding of GDM in a young and previously healthy mother highlights the potential maternal-fetal interaction between GDM and GKD previously noted [20].

In conclusion, this case highlights the diagnostic challenges of pseudohypertriglyceridemia, presents a novel mutation that leads to isolated GKD, and discusses the expected course, management, and prognosis of GKD, while emphasizing the importance of glycerol blanking and the addition of *GK* gene to chylomicronemia or hypertriglyceridemia gene sequencing panels. Additionally, this case underscores the need for further investigation into the maternal-fetal interaction between GDM and GKD.

Abbreviations

GKD: Glycerol kinase deficiency
WHO: World Health Organization
MCT: Medium-chain triglycerides
GDM: Gestational diabetes mellitus.

Authors' Contributions

AR wrote the case presentation. AR, MM, JM, and JT di-

agnosed the case and were involved in the care of the patient. KB provided laboratory technique expertise. HP provided genetics expertise. All authors contributed to the review of the manuscript. All authors have read and approved the final version of the manuscript.

Acknowledgments

The authors thank Dr. Piers Blackett and Dr. Don Wilson for their helpful suggestions during the workup leading to the patient's diagnosis.

References

[1] J. Backes, T. D. Dayspring, D. M. Hoefner, J. H. Contois, J. P. McConnell, and P. M. Moriarty, "Identifying pseudo-hypertriglyceridemia in clinical practice," *Clinical Lipidology*, vol. 9, no. 6, pp. 625–641, 2014.

[2] G. R. Warnick, M. M. Kimberly, P. P. Waymack, E. T. Leary, and G. L. Myers, "Standardization of measurements for cholesterol, triglycerides, and major lipoproteins," *Laboratory Medicine*, vol. 39, no. 8, pp. 481–490, 2008.

[3] R. H. Jessen, C. J. Dass, and J. H. Eckfeldt, "Do enzymatic analyses of serum triglycerides really need blanking for free glycerol?" *Clinical Chemistry*, vol. 36, no. 7, pp. 1372–1375, 1990.

[4] J. M. Backes, T. D Dayspring, D. M Hoefner, and P. M Moriarty, "Hypertriglyceridaemia unresponsive to multiple treatments," *BMJ Case Reports*, vol. 2015, Article ID bcr2015210788, 2015.

[5] *GK Glycerol Kinase [Homo sapiens], Gene ID: 2710*, National Center for Biotechnology Information (US), Bethesda, MD, USA, 2019.

[6] D. R. Sjarif, J. K Ploos Van Amstel, M Duran, F. A Beemer, and B. T Poll-The, "Isolated and contiguous glycerol kinase gene disorders: a review," *Journal of Inherited Metabolic Disease*, vol. 23, no. 6, pp. 529–547, 2000.

[7] T. G. Cole, "Glycerol blanking in triglyceride assays: is it necessary?" *Clinical Chemistry*, vol. 36, no. 7, pp. 1267-1268, 1990.

[8] R. Vaser, S. Adusumalli, S. N. Leng, M. Sikic, and P. C. Ng, "SIFT missense predictions for genomes," *Nature Protocols*, vol. 11, no. 1, pp. 1–9, 2016.

[9] J. M. Schwarz, D. N. Cooper, M. Schuelke, and D. Seelow, "MutationTaster2: mutation prediction for the deep-sequencing age," *Nature Methods*, vol. 11, no. 4, pp. 361-362, 2014.

[10] I. A. Adzhubei, S. Schmidt, L. Peshkin et al., "A method and server for predicting damaging missense mutations," *Nature Methods*, vol. 7, no. 4, pp. 248-249, 2010.

[11] J. M. Backes, T. Dayspring, T. Mieras, and P. M. Moriarty, "Pseudohypertriglyceridemia: two cases of probable glycerol kinase deficiency," *Journal of Clinical Lipidology*, vol. 6, no. 5, pp. 469–473, 2012.

[12] S. Daniels and S. C. Couch, "Lipid disorders in children and adolescents," in *Pediatric Endocrinology*, M. A. Sperling, Ed., Elsevier Saunders, Philadelphia, PA, USA, 2014.

[13] L. G. Lara, A. V. Villa, M. M. O. Rivas, M. S. Capella, F. Prada, and M. A. G. Enseñat, "Subcutaneous fat necrosis of the newborn: report of five cases," *Pediatrics & Neonatology*, vol. 58, no. 1, pp. 85–88, 2017.

[14] K. M. Dipple and E. R. B. McCabe, "Disorders of glycerol metabolism," in *Physician's Guide to the Laboratory Diagnosis*

of Metabolic Diseases, N. Blau et al., Ed., pp. 369–376, Springer Berlin Heidelberg, Berlin, Heidelberg, Germany, 2003.

[15] C. I. Rose and D. S. Haines, "Familial hyperglycerolemia," *Journal of Clinical Investigation*, vol. 61, no. 1, pp. 163–170, 1978.

[16] A. Scheuerle, F. Greenberg, and E. R. B. McCabe, "Dysmorphic features in patients with complex glycerol kinase deficiency," *The Journal of Pediatrics*, vol. 126, no. 5, pp. 764–767, 1995.

[17] C. Hellerud, N. Wramner, A. Erikson, Å. Johansson, G. Samuelson, and S. Lindstedt, "Glycerol kinase deficiency: follow-up during 20 years, genetics, biochemistry and prognosis," *Acta Paediatrica*, vol. 93, no. 7, pp. 911–921, 2004.

[18] W. T. Friedewald, R. I. Levy, and D. S. Fredrickson, "Estimation of the concentration of low-density lipoprotein cholesterol in plasma, without use of the preparative ultracentrifuge," *Clinical Chemistry*, vol. 18, no. 6, pp. 499–502, 1972.

[19] L. Rahib, N. K. MacLennan, S. Horvath, J. C. Liao, and K. M. Dipple, "Glycerol kinase deficiency alters expression of genes involved in lipid metabolism, carbohydrate metabolism, and insulin signaling," *European Journal of Human Genetics*, vol. 15, no. 6, pp. 646–657, 2007.

[20] Y. H. Zhang, J. L. Van Hove, E. R. B. McCabe, and K. M. Dipple, "Gestational diabetes associated with a novel mutation (378-379insTT) in the glycerol kinase gene," *Molecular Genetics and Metabolism Reports*, vol. 4, pp. 42–45, 2015.

[21] J. A. Ibdah, M. J. Bennett, P. Rinaldo et al., "A fetal fatty-acid oxidation disorder as a cause of liver disease in pregnant women," *New England Journal of Medicine*, vol. 340, no. 22, pp. 1723–1731, 1999.

43

Carglumic Acid Contributes to a Favorable Clinical Course in a Case of Severe Propionic Acidemia

Jun Kido (ID), **Shirou Matsumoto** (ID), and **Kimitoshi Nakamura** (ID)

Department of Pediatrics, Graduate School of Medical Sciences, Kumamoto University, Kumamoto, Japan

Correspondence should be addressed to Jun Kido; kidojun@kuh.kumamoto-u.ac.jp

Academic Editor: Maria Moschovi

Propionic acidemia (PA) is manifested as an abnormal accumulation of propionic acid and its metabolites, including methylcitrate, 3-hydroxypropionic acid, and propionylglycine, and is caused by a defect of propionyl-CoA carboxylase. PA is complicated by acute life-threatening metabolic crises, which are precipitated by a catabolic state and result in multiple organ failure or even death, if untreated. A neonate with PA recovered from the first metabolic crisis 3 days after birth but developed a second metabolic crisis during the recovery phase. This patient was considered to have severe PA and was accordingly given carglumic acid treatment in combination with carnitine supplementation and protein restriction, which was expected to prevent a recurrent metabolic attack. The patient did not develop hyperammonemia after receiving carglumic acid and was never hospitalized. Moreover, she did not present with acidosis even during viral infection. At 26 months of age, she led a stable life while receiving carglumic acid and regular rehabilitation. Carglumic acid treatment in combination with carnitine supplementation and protein restriction prevented metabolic decompensation, which would have otherwise required hospitalization, and resulted in improved quality of life and developmental outcomes.

1. Introduction

Propionic acidemia (PA) (MIM number: 606054) is an autosomal recessive genetic disease that affects the catabolic pathways of the branched-chain amino acids valine and isoleucine, methionine, threonine, thymine, odd-chain fatty acids, and the side chain of cholesterol. It is characterized by an abnormal accumulation of propionic acid and its metabolites, including 3-hydroxypropionic acid, propionylglycine, and methylcitrate, and is caused by a defect of propionyl-CoA carboxylase (PCC) (EC: 6.4.1.3) that converts propionyl-CoA to methylmalonyl-CoA [1].

Acute life-threatening metabolic crises complicate PA. These are precipitated by a catabolic state and result in multiple organ failure or even death, if untreated [1]. The age of onset and clinical course vary among patients, with symptoms including neonatal metabolic encephalopathy, recurrent ketoacidotic coma or Reye-like syndromes, psychomotor retardation, and failure to thrive, in the absence of acute crises.

Prevention of catabolism in the body via the administration of intravenous fluids containing glucose is critical in managing PA metabolic crises. In hyperammonemia, protein intake is restricted, and medications used in urea cycle disorders including L-arginine-HCl, sodium phenylbutyrate, sodium benzoate, and carglumic acid are administered. Persistent hyperammonemia, metabolic acidosis, and severe electrolyte imbalances are indications for extracorporeal detoxification such as plasma exchange and continuous hemodiafiltration (CHDF) [2].

Here, we describe the case of a neonate with PA who recovered from the first metabolic crisis 3 days after birth and developed a second crisis during the recovery phase. We describe the clinical course of the patient following the administration of carglumic acid and discuss its role in her treatment.

2. Case Presentation

A 6-day-old female neonate was admitted to our institution with metabolic acidosis and hyperammonemia. She was born at 40 weeks and 2 days' gestation and weighed 2828 g. Her APGAR scores at 1 and 5 minutes after birth were 9 and

10, respectively. There were no fetal or maternal medical problems during pregnancy. From day 3 after birth, her feeding gradually decreased, she could not feed on breast milk, and she developed metabolic acidosis (pH: 7.26, HCO_3^-: 13.3 mmol/L, BE: −12.3 mmol/L, anion gap (AG): 19.7) and hyperammonemia (881 μmol/L). She accordingly underwent CHDF and treatment for hyperammonemia, including the administration of arginine, sodium benzoate, L-carnitine, biotin, and multiple vitamins such as vitamins B1, B6, B12, C, and coenzyme Q10 in the intensive care unit. Her blood ammonia level decreased to 435 μmol/L six hours after undergoing CHDF but increased to 739 μmol/L 12 hours after undergoing CHDF. Additional treatment was, therefore, needed, and citrulline and sodium butyrate were administered. Her blood ammonia levels decreased with time, and CHDF was discontinued after 74 hours. The blood ammonia levels did not exceed 60 μmol/L thereafter, and she recovered from the metabolic crisis. We diagnosed her with PA owing to the large quantities of 3-hydroxypropionic acid, methyl citric acid, propionylglycine, and 2-methyl-3-hydroxybutyric acid excreted in the urine. Ten days after withdrawal of CHDF, she developed a second metabolic crisis with severe acidosis and apnea (pH: 6.73, pCO2: 89.9 mmHg, HCO_3^-: 11.5 mmol/L, BE: −24.6 mmol/L, AG: 33.1, lactate: 9.00 mmol/L, pyruvate: 0.46 mmol/L, lactate/pyruvate ratio: 19.6) without hyperammonemia (54 μmol/L). We administered carglumic acid (100 mg/kg/day) to prevent secondary hyperammonemia. She recovered from the second metabolic crisis after 3 days without CHDF on infusion of glucose, L-carnitine, carglumic acid, multivitamins, potassium citrate, and sodium citrate. We continued administering these medicines and special formulas for protein restriction after she recovered from the crisis.

She did not develop hyperammonemia after discharge and was never hospitalized under carglumic acid treatment. Moreover, she did not present with acidosis even during a viral infection (Table 1). Her genetic analysis revealed a c.923dupT (p.Leu308fs) homozygous mutation in the PCCA gene. Analysis of her blood acylcarnitine and amino acids using tandem mass spectrometry while receiving combination therapy with carglumic acid, L-carnitine, and a restricted protein diet demonstrated a lowered blood propionylcarnitine (C3) level, C3/acetylcarnitine (C2) ratio, and valine and isoleucine + leucine levels (Tables 2 and 3). Brain magnetic resonance imaging at the age of 2 months revealed mild atrophy in the frontal lobe; however, imaging at the age of 23 months did not reveal brain atrophy (Figure 1). At the age of 24 months, her development quotient (DQ) on the Kyoto Scale of Psychological Development corresponded to that at the age of 12 months in a healthy control (total DQ: 49). At 26 months of age, she was leading a stable life while receiving carglumic acid (50 mg/kg/day) and regular rehabilitation.

3. Discussion

We presented a case of severe PA in a neonate, who developed a metabolic crisis with severe hyperammonemia and

acidosis. The c.923dupT (p.Leu308fs) homozygous mutation in the PCCA gene resulted in null propionyl-CoA carboxylase activity and led to the development of a severe type of PA [3, 4].

Hyperammonemia ≥360 μmol/L has a significant adverse effect on the brain and is likely to result in mental retardation [5]. Therefore, in PA with metabolic decompensation, any excess toxic metabolites and ammonia should be removed from the body as soon as possible. Moreover, it is important to manage patients with PA to prevent metabolic acidosis and hyperammonemia in the long term, as far as practicable [2].

In patients with PA, excessive propionyl-CoA inhibits N-acetylglutamate synthase (NAGS) [6], which catalyzes the formation of NAG, an activator of carbamoyl phosphate synthetase I (CPSI). CPSI is a key enzyme in the first step of the urea cycle. Propionyl-CoA also inhibits the pathway by depleting hepatic acetyl CoA, which is responsible for NAG synthesis. Carglumic acid is a synthetic structural analogue of NAG and is, therefore, specifically indicated for treating hyperammonemia in patients with PA. In 2016, the Ministry of Health, Labour and Welfare approved its clinical use in Japan for the treatment of hyperammonemia owing to primary NAGS deficiency and organic acidemia. Carglumic acid accelerates ammonia detoxification by mimicking the effects of NAG on CPSI, thereby driving the urea cycle forward independent of other mechanisms that detoxify organic acids.

There are some reports on the long-term treatment of NAGS deficiency, and the short- and acute-term treatment of organic acidemia for hyperammonemia [7, 8]. However, the long-term effect of treatment in patients with organic acidemia remains unknown. The clinical course, blood C3 level, and C2/C3 ratio in this case suggested the effectiveness of long-term carglumic acid treatment in patients with severe PA. Blood acylcarnitine or amino acid levels exceeding the cutoff values indicate metabolic disorders of fatty, amino, and organic acids [9, 10], and the blood C3 level and C3/C2 ratio significantly increase in severe PA.

The urea cycle is linked to the tricarboxylic acid (TCA) cycle. Fumarate, synthesized form argininosuccinate in the urea cycle, is utilized in the TCA cycle. Impaired ammonia detoxification in the urea cycle leads to impaired function of enzymes in the TCA cycle owing to ammonia toxicity [11] and a shortage of substrates in the TCA cycle.

Regulation of the urea cycle, therefore, prevents dysfunction in the TCA cycle. Moreover, carglumic acid may be converted to α-ketoglutaric acid, which is utilized in the TCA cycle via anaplerosis. Although carglumic acid is considered to increase substrates in the TCA cycle via anaplerosis, succinyl-CoA may not be necessarily decreased. Furthermore, the reverse conversion of succinyl-CoA to propionyl-CoA is minimal. The beneficial impact of carglumic acid on the TCA cycle could result from compensatory anaplerosis following the lack of anaplerotic contribution from propionyl-CoA in PA. Carglumic acid, therefore, contributes to the regulation of urea and TCA cycles and prevents the excessive production and

TABLE 1: Venous blood gas analysis at the time of discharge and at 1, 3, 6, and 12 months after discharge.

	At the time of discharge	1 month	3 months	6 months	12 months
PH	7.35	7.39	7.40	7.36	7.43
BE (mmol/L)	−2.1	−2.7	−5.1	−0.9	−3.3
HCO$_3^-$ (mmol/L)	23.4	22.0	19.0	23.8	20.2
NH$_3$ (μmol/L)	25	41	33	36	59

TABLE 2: Blood acylcarnitine analysis before and after carglumic acid and carnitine treatment.

	At the onset time (before carglumic treatment)	3 months after carglumic treatment	Cutoff values (μmol/L)
C0	23.96	42.78	<10.00
C2	10.76	24.91	
C3	73.85	9.78	≥3.50
C3/C2	6.86	0.39	≥0.25
C4	0.32	0.29	≥0.60
C5	0.21	0.2	≥1.00
C5:1	0.04	0.01	≥0.025
C5DC	0.08	0.06	≥0.25
OH-C5	0.19	0.24	≥0.60
C6	0.08	0.08	
C8	0.09	0.06	≥0.30
C8/C10	1	0.79	≥1.00
C10	0.09	0.07	≥0.40
C12	0.09	0.11	
C14	0.1	0.28	
C14:1	0.07	0.05	≥0.40
C16	0.97	1.73	≥3.00
OH-C16	0.01	0.02	≥0.05
C0/(C16+C18)	18.75	17.25	≥100.00
C18	0.31	0.76	
C18:1	0.47	1.02	
OH-C18:1	0.01	0.01	≥0.05

C0: free carnitine; C2: acetylcarnitine; C3: propionylcarnitine; C4: butyrylcarnitine; C5: isovalerylcarnitine; C5:1: tiglylcarnitine; C5-DC: glutarylcarnitine; OH-C5: 3-hydroxy isovalerylcarnitine; C6: hexanoylcarnitine; C8: octanoylcarnitine; C10: decanoylcarnitine; C12: lauroylcarnitine; C14: myristoylcarnitine; C14:1: myristoylcarnitine; C16: palmitoylcarnitine; OH-C16: 3-hydroxy palmitoylcarnitine; C18: octadecanoylcarnitine C18:1: octadecenoylcarnitine; OH-C18:1: 3-hydroxy octadecenoylcarnitine.

TABLE 3: Blood amino acids analysis before and after carglumic acid and carnitine treatment.

	At onset (before carglumic treatment)	3 Months after carglumic treatment	Cutoff values (mg/dL)
Valine	1.62	0.25	≥2.93
Methionine	0.21	0.07	≥1.20
Isoleucine + leucine	1.14	0.58	≥4.59
Tyrosine	0.77	0.26	≥8.00
Phenylalanine	0.48	0.33	≥3.00
Citrulline	0.13	0.18	≥0.88
Arginine	0.24	0.2	≥2.61

accumulation of propionic acid and its metabolites. In this report, we described the outcome of treatment of severe PA with carglumic acid for 2 years. It was considered that her good clinical course and blood C3 level and C3/C2 ratio could be ascribed to carglumic acid in combination with protein restriction and L-carnitine. Protein restriction, L-carnitine supplementation, or carglumic acid treatment alone may not achieve good clinical outcomes in severe cases of PA. Cumulative evidence from further cases is needed to evaluate the effects of carglumic acid treatment for longer duration in PA.

In conclusion, carglumic acid combined with the standard treatments such as protein restriction and L-carnitine prevents metabolic decompensation, which would otherwise require hospitalization, and results in improved quality of life and developmental outcomes. The effects of carglumic acid should be given serious consideration, and possible indications for its long-term

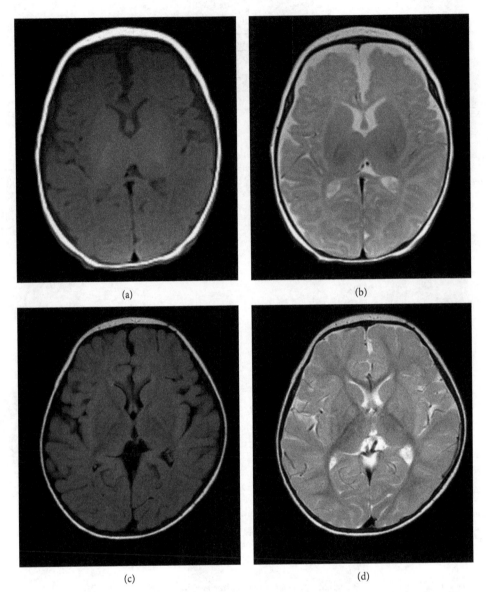

(a)

(b)

(c)

(d)

FIGURE 1: Brain magnetic resonance imaging in the patient with severe propionic acidemia. (a) T1-weighted imaging at the age of 2 months, (b) T2-weighted imaging at the age of 2 months, (c) T1-weighted imaging at the age of 23 months, and (d) T2-weighted imaging at the age of 23 months.

administration in severe organic acidemias should be explored.

Consent

Written informed consent was obtained from the patient's family.

Acknowledgments

The authors thank all the staff at Kumamoto University Hospital, Department of Pediatrics and Department of Intensive Care Medicine for their clinical contributions. This study was supported in part by a Grant-in-Aid for Research on Rare and Intractable Diseases, Health and Labor Sciences Research; a Grant-in-Aid for Pediatric Research from the Ministry of Health, Labour and Welfare; a Grant-in-Aid from Japan Agency for Medical Research and Development; and a Grant-in-Aid for Scientific Research from the Ministry of Education, Culture, Sports, Science, and Technology.

References

[1] W. A. Fenton, R. A. Gravel, and D. S. Rosenblatt, "Disorders of propionate and methylmalonate metabolism.," in *The Metabolic and Molecular Bases of Inherited Disease*, C. R. Scriver, A. L. Beaudet, W. S. Sly et al., Eds., pp. 2165–2193, McGraw-Hill, New York, NY, USA, 8th edition, 2001.

[2] M. R. Baumgartner, F. Hörster, C. Dionisi-Vici et al., "Proposed guidelines for the diagnosis and management of methylmalonic and propionic acidemia," *Orphanet Journal of Rare Diseases*, vol. 9, p. 130, 2014.

[3] B. Pérez, L. R. Desviat, P. Rodríguez-Pombo et al., "Propionic

acidemia: identification of twenty-four novel mutations in Europe and North America," *Molecular Genetics and Metabolism*, vol. 78, no. 1, pp. 59–67, 2003.

[4] L. Gallego-Villar, C. Pérez-Cerdá, B. Pérez et al., "Functional characterization of novel genotypes and cellular oxidative stress studies in propionic acidemia," *Journal of Inherited Metabolic Disease*, vol. 36, no. 5, pp. 731–740, 2013.

[5] J. Kido, K. Nakamura, H. Mitsubuchi et al., "Long-term outcome and intervention of urea cycle disorders in Japan," *Journal of Inherited Metabolic Disease*, vol. 35, no. 5, pp. 777–785, 2012.

[6] F. X. Coude, L. Sweetman, and W. L. Nyhan, "Inhibition by propionyl-coenzyme A of N-acetylglutamate synthetase in rat liver mitochondria. A possible explanation for hyperammonemia in propionic and methylmalonic acidemia," *Journal of Clinical Investigation*, vol. 64, no. 6, pp. 1544–1551, 1979.

[7] V. Valayannopoulos, J. Baruteau, M. B. Delgado et al., "Carglumic acid enhances rapid ammonia detoxification in classical organic acidurias with a favourable risk-benefit profile: a retrospective observational study," *Orphanet Journal of Rare Diseases*, vol. 11, p. 32, 2016.

[8] J. Häberle, "Role of carglumic acid in the treatment of acute hyperammonemia due to N-acetylglutamate synthase deficiency," *Therapeutics and Clinical Risk Management*, vol. 7, pp. 327–332, 2011.

[9] G. Tajima, N. Sakura, H. Yofune et al., "Enzymatic diagnosis of medium-chain acyl-CoA dehydrogenase deficiency by detecting 2-octenoyl-CoA production using high-performance liquid chromatography: a practical confirmatory test for tandem mass spectrometry newborn screening in Japan," *Journal of Chromatography B*, vol. 823, no. 2, pp. 122–130, 2005.

[10] P. Rinaldo, T. M. Cowan, and D. Matern, "Acylcarnitine profile analysis," *Genetics in Medicine*, vol. 10, no. 2, pp. 151–156, 2008.

[11] N. Katunuma, M. Okada, and Y. Nishii, "Regulation of the urea cycle and TCA cycle by ammonia," *Advances in Enzyme Regulation*, vol. 4, pp. 317–335, 1966.

44

Presumptive *Dipylidium caninum* Infection in a Toddler

Hannah F Chong,[1] **Roukaya Al Hammoud** (ID)**,**[2] **and Michael L Chang**[2]

[1]*Memorial Hermann Hospital, Houston, TX, USA*
[2]*The University of Texas Health Science Center, McGovern Medical School, Pediatric Infectious Diseases Division, 6431 Fannin, MSB 3.126, Houston, TX 77030, USA*

Correspondence should be addressed to Roukaya Al Hammoud; roukaya.alhammoud@uth.tmc.edu

Academic Editor: Miguel O'Ryan

We report a female toddler who presented repetitively with a chief complaint of motile white worms seen in her diapers. Symptoms of perianal itching and visualization of visible motile worms persisted for 6 months despite being treated with multiple courses of albendazole causing a lot of frustration and distress to the caregivers. The characteristics of the worms by inspection along with the presence of 3 pet dogs are consistent with *Dipylidium caninum*.

1. Introduction

A previously healthy 2-year-old girl presented with numerous small, white, visibly moving worms in her stool daily for 6 months. She had perianal pruritus but no fever, diarrhea, vomiting, or abnormal weight gain. Her pediatrician prescribed 2 doses of albendazole for suspected diagnosis of pinworms. Stool specimens were sent on six separate occasions for microscopic examination for ova and parasites and were reported as negative each time. Fecal occult blood testing and stool cultures for bacterial pathogens were also negative. All family members were prescribed albendazole, under the presumption of recurring pinworm infection. Despite negative testing and multiple courses of albendazole, the mother continued to see live worms, and the patient developed increased irritability and night-time fussiness. The mother became frustrated with her pediatrician. She then was referred to a pediatric infectious diseases specialist.

The patient lived with both parents in a rural area near Houston, Texas, and had no siblings. The patient did attend daycare. The family had no history of travel outside the Houston area. No other family members had similar symptoms. The family denied eating undercooked meat or seafood. They had three dogs which had access to outdoors and one cat inside the house. No history of fleas on pets or in the house or regular treatment of the pets for fleas.

Physical examination was normal except for mild dermatitis in the perineal area with linear excoriations thought to be secondary to the patient scratching. No obvious worms were visualized. The mother presented video footage and pictures of the worms in the stool from her smartphone. The video revealed motile, white worms about 1 centimeter in length (see Supplementary Materials). Based on the history and visual footage, the child was presumptively treated with one dose of praziquantel (10 mg/kg) for *Dipylidium caninum* infection followed by complete resolution of her symptoms.

2. Discussion

Dipylidium caninum, also known as flea tapeworm, is the most common cestode (tapeworm) of dogs and cats in the United States. Infection rates range from 0.1 to 4.0% for dogs in the North America [1]. One study identified *Dipylidium caninum* in 49.5% of nontreated dogs in animal shelters in Northern Oklahoma [1]. Using a new PCR method that identifies *Dipylidium caninum* rDNA inside single fleas in pet dogs and cats, out of 1969 *Ctenocephalides felis* from cats, 2.23% were found to be infected with *Dipylidium* and from

396 dogs infested with *Ctenocephalides canis*, 9.1% were infested with the *Dipylidium*-infected fleas [2]. The life cycle of this cestode starts with gravid proglottids that are passed in the feces or emerges from the perianal region of the host. The proglottids release egg packets which are consumed by flea larvae, the intermediate host. Eggs mature into infective cysticercoid larvae within the flea larvae as they mature to adults. Adult fleas containing cysticercoids are then ingested by dogs, the principal definitive hosts. Humans are usually infected via accidental ingestion of the intermediate host, cysticercoid-infected fleas. In the small intestine of the host (humans or dogs/cats), the cysticercoid develops into an adult tapeworm that produces proglottids which are later released into feces completing the life cycle [3]. Proglottids of the *Dipylidium caninum* are usually 12 mm in length and similar in appearance to rice grains.

Human infections, mostly in infants and children, occur worldwide but are uncommonly reported, likely representing under-reporting. In 2008, Samkari et al. reported one pediatric case and reviewed cases reported in the English-language literature which revealed a total of 34 cases since 1950s [4]. Since that publication, a total of 9 individual pediatric cases have been reported in journals indexed by PubMed, though only 4 are in English language [5–13]. An additional case series of 10 pediatric patients were reported in Greece [14]. Most *Dipylidium* infections are asymptomatic and self-limited, though abdominal pain, restlessness, and agitation can occur. The most notable sign is the presence of proglottids in the stool, diapers, or on the perineum. The duration of symptoms in our patient appears unusual, and it is possible that she had multiple reinoculations.

The gold standard diagnosis of *Dipylidium caninum* is made by visualizing the distinctive characteristics of proglottids which are usually highly motile when freshly passed. Unlike proglottids of *Taenia* species which are more square in shape, they are longer than they are wide (average mature size 12 mm × 3 mm), appears as rice grains or cucumber seeds, and have two sets of male and female reproductive organs. They therefore demonstrate two genital pores that lead to their name as the "double-pored" tapeworm. Proglottids of different *Taenia* species can be identified by their uterine branches. Within the gravid proglottids of *Dipylidium caninum* are egg packets. These eggs are round to ovoid, and their numbers can range from 5 to 30. Stool examination for ova is typically negative as eggs are rarely released from the proglottids within humans. Patient did not have risk factors (eating undercooked meat or fish) for other tapeworms that may infect humans as *Taenia saginata*, *Taenia solium*, *Diphyllobothrium latum* or others.

Affected children are often treated multiple times for *Enterobius* infection with albendazole, which is ineffective against *Dipylidium*. Families and primary care providers who are unfamiliar with the infection can become frustrated when the treatment seems to fail repeatedly which occurred in our case. The treatment of choice in the United States is a single dose of praziquantel (5 to 10 mg/kg). Praziquantel resistance in unresolving *Dipylidium* infection in dogs has been recently reported. These dogs were later successfully treated with nitroscanate or a compounded pyrantel/praziquantel/oxantel product [15]. Importantly, prevention of human cases should include primarily prompt parasitic treatment of the pets and flea control in their indoor and outdoor environments along with appropriate disposal of their feces, discouraging children to play in areas soiled with pets' feces, and good hand hygiene after playing with animals or outdoors.

In conclusion, we present a 2 year-old infected with *Dipylidium caninum* presumptively diagnosed by visualizing the characteristic motile proglottids from the video provided by the mother. We bring attention to this case in order to facilitate diagnosis and minimize provider and parent frustration when persistent pinworm infection is being considered.

References

[1] C. Adolph, S. Barnett, M. Beall et al., "Diagnostic strategies to reveal covert infections with intestinal helminths in dogs," *Veterinary Parasitology*, vol. 247, pp. 108–112, 2017.

[2] F. Beugnet, M. Labuschagne, J. Fourie et al., "Occurrence of Dipylidium caninum in fleas from client-owned cats and dogs in Europe using a new PCR detection assay," *Veterinary Parasitology*, vol. 205, no. 1-2, pp. 300–306, 2014.

[3] https://www.cdc.gov/dpdx/dipylidium.

[4] A. Samkari, D. L. Kiska, S. W. Riddell, K. Wilson, L. B. Weiner, and J. B. Domachowske, "*Dipylidium caninum* mimicking recurrent *Enterobius vermicularis* (pinworm) infection," *Clinical Pediatrics*, vol. 47, no. 4, pp. 397–399, 2008.

[5] O. P. Neira, M. L. Jofre, and S. N. Munoz, "*Dipylidium caninum* infection in a 2 year old infant: case report and literature review," *Revista chilena de infectología*, vol. 25, no. 6, pp. 465–471, 2008.

[6] B. Szwaja, L. Romanski, and M. Zabczyk, "A case of *Dipylidium caninum* infection in a child from the southeastern Poland," *Wiadomości Parazytologiczne*, vol. 57, no. 3, pp. 175–178, 2011.

[7] R. R. Cabello, A. C. Ruiz, R. R. Feregrino, L. C. Romero, R. R. Feregrino, and J. T. Zavala, "*Dipylidium caninum* infection," *BMJ Case Reports*, vol. 2011, Article ID bcr0720114510, 2011.

[8] M. Narasimham, P. Panda, I. Mohanty, S. Sahu, S. Padhi, and M. Dash, "*Dipylidium caninum* infection in a child: A rare case report," *Indian Journal of Medical Microbiology*, vol. 31, no. 1, pp. 82–84, 2013.

[9] H. Li, Y. N. Zhang, and S. H. Chen, "*Dipylidium caninum* infection in a toddler," *Zhongguo Ji Sheng Chong Xue Yu Ji Sheng Chong Bing Za Zhi*, vol. 32, no. 5, p. 333, 2014.

[10] I. Sahin, S. Köz, M. Atambay, U. Kayabas, T. Piskin, and B. Unal, "A rare cause of diarrhea in a kidney transplant recipient: *Dipylidium caninum*," *Transplantation Proceedings*, vol. 47, no. 7, pp. 2243-2244, 2015.

[11] P. Jiang, X. Zhang, R. D. Liu, Z. Q. Wang, and J. Cui, "A human case of zoonotic dog tapeworm, *Dipylidium caninum* (Eucestoda: dilepidiidae), in China," *The Korean Journal of Parasitology*, vol. 55, no. 1, pp. 61–64, 2017.

[12] P. Xaplanteri, D. Gkentzi, V. Stamouli et al., "Rare worm in an infant's nappy," *Archives of Disease in Childhood*, vol. 103, no. 2, p. 199, 2018.

[13] T. Taylor and M. Zitzmann, "*Dipylidium caninum* in a 4-month old male," *American Society for Clinical Laboratory Science*, vol. 24, no. 4, pp. 212–214, 2011.

[14] S. Portokalidou, D. Gkentzi, V. Stamouli et al., "*Dipylidium caninum* infection in children: clinical presentation and therapeutic challenges," *The Pediatric Infectious Disease Journal*, vol. 38, no. 7, pp. e157–e159, 2019.

[15] J. Jesudoss Chelladurai, T. Kifleyohannes, J. Scott, and M. T. Brewer, "Praziquantel resistance in the zoonotic cestode Dipylidium caninum," *The American Journal of Tropical Medicine and Hygiene*, vol. 99, no. 5, pp. 1201–1205, 2018.

45

Challenges of Diagnosing Viral Myocarditis in Adolescents in the Era of COVID-19 and MIS-C

Hemali P. Shah ⓘ**, Richard Frye, Sunny Chang, Erin Faherty** ⓘ**, Jeremy Steele** ⓘ**, and Ruchika Karnik** ⓘ

Department of Pediatrics, Section of Pediatric Cardiology, Yale University School of Medicine, New Haven, CT, USA

Correspondence should be addressed to Hemali P. Shah; hemali.shah@yale.edu

Academic Editor: Bibhuti Das

Myocarditis has a wide array of clinical presentations ranging from asymptomatic to sudden cardiac death. Pediatric myocarditis is a rare disease, with an estimated annual incidence of 1 to 2 per 100,000 children though its true prevalence remains unknown due to its variable and often subclinical presentation. The diagnosis of myocarditis is challenging in the era of COVID-19 and Multisystem Inflammatory Syndrome in Children (MIS-C), which can have overlapping clinical conundrum. Here, we present a case of a 17-year-old male presenting with chest tightness, shortness of breath, and electrocardiogram (EKG) findings concerning for myocardial injury along with elevated inflammatory markers such as D-dimer, ESR (Erythrocyte Sedimentation Rate), and CRP (C-Reactive Protein). We discuss the key elements of our clinical experience with this case and review the literature for pediatric myocarditis, with a focus on differentiating it from MIS-C in the current COVID-19 pandemic era.

1. Introduction

Myocarditis is a rare diagnosis in pediatrics and has a heterogeneous clinical course ranging from asymptomatic, gradual-onset congestive heart failure (CHF) to fulminant myocarditis complicated by cardiogenic shock and sudden death [1,2]. This range of presentations makes the diagnosis of myocarditis exceptionally challenging, especially in the pediatric population and in the current era of the COVID-19 pandemic. The possibility of COVID-19 and MIS-C with their own breadth of clinical presentations adds another layer of nuance to diagnosing myocarditis.

In children ultimately diagnosed with myocarditis, tachycardia, tachypnea, and an abnormal respiratory examination are among the most frequently reported presenting symptoms in the emergency department [2,3]. Other presenting symptoms include chest pain, syncope, palpitations, and isolated gastrointestinal symptoms (e.g., abdominal pain and vomiting). A pathological confirmation is required for definitive diagnosis of myocarditis. However, given the invasive nature of endomyocardial biopsies, cardiac MRI is currently the gold standard noninvasive modality for diagnosis [1].

Beyond varying symptomatology, the clinical outcomes of children with myocarditis are also widely variable. The overall mortality rate of myocarditis has been reported to be 7–15% in the pediatric population; of those that survive, many develop long-term sequelae such as dilated cardiomyopathy and CHF [1–4]. Furthermore, it is difficult to predict which children may have poor outcomes and are at risk for developing the aforementioned long-term sequelae; studies have not yet found definitive predictors for prognosis [1,2,4]. Given these consequences and prognostic uncertainty, pediatric myocarditis warrants timely assessment and supportive measures, which are the mainstay of treatment.

2. Case Presentation

A 17-year-old male with a history of asthma presented to an outside adult emergency department (ED) with 24 hours of progressively worsening shortness of breath and chest tightness at rest that was unresponsive to bronchodilators. No recent illness was reported. He had a dental cleaning visit 3 days prior. He had no significant family history of cardiac disease, sudden cardiac death, or coagulopathies.

On presentation, he was well appearing. Vital signs were BP 107/56, heart rate 97, temperature 99.4°F, respiratory rate 18, and O_2 saturation 95% on room air. Cardiac exam was unremarkable. Lungs were clear to auscultation bilaterally without wheezing, rhonchi, and crackles. There was no jugular venous distension, hepatomegaly, or pedal edema. Extremities were well perfused, and pulses were 2+ and symmetric throughout. Complete metabolic panel and blood count with differential were unremarkable. A drug toxicology panel screening for nine drugs, which tested for cocaine, amphetamines, etc., was completely negative. EKG demonstrated ST elevations in leads I and aVL and T-wave inversions in the inferior and lateral leads (Figure 1). Additional clinical laboratory tests revealed elevated cardiac and inflammatory markers (Table 1). Given the patient's age, both adult and pediatric cardiology were consulted; further management decisions were made jointly between these teams. A bedside transthoracic echocardiogram revealed regional wall motion abnormalities in the inferior left ventricular (LV) segments with preserved global LV systolic function.

Two hours into his presentation, the patient became hypoxic to 91% on pulse oximetry and was placed on 4L nasal cannula 100% FiO_2 with improvement in O_2 saturations to 96%. Chest X-ray (CXR) showed scattered bilateral hazy opacities (Figure 2). These additional clinical changes prompted a computed tomographic angiogram (CTA) to rule out pulmonary embolism (PE). Chest CTA was notable for multifocal consolidated ground-glass opacities in the lungs bilaterally (Figure 3). These imaging findings raised a significant concern for COVID-19. The decision was made to not pursue cardiac catheterization at this time.

He was transferred to the pediatric ED and subsequently admitted to the Pediatric Intensive Care Unit (PICU) for further evaluation with differential diagnosis including COVID-19-related myocarditis, non-COVID-19 myocarditis, and MIS-C. The patient had not received any doses of any COVID-19 vaccines. Further laboratory studies were notable for negative SARS-CoV-2 RNA and elevated levels of ESR (68 mm/hr) and CRP (201.3 mg/L) (Table 1). Formal echocardiogram performed the next morning revealed mild-to-moderate mitral valve regurgitation, low-to-normal left ventricular systolic function with an ejection fraction of 52%, regional wall motion abnormalities of the inferolateral LV wall, and normal origin of both coronary arteries with no dilation or aneurysms. Our institutional multidisciplinary MIS-C protocol was activated. Our patient was treated with 1 mg/kg methylprednisolone every 12 hours and heparin while undergoing evaluation for MIS-C. IVIg was not given due to the patient's depressed cardiac function, mild disease, and normal coronary arteries on the echocardiogram. Our institutional protocol recommends steroids and anticoagulation for MIS-C with addition of IVIg if there is clinically moderate-to-severe disease or if criteria are met for Kawasaki Disease (including coronary artery abnormalities). The LIAISON® SARS-CoV-2 S1/S2 IgG test was conducted to detect IgG against SARS-CoV-2; this test has been found to have a false positive rate of up to 1.1% and a false negative rate of up to 1.9% [5]. SARS-CoV-2 IgG and repeat PCR were subsequently negative.

The patient remained afebrile throughout his hospitalization; as fever is a key manifestation of MIS-C, this further made a diagnosis of MIS-C unlikely. At this time, non-COVID-19 myocarditis was thought to be the most likely diagnosis and further work up was pursued in that direction. His work up was negative for autoimmune etiologies of myocarditis, including systemic lupus erythematosus and sarcoidosis, as well as for viruses commonly known to cause myocarditis: adenovirus, herpesviruses (cytomegalovirus, Epstein–Barr virus, and HHV-6), and parvovirus B19. Another pathogen associated with myocarditis is *Mycoplasma pneumoniae*, which the patient tested negative for by PCR, as well.

A cardiac MRI was performed to assess the diagnostic MRI criteria for myocarditis. Cardiac MRI is considered the gold standard noninvasive modality for diagnosis of myocarditis. His MRI was positive for subacute myopericarditis demonstrating patchy and extensive subepicardial and transmural myocardial late gadolinium enhancement of the LV lateral and inferior walls extending from the base to midventricle, along with enhancement of the pericardium with normal T2 relaxation times (Figure 4). Between hospital days 2 and 3, he was weaned off supplemental oxygen. Cardiac and inflammatory markers gradually improved (Table 1). The day before discharge, he developed new asymptomatic, isolated premature ventricular contractions without sustained arrhythmias. He was discharged home with a diagnosis of myopericarditis of unclear etiology on a prednisone taper. At 8-week follow-up, he remained clinically asymptomatic. Repeat cardiac MRI revealed persistent, extensive fibrosis in different LV segments, similar to his initial MRI. Based on the American Heart Association myocarditis guidelines for return to competitive sports, he is currently restricted for at least 3–6 months, pending follow-up testing [6].

3. Discussion

Myocarditis has a broad spectrum of clinical presentations, ranging from asymptomatic to acute fulminant disease and sudden cardiac death, with continuously evolving diagnostic criteria; this makes the diagnosis quite challenging [3]. Pediatric myocarditis is considered a rare disease that accounts for about 0.05% of pediatric hospital discharges [4]. However, given its variable, often subclinical presentation, its true prevalence remains unknown and may be greater than documented [1]. Retrospective cohort studies have delineated a bimodal distribution for acute myocarditis in the pediatric population with most cases occurring in infants and adolescents [1,7].

Classically, myocarditis presents with a preceding viral prodrome. Many viruses are recognized as the underlying etiology with enteroviruses (e.g., coxsackieviruses A and B), parvovirus B19, and human herpesvirus 6 (HHV-6) being most common in the current era [3,8,9]. Myocarditis and associated symptoms can also be caused by substances such as cocaine and amphetamines, for which our patient tested negative [3,8]. Resting tachycardia, ventricular arrhythmias, chest pain, respiratory distress, abdominal pain, and

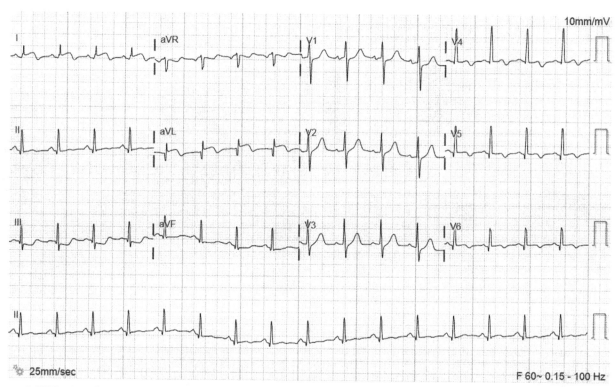

FIGURE 1: EKG at initial presentation to adult ED. Sinus rhythm with ST elevations in leads I and aVL, T-wave inversions in the inferior and lateral leads, and prolonged QT interval.

TABLE 1: Laboratory values from the time of presentation and at the time of discharge.

	Initial presentation	At discharge
Troponin T	1.11 ng/mL (normal reference <0.01)	0.10 ng/mL
N-terminal pro-B-type natriuretic peptide (NT-proBNP)	2,312 pg/mL (<125)	796 pg/mL
D-dimer	2.29 mg/L FEU (<0.50)	0.73 mg/L FEU
Fibrinogen	851 mg/dL (194–448)	
CRP	201.3 mg/L[a]	8.2 mg/L
ESR	68 mm/hr (0–20)	12 mm/hr[b]
Ferritin	121 ng/mL (30–400)	51 ng/mL
Angiotensin-converting enzyme	31 U/L (8–52)	20 U/L
Interleukin-6	65.2 pg/mL (<5)	-

[a]CRP <1.0 indicates lower relative cardiovascular (CV) risk, 1.0–3.0 = average relative CV risk, 3.0–10.0 = higher relative CV risk, and >10.0 may be associated with infection and inflammation. [b]ESR value is from follow-up appointment, which was 3 days after discharge.

vomiting are common presenting symptoms of pediatric viral myocarditis [2,8,9]. Chest pain has been found to be a typical symptom of acute myocarditis in adolescents [10]. ECG abnormalities are found in approximately 90% of children with myocarditis: nonspecific ST-T wave abnormalities, ST-segment elevation, low-voltage QRS complexes, and atrioventricular conduction delays [2,8,9]. Cardiac biomarker abnormalities, such as troponin T and I, are commonly elevated in children with myocarditis [2,8]. Elevated troponin T levels have been observed in up to 65% of pediatric myocarditis cases [2]. Importantly, these ST changes can mimic acute MI, as in the case of our patient, making diagnosis difficult and prone to cognitive bias [3,10]. Reports have shown that cases of adolescents initially diagnosed with acute MI may have been myocarditis with an infarct-like presentation [10,11]. Though acute MI is

extremely rare among adolescents, it has been described in association with the anomalous origin of coronary arteries [10,11].

The differential diagnosis based on presentation with respiratory symptoms, CXR findings, EKG abnormalities and elevated troponin level was broad including PE, myocarditis, and acute MI. However, during the COVID-19 pandemic, the differential for this patient's presentation would be incomplete without COVID-19-related myocarditis and MIS-C. Key diagnostic features of myocarditis, MI, MIS-C, and COVID-19-related myocarditis are summarized (Table 2). CTA in our case helped rule out the anomalous coronary artery origin, which would be the most likely cause for MI in a young adult, and PE. The diagnostic challenge was then refocused on differentiating COVID-19-related cardiac disease versus non-COVID-19-related myocarditis.

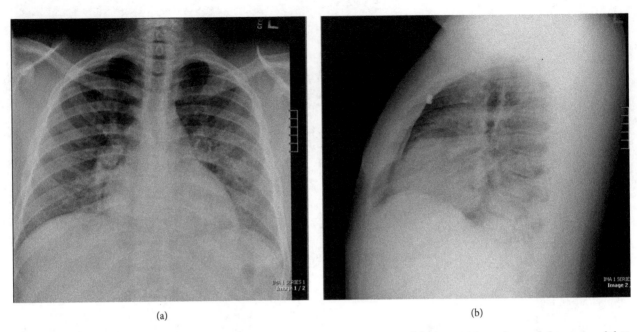

(a)   (b)

FIGURE 2: Chest X-ray at presentation with PA (a) and lateral (b) views with scattered hazy opacities and no confluent consolidation, pulmonary edema, pleural effusions, or pneumothorax. The cardiac silhouette is within normal limits. Findings are suggestive of an acute inflammatory process.

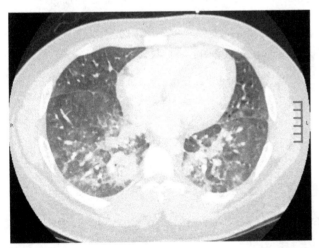

FIGURE 3: Chest CTA (lung window) at presentation showing multifocal consolidated and ground-glass opacities in the bilateral lungs.

Myocardial injury defined by elevated cardiac biomarkers has been reported in multiple reviews of adult patients hospitalized with COVID-19 [18–20]. Myocardial injury is rare in children with acute COVID-19 compared to adults; however, children with MIS-C can have significant myocardial involvement [13–15,21]. The understanding of MIS-C is still evolving. Cardiac findings of MIS-C encountered in the pediatric population include myocardial dysfunction, acute myocarditis or myocarditis-like clinical picture, and coronary artery dilation or aneurysms [21–23]. Dufort et al. reported that prevalence of myocarditis was the highest among adolescents, relative to other pediatric age groups, with MIS-C [23]. In the pediatric population, case

series and case reports describing myocarditis in the setting of COVID-19 and MIS-C have been recently published; these patients tended to be critically ill, presenting with severe abdominal pain, vomiting, and fever [24–26].

Cardiac MRI is considered the gold standard noninvasive modality for diagnosis of myocarditis. We are still learning about the cardiac changes on MRI in patients with MIS-C. One published case series found evidence of myocardial injury on cardiac MRI in pediatric patients with MIS-C to be dissimilar to those with myocarditis in the acute phase; in this series, cardiac MRI in patients with MIS-C showed diffuse myocardial edema without evidence of focal late gadolinium enhancement [27]. On echocardiography, systolic dysfunction can be seen in both myocarditis and MIS-C [16]. However, in MIS-C, diastolic dysfunction has been shown to persist even after systolic dysfunction resolves [16]. Our patient did not have any evidence of diastolic dysfunction.

Most recently, with the approval of the Pfizer-BioNTech COVID-19 vaccine for children 12 years of age and older in the U. S., there have been rare cases of myocarditis and myopericarditis reported in adolescent males within 4 days of receiving the second vaccine dose [28]. The seven adolescent males presented with chest pain and evidence of myocarditis on cardiac MRI [28]. This series of cases presents an additional layer of complexity to the diagnosis of pediatric myocarditis in the current era. Of note, our patient presented prior to the approval and availability of the Pfizer-BioNTech COVID-19 vaccine and, therefore, had not received any doses. Though a causal relationship between the vaccine and myocarditis has not yet been established in the pediatric population, healthcare providers' awareness of myocarditis as a possibility after COVID-19 vaccination is crucial for appropriate referral to pediatric cardiology and

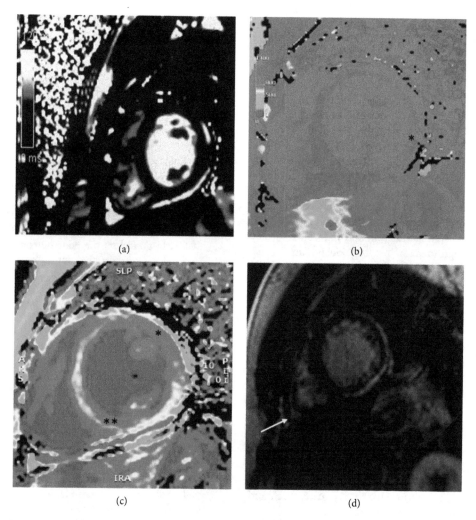

FIGURE 4: Parametric mapping and tissue characterization in myocarditis on cardiac MRI. (a) Short-axis midmyocardial T2 map with normal relaxation time and no evidence of acute edema. (b) Precontrast native midmyocardial T1 map showing diffusely elevated T1 relaxation time specifically along the lateral wall (*). (c) Midmyocardial extracellular volume (ECV) map indicating increased ECV along the anterior and lateral walls (*) and the inferoseptal wall (**). (d) Postcontrast pulse sequence inversion recovery image of the midmyocardium with increased pericardial signal (**), evidence of diffuse subepicardial late gadolinium enhancement along the entirety of the lateral wall (*), and mild pericardial effusion (arrow).

TABLE 2: Comparison of key features of pediatric myocarditis, myocardial infarction, MIS-C (focusing on cardiovascular manifestations), and COVID-19-related myocarditis.

	Acute myocarditis [8–10]	Acute myocardial infarction [10–12]	MIS-C [13–16]	COVID-19-related myocarditis* [17]
Fever	May be present	Unlikely	Persistent	Common
Clinical symptoms	Resting tachycardia, chest pain, palpitations, shortness of breath, respiratory distress, abdominal pain, and vomiting	Can present with chest pain	Multisystem involvement, including rash, tachycardia, abdominal pain, vomiting, diarrhea, and conjunctivitis	Shortness of breath, respiratory distress, chest pain, abdominal pain, vomiting, diarrhea, etc.
Cardiac biomarkers (troponin I or T)	Elevated	Elevated	Elevated (mild to moderate)	Elevated
Inflammatory markers (CRP, ESR, ferritin, etc.)	Often elevated	Normal	Elevated	Elevated
Echocardiogram findings	Regional wall motion abnormalities; decreased LV systolic function	Coronary arteries may be normal or anomalous	Coronary artery dilatation; systolic dysfunction that resolves; and persistent diastolic dysfunction	Reduced LV ejection fraction and pericardial effusion

*COVID-19-related myocarditis features include data from adults.

further management. This awareness may also spare otherwise healthy adolescents presenting with chest pain, like our patient, from invasive procedures such as cardiac catheterization.

The management of acute myocarditis is mainly supportive [3]. The use of IVIg, which has antiviral, anti-inflammatory, and immunomodulatory effects, remains controversial; IVIg has been shown to provide meaningful benefit in some pediatric patients, though not definitively [3,8,29]. The role of steroids for treatment of myocarditis also remains controversial [29]. Despite this controversy, prednisone is used in about 25–30% of acute myocarditis cases in the United States [3,8]. In MIS-C, there is some evidence suggesting that combination therapy with IVIg and steroids is associated with reduction in recovery time of LV systolic function and reduced ICU stay [14]. Currently, though there are broad guidelines and expert consensus, management of MIS-C and myocarditis remains dependent on institutional protocols.

Acute pediatric myocarditis is often associated with heart failure [3]. Heart failure in the setting of adult myocarditis is managed with diuretics, angiotensin-converting enzyme inhibitors, or angiotensin receptor blockers and β-blockers. However, in pediatrics, a conventional heart failure regimen has not yet been established [8]. Many pediatric myocarditis patients receive supportive care in an ICU at presentation, like our patient. Inotropic agents are used with or without extracorporeal membrane oxygenation for patients with cardiogenic shock or patients who deteriorate despite medical treatment [3,8]. Pediatric myocarditis can deteriorate into fulminant myocarditis and continues to have significant morbidity and mortality [1,9]. Thus, myocarditis is a must-not-miss diagnosis that is important to recognize, treat, and monitor closely with serial echocardiograms.

The current case highlights how challenging the diagnosis of myocarditis can be in the pediatric population, especially in the era of COVID-19. Adolescents are a unique cohort where collaboration between pediatric and adult specialists is essential for optimal clinical care. With this case, we illustrate a wide range of differential diagnoses that have overlapping features of classic myocarditis. As our knowledge of the cardiac manifestations of COVID-19 and MIS-C evolves, it is crucial that myocarditis continues to be part of clinicians' diagnostic thinking.

Consent

No written consent has been obtained from the patient/patient's guardian as there are no patient-identifiable data included in this case report.

Authors' Contributions

Hemali P. Shah and Ruchika Karnik conceived and designed the study, and performed acquisition of data, analysed and interpreted data, drafted the manuscript, and made critical revisions. Richard Frye and Sunny Chang performed acquisition of data, analysis and interpretation of data, and

critical revision. Erin Faherty conceived and designed the study, performed data acquisition, analysed and interpreted data, and made critical revisions. Jeremy Steele performed data acquisition, analysed and interpreted of data, and done critical revision.

References

[1] S. J. Ghelani, M. C. Spaeder, W. Pastor, C. F. Spurney, and D. Klugman, "Demographics, trends, and outcomes in pediatric acute myocarditis in the United States, 2006 to 2011," *Circulation: Cardiovascular Quality and Outcomes*, vol. 5, no. 5, pp. 622–627, 2012.

[2] M. Rodriguez-Gonzalez, M. I. Sanchez-Codez, M. Lubian-Gutierrez, and A. Castellano-Martinez, "Clinical presentation and early predictors for poor outcomes in pediatric myocarditis: a retrospective study," *World Journal of Clinical Cases*, vol. 7, no. 5, pp. 548–561, 2019.

[3] C. E. Canter and K. E. Simpson, "Diagnosis and treatment of myocarditis in children in the current era," *Circulation*, vol. 129, no. 1, pp. 115–128, 2014.

[4] D. Klugman, J. T. Berger, C. A. Sable, J. He, S. G. Khandelwal, and A. D. Slonim, "Pediatric patients hospitalized with myocarditis: a multi-institutional analysis," *Pediatric Cardiology*, vol. 31, no. 2, pp. 222–228, 2010.

[5] M. Ainsworth, M. Andersson, K. Auckland et al., "Performance characteristics of five immunoassays for SARS-CoV-2: a head-to-head benchmark comparison," *The Lancet Infectious Diseases*, vol. 20, no. 12, pp. 1390–1400, 2020.

[6] B. J. Maron, J. E. Udelson, R. O. Bonow et al., "Eligibility and disqualification recommendations for competitive athletes with cardiovascular abnormalities: task force 3: hypertrophic cardiomyopathy, arrhythmogenic right ventricular cardiomyopathy and other cardiomyopathies, and myocarditis: a scientific statement from the American heart association and American college of cardiology," *Circulation*, vol. 132, no. 22, pp. e273–80, 2015.

[7] R. J. Butts, G. J. Boyle, S. R. Deshpande et al., "Characteristics of clinically diagnosed pediatric myocarditis in a contemporary multi-center cohort," *Pediatric Cardiology*, vol. 38, no. 6, pp. 1175–1182, 2017.

[8] S. Dasgupta, G. Iannucci, C. Mao, M. Clabby, and M. E. Oster, "Myocarditis in the pediatric population: a review," *Congenital Heart Disease*, vol. 14, no. 5, pp. 868–877, 2019.

[9] R. Bejiqi, R. Retkoceri, A. Maloku, A. Mustafa, H. Bejiqi, and R. Bejiqi, "The diagnostic and clinical approach to pediatric myocarditis: a review of the current literature," *Open Access Macedonian Journal of Medical Sciences*, vol. 7, no. 1, pp. 162–173, 2019.

[10] M. Martinez-Villar, F. Gran, A. Sabaté-Rotés et al., "Acute myocarditis with infarct-like presentation in a pediatric population: role of cardiovascular magnetic resonance," *Pediatric Cardiology*, vol. 39, no. 1, pp. 51–56, 2018.

[11] A. Desai, S. Patel, and W. Book, ""Myocardial infarction" in adolescents: do we have the correct diagnosis?" *Pediatric Cardiology*, vol. 26, no. 5, pp. 627–631, 2005.

[12] W. T. Mahle, R. M. Campbell, and J. Favaloro-Sabatier, "Myocardial infarction in adolescents," *The Journal of Pediatrics*, vol. 151, no. 2, pp. 150–154, 2007.

[13] I. Valverde, Y. Singh, J. Sanchez-de-Toledo et al., "Acute cardiovascular manifestations in 286 children with multisystem inflammatory syndrome associated with COVID-19 infection in europe," *Circulation*, vol. 143, no. 1, pp. 21–32, 2021.

[14] Z. Belhadjer, M. Méot, F. Bajolle et al., "Acute heart failure in multisystem inflammatory syndrome in children in the context of global SARS-CoV-2 pandemic," *Circulation*, vol. 142, no. 5, pp. 429–436, 2020.

[15] T. Alsaied, A. H. Tremoulet, J. C. Burns et al., "Review of cardiac involvement in multisystem inflammatory syndrome in children," *Circulation*, vol. 143, no. 1, pp. 78–88, 2021.

[16] D. Matsubara, H. L. Kauffman, Y. Wang et al., "Echocardiographic findings in pediatric multisystem inflammatory syndrome associated with COVID-19 in the United States," *Journal of the American College of Cardiology*, vol. 76, no. 17, pp. 1947–1961, 2020.

[17] K. Sawalha, M. Abozenah, A. J. Kadado et al., "Systematic review of COVID-19 related myocarditis: insights on management and outcome," *Cardiovascular Revascularization Medicine*, vol. 23, pp. 30497-30498, 2020.

[18] A. Pirzada, A. T. Mokhtar, and A. D. Moeller, "COVID-19 and myocarditis: what do we know so far?" *CJC Open*, vol. 2, no. 4, pp. 278–285, 2020.

[19] B. Siripanthong, S. Nazarian, D. Muser et al., "Recognizing COVID-19-related myocarditis: the possible pathophysiology and proposed guideline for diagnosis and management," *Heart Rhythm*, vol. 17, no. 9, pp. 1463–1471, 2020.

[20] F. Tahir, T. Bin Arif, J. Ahmed, F. Malik, and M. Khalid, "Cardiac manifestations of coronavirus disease 2019 (COVID-19): a comprehensive review," *Cureus*, vol. 12, no. 5, Article ID e8021-e, 2020.

[21] T. Niaz, K. Hope, M. Fremed et al., "Role of a pediatric cardiologist in the COVID-19 pandemic," *Pediatric Cardiology*, vol. 42, no. 1, pp. 19–35, 2020.

[22] F. Sperotto, K. G. Friedman, M. B. F. Son, C. J. VanderPluym, J. W. Newburger, and A. Dionne, "Cardiac manifestations in SARS-CoV-2-associated multisystem inflammatory syndrome in children: a comprehensive review and proposed clinical approach," *European Journal of Pediatrics*, vol. 180, no. 2, pp. 307–322, 2020.

[23] E. M. Dufort, E. H. Koumans, E. J. Chow et al., "Multisystem inflammatory syndrome in children in New York state," *New England Journal of Medicine*, vol. 383, no. 4, pp. 347–358, 2020.

[24] M. Grimaud, J. Starck, M. Levy et al., "Acute myocarditis and multisystem inflammatory emerging disease following SARS-CoV-2 infection in critically ill children," *Annals of Intensive Care*, vol. 10, no. 1, p. 69, 2020.

[25] B. Trogen, F. J. Gonzalez, and G. F. Shust, "COVID-19-Associated myocarditis in an adolescent," *The Pediatric Infectious Disease Journal*, vol. 39, no. 8, pp. e204–e205, 2020.

[26] J. T. Beaudry, B. Dietrick, D. B. Lammert et al., "Fatal SARS-CoV-2 inflammatory syndrome and myocarditis in an adolescent: a case report," *The Pediatric Infectious Disease Journal*, vol. 40, no. 2, p. e72, 2021.

[27] E. Blondiaux, P. Parisot, A. Redheuil et al., "Cardiac MRI of children with multisystem inflammatory syndrome (MIS-C) associated with COVID-19," *Radiology*, vol. 297, no. 3, pp. E283–E288, Article ID 202288, 2020.

[28] M. Marshall, I. D. Ferguson, P. Lewis et al., "Symptomatic acute myocarditis in seven adolescents following pfizer-BioNTech COVID-19 vaccination," *Pediatrics*, vol. 148, no. 3, Article ID e2021052478, 2021.

[29] M.-S. Lin, Y.-H. Tseng, M.-Y. Chen et al., "In-hospital and post-discharge outcomes of pediatric acute myocarditis underwent after high-dose steroid or intravenous immunoglobulin therapy," *BMC Cardiovascular Disorders*, vol. 19, no. 1, p. 10, 2019.

46

Fecal Impaction in the Rectum and Rectosigmoid Colon Secondary to Sunflower Seed Ingestion

Alexander Lyons [ID],[1] Jamie Lee,[2] and Kristen Cares[2]

[1]*Children's Hospital of Michigan, Detroit, MI, USA*
[2]*Division of Pediatric Gastroenterology, Children's Hospital of Michigan, Detroit, MI, USA*

Correspondence should be addressed to Alexander Lyons; alyons@dmc.org

Academic Editor: Alexander K. C. Leung

A 35-month-old male who had eaten a bag of sunflower seeds initially presented to the emergency department (ED) with visible seeds in the anus and was discharged home with a stool softener after manual disimpaction. He then returned to the hospital 2 days later, and abdominal radiographs confirmed significant fecal material within the rectum and rectosigmoid colon. After failed oral and rectal laxative therapy attempts, subsequent disimpaction under anesthesia revealed an undigested sunflower seed bezoar in the rectum extending to the distal segment of his sigmoid colon. This case highlights the dangers and possible complications of seed ingestion even in small quantities in children along with the pathophysiology of impaction. This is one of the youngest cases reported in the United States involving the rectum and rectosigmoid colon with a sunflower bezoar.

1. Introduction

Fecal impaction, an accumulation of hard stool in the anorectum or distal colon, may occur due to a variety of primary causes, with the most common being a diet consisting of inadequate intake of fiber and fluids [1, 2]. Although seeds are a source of fiber, there is a crucial difference between soluble and insoluble fiber. Soluble fiber absorbs water when exposed to gastrointestinal fluids, forming a gel-like substance that is subsequently digested by bacteria in the large intestine, ultimately releasing gas. However, seeds are a source of insoluble fiber; therefore, they pass through the intestinal tract without being digested, which can lead to a bezoar [3]. The different types of bezoars include phytobezoars (fruit and vegetable fibers), trichobezoars (hair), lactobezoars (milk concretions), and pharmacobezoars (medications) [4]. In a majority of children, fecal impaction of seeds is found in the rectum followed by the ileum [1, 5].

2. Case Report

A previously healthy 35-month-old male (16.8 kg) initially presented to the emergency department (ED) with complaints of abdominal pain and difficulty passing stool for 2 days. Two days prior to the ED visit, the mother noted that the patient had consumed an entire bag of sunflower seeds. Following this, he developed constipation with straining during defecation, and sunflower seeds were seen protruding from the rectum, prompting his mother to bring him to the ED. In the ED, an abdominal X-ray revealed a nonobstructive bowel gas pattern with a moderate amount of stool seen in the colon and rectum (Figure 1). During an attempt to administer an enema, sunflower seeds were protruding from the rectum; therefore, several seeds were manually removed. He subsequently passed a small amount of stool and was then discharged home on a stool softener.

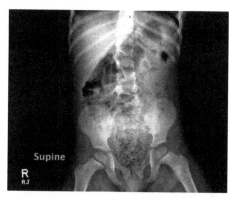

FIGURE 1: Abdominal X-ray, supine view. There is a nonobstructive gas pattern with moderate stool burden, primarily in the rectosigmoid colon and to a lesser extent in the ascending colon.

Two days following his discharge, the patient returned to the ED with persistent constipation, abdominal pain with straining, vomiting, as well as decreased appetite. His mother reported nonbloody liquid stools. An abdominal X-ray revealed gaseous distention of the colon with a moderate degree of fecal material in the rectum and rectosigmoid colon (Figure 2). A mineral oil enema was administered; however, it failed to produce any stool. The patient was admitted for an exam under anesthesia and manual disimpaction.

Upon the digital rectal exam, a large number of sunflower seeds were palpable in the rectal vault with significant distention. Whole sunflower seeds were then evacuated from the rectum (Figure 3). There was minimal fecal material in the rectum. The sharp edges of the sunflower seeds also created mucosal trauma from within the rectum. All of the sunflower seeds within reach were removed. The patient was later discharged from the hospital on daily MiraLAX and Calmoseptine cream for any possible anorectal pain. He was subsequently lost to follow-up.

3. Discussion

Seeds can produce phytobezoars, which are accumulations of indigestible vegetables or fruit seeds in the intestinal tract. Unlike dietary fiber bezoars contained in fruits and vegetables, which more often accumulate in the stomach, seed bezoars are able to pass the pylorus and subsequently the ileocecal valve and accumulate in the colon and rectum due to their small size. Seed bezoars typically form an impaction in the rectum due to the decreased water absorption [4–6].

A systematic review of cases of gastrointestinal bezoars spanning from 1980 to 2018 revealed that the most common ethnicity groups affected were from the Eastern Mediterranean and Middle Eastern regions likely due to diets containing more fruits and vegetables, followed by Western Europe and the Americas. Affected children were predominately male (65%) with ages ranging from 2 to 16 years old with a median age of 10. Common locations of bezoar impaction included the rectum, which would explain the most common symptoms of abdominal and rectal pain. Other symptoms reported include tenesmus and loose

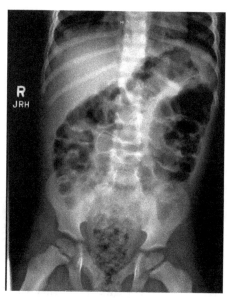

FIGURE 2: Abdominal X-ray, supine view. Following 2 days on stool softener and representation to the ED, there is mild gaseous distention of the visualized large colon with a moderate degree of fecal material within the rectum and rectosigmoid colon, not subsequently moved by mineral oil enema.

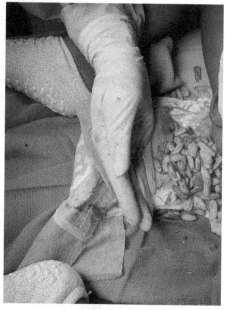

FIGURE 3: Sunflower seeds removed by manual disimpaction from the rectum and rectosigmoid colon. There is minimal fecal material with some specks of blood secondary to trauma. Photo was obtained with signed and informed consent.

stools. There were few case reports in children that presented with mildly elevated temperature and leukocytosis mimicking acute appendicitis, one of which involved a 3-year-old child that presented with fever, leukocytosis, and signs of colitis [7]. Of the different seed types found in bezoars, watermelon seeds comprised the majority (54%) followed by sunflower seeds (21%) [6]. Among reported cases, this is the second reported case in the United States with rectal and rectosigmoid colon involvement due to sunflower seeds.

Based on the 2014 recommendations from ESPGHAN and NASPGHAN, diagnosis of fecal impaction should be based upon the clinical history and digital rectal examination. Plain abdominal radiography may be used in children where fecal impaction is suspected and physical examination is unreliable or impossible [1]. The patient in our case met the diagnostic criteria for fecal impaction based on the physical examination and history. This highlights the importance of obtaining a sufficient dietary history and physical exam prior to getting abdominal X-rays. In instances where a bezoar causes obstruction in the small bowel, complications such as pancreatitis and rarely bowel perforation may occur and require computerized tomography for diagnosis and referral to surgery [6, 8, 9].

In patients with rectal seed impaction, manual disimpaction under general anesthesia has been the preferred treatment to minimize patient discomfort [6, 8, 9]. Initial conservative measures of intervention failed in our patient, which is a common occurrence in patients with fecal impaction, as only 6% of seed bezoars are typically removed with Fleet enemas and stool softeners [6].

4. Conclusion

Rectal bezoars should be diagnosed using a dietary history and physical exam. Given that the initial treatment in our patient was manual disimpaction without anesthesia, it partially removed the seed impaction. However, it could not remove any further impaction secondary to pain in the child. Understanding the pathophysiology of rectal bezoars and the success of manual disimpaction under general anesthesia will prove beneficial, as it should be used as a first-line treatment in children with a history of seed ingestion or visualization of seeds on rectal exam as in our patient, minimizing treatment failure.

References

[1] D. K. Manatakis, V. Acheimastos, M. I. Antonopoulou, D. Balalis, and D. P. Korkolis, "Gastrointestinal seed bezoars: a systematic review of case reports and case series," *Cureus*, vol. 11, no. 5, Article ID e4686, 2019.

[2] M. M. Tabbers, C. DiLorenzo, M. Y. Berger et al., "Evaluation and treatment of functional constipation in infants and children," *Journal of Pediatric Gastroenterology and Nutrition*, vol. 58, no. 2, pp. 258–274, 2014.

[3] C. Axelrod and M. Saps, "The role of fiber in the treatment of functional gastrointestinal disorders in children," *Nutrients*, vol. 10, no. 11, Article ID 1650, 2018.

[4] K. Eng and M. Kay, "Gastrointestinal bezoars: history and current treatment paradigms," *Gastroenterology and Hepatology*, vol. 8, pp. 776–778, 2012.

[5] A. Eitan, I. M. Katz, Y. Sweed, and A. Bickel, "Fecal impaction in children: report of 53 cases of rectal seed bezoars," *Journal of Pediatric Surgery*, vol. 42, no. 6, pp. 1114–1117, 2007.

[6] M. Iwamuro, H. Okada, K. Matsueda et al., "Review of the diagnosis and management of gastrointestinal bezoars," *World Journal of Gastrointestinal Endoscopy*, vol. 7, no. 4, pp. 336–345, 2015.

[7] Y. Efrati, E. Freud, F. Serour, and B. Klin, "Phytobezoar-induced ileal and colonic obstruction in childhood," *Journal of Pediatric Gastroenterology and Nutrition*, vol. 25, no. 2, pp. 214–216, 1997.

[8] Y.-C. Chen, C.-H. Liu, H.-H. Hsu et al., "Imaging differentiation of phytobezoar and small-bowel faeces: CT characteristics with quantitative analysis in patients with small-bowel obstruction," *European Radiology*, vol. 25, no. 4, pp. 922–931, 2015.

[9] R. D. Lane and J. E. Schunk, "Sunflower rectal bezoar presenting with an acute abdomen in a 3-year-old child," *Pediatric Emergency Care*, vol. 26, no. 9, pp. 662–664, 2010.

47

Septo-Optic Dysplasia Diagnosed in a Newborn Infant with Normoglycemia: The Importance of Thorough Physical Examination

Aishwarya Palorath ⑩¹ and **Ishita Kharode** ⑩²

¹*Department of Pediatric Gastroenterology, University of Miami-Jackson Health System, 1601 NW 12th Ave, Miami, FL 33137, USA*
²*Department of Pediatrics, Division of Pediatric Endocrinology, Richmond University Medical Center, 355 Bard Ave, Staten Island, New York, NY 10310, USA*

Correspondence should be addressed to Ishita Kharode; ikharode@rumcsi.org

Academic Editor: Ozgur Kasapcopur

A newborn male infant was admitted to the neonatal intensive care unit due to suspected sepsis. He was clinically stable with normal electrolyte levels on admission. However, he was noted to have micropenis and bilateral nonpalpable testes. Ultrasound imaging confirmed the presence of both gonads in the inguinal canal, with no Müllerian structures visualized. Laboratory examination revealed an undetectable random plasma cortisol level; subsequent ACTH stimulation testing confirmed adrenal insufficiency. Further testing revealed additional pituitary hormone deficiencies, and the infant was started on multiple hormone replacement therapies. Magnetic resonance imaging identified absent septum pellucidum, pointing of the frontal horns, and optic nerve hypoplasia. A diagnosis of septo-optic dysplasia was made based on this combination of findings. This case highlights the importance of thorough physical examination in newborn infants, which may reveal the only sign of underlying pathology in the absence of other concerning findings.

1. Introduction

Formerly known as de Morsier's syndrome, septo-optic dysplasia (SOD) occurs in 1 out of every 10,000 live births. It is a clinical diagnosis involving at least two of the following: midline brain defects (e.g., septum pellucidum and/or corpus callosum agenesis), optic nerve hypoplasia, and hypopituitarism. The phenotype is variable as most patients do not exhibit all three findings [1].

Hypopituitarism is the most common clinical finding in SOD, observed in 62–80% of patients [2]. Suggestive features include hypoglycemia, cleft lip and/or palate, micropenis, undescended testes, and prolonged jaundice [3].

We report a case of SOD diagnosed in a newborn infant who presented with micropenis and bilateral undescended testes. The infant was otherwise clinically well with persistently normal electrolytes, including normal blood glucose levels. However, his exam findings prompted an extensive diagnostic evaluation, and he was ultimately diagnosed with SOD based on laboratory and magnetic resonance imaging (MRI) results. This case report underscores the importance of a full physical examination in newborn infants, including a genital exam as atypical genitalia may be the only presenting sign of hypopituitarism and SOD.

2. Case Presentation

A newborn male infant was born at our institution at 41 weeks of gestation via normal spontaneous vaginal delivery to a 20-year-old G1P0 mother with negative prenatal

TABLE 1: Pertinent laboratory findings.

	Patient's age in days at the time of blood draw	Value	Units	Reference ranges for age
Plasma glucose	2	4.5	mmol/L	3.9–5.6
Random cortisol	4	<13.8	nmol/L	46.9–386
TSH	13	3.704	μIU/mL	1.3–16
Free T4	13	11.6	pmol/L	10.8–63.9
IGF-1	5	<4.2	nmol/L	1.9–14.3
IGFBP-3	7	0.8	mg/L	1.11–3.18
LH	3	0.09	mIU/mL	0.02–7
FSH	3	0.0	mIU/mL	0.16–4.1
Total testosterone	3	2.1	nmol/L	2.6–3.5
Total testosterone (repeated level)	89	0.72	nmol/L	2.5–11.9
Karyotype	3		46, XY	

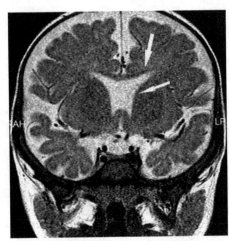

FIGURE 1: Absence of the septum pellucidum (white arrow) and pointing of frontal horns (yellow arrow) seen on MRI of the brain.

serologies and normal prenatal ultrasounds. There was no known family history of endocrine conditions or midline defects or history of consanguinity between the parents. Birth weight was 3.71 kg. The patient was vigorous after birth, with Apgar scores of 9 at 1 minute and 9 at 5 minutes. However, due to maternal fever, the infant was admitted to the neonatal intensive care unit for suspected sepsis.

On physical exam, the infant was noted to have stretched penile length of 1.5 cm. Neither testis was palpable in the scrotum or inguinal canal. The remainder of the exam was unremarkable, with no cleft lip, cleft palate, or other dysmorphic features.

Initial laboratory evaluation showed normal electrolytes (sodium 137 mmol/L, potassium 3.5 mmol/L, and glucose 4.5 mmol/L). Scrotal ultrasound confirmed that both testes were present in the inguinal canal. No uterus or ovaries were seen. Pediatric endocrinology was consulted, and multiple laboratory tests were ordered to evaluate pituitary, adrenal, and gonadal functions. Pertinent results are presented in Table 1.

The patient's cortisol level resulted first as undetectably low, which prompted an ACTH stimulation test. A high-dose stimulation test was performed as it was unclear at that time whether cortisol deficiency was primary or secondary. Cortisol levels drawn at 30 and 60 minutes were both

24.8 nmol/L, consistent with suboptimal response and adrenal insufficiency. Within this context, the low insulin-like growth factor 1 and insulin-like growth factor-binding protein levels were suggestive of growth hormone deficiency. Growth hormone stimulation testing was not performed due to patient's young age. Thyroid function tests revealed central hypothyroidism, with inappropriately normal thyroid-stimulating hormone (TSH) level in the setting of borderline low free thyroxine (T4) level. There was no evidence of diabetes insipidus. The patient's sodium levels ranged 137–143 mmol/L, and mean urine output was 1.3 mL/kg/hour.

Given these findings, the patient was started on growth hormone, levothyroxine, and hydrocortisone therapy. Subsequent MRI revealed a small pituitary gland, absent septum pellucidum, and pointing of the frontal horns, consistent with a diagnosis of septo-optic dysplasia (Figure 1). Laboratory evaluation at three months of age, during minipuberty of infancy, again showed low total testosterone level (0.73 nmol/L).

Starting at six months of age, the patient underwent a short course of intramuscular testosterone therapy for micropenis, receiving 25 mg testosterone once monthly for a total of three doses. Stretched penile length after treatment completion was 3 cm, within 2.5 standard deviations for age. Our patient also underwent orchiopexy at 8 and 11 months of age, receiving perioperative hydrocortisone stress dosing for both surgeries.

Our patient has been evaluated by a pediatric ophthalmologist, who confirmed the presence of optic nerve hypoplasia. As of 18 months of age, he is tracking well with full extraocular muscle movements and has not, thus far, required eyeglasses. He has been receiving occupational and physical therapy since 9 months of age. The patient has been referred for genetic analysis but has not yet undergone evaluation.

3. Discussion

The presence of bilateral undescended testes in a genetically 46, XY male infant suggests either a defect in androgen action (such as partial 5-α reductase deficiency or partial androgen insensitivity syndrome) or a defect in androgen production, also known as hypogonadism [4].

Hypogonadism, in turn, can occur at either the central or peripheral level. Causes of congenital central, or hypogonadotropic, hypogonadism include pituitary defects such as Kallmann syndrome, septo-optic dysplasia, and adrenal hypoplasia congenita. The presence of midline defects such as cleft lip, cleft palate, solitary central incisor, and omphalocele makes a pituitary defect more likely [5]. Conversely, differential diagnoses for congenital hypergonadotropic hypogonadism include Klinefelter syndrome, partial gonadal dysgenesis, and enzymatic defects in adrenal testosterone biosynthesis [6].

Our patient presented with both undescended testes and micropenis, which is also associated with hypogonadism. Micropenis is defined as penile length less than 2.5 standard deviations below the mean. A stretched penile length measurement is vital in order to distinguish true micropenis from situations where the penile base is obscured [4].

Infants with suspected hypogonadotropic hypogonadism should undergo full pituitary hormone evaluation. Hypoglycemia, which is associated with both growth hormone and cortisol deficiencies, can be an additional suggestive finding. Interestingly, our patient was normoglycemic throughout his hospitalization, despite having multiple pituitary hormone deficiencies. The presence of low growth hormone and/or cortisol levels during hypoglycemia can assist in diagnosing deficiencies of these hormones [7, 8]. ACTH stimulation testing with cosyntropin is often used to confirm cortisol deficiency [3]. Thyroid function tests and serum/urine osmolality should also be monitored to assess for central hypothyroidism and diabetes insipidus, respectively [9, 10]. Importantly, pituitary hormone deficiencies can develop over time, so close endocrine follow-up is essential [1].

Hypogonadism itself can be confirmed during minipuberty of infancy, which occurs in boys up to age 6 months and in girls up to age 3 years [11]. Along with laboratory testing, MRI of the brain should be obtained to evaluate the morphology of the pituitary gland (including the presence of the posterior pituitary bright spot), corpus callosum, septum pellucidum, optic nerves, and optic chiasm [2].

Patients with hypopituitarism should receive replacement of any deficient hormones. Families of patients with adrenal insufficiency should be counseled on steroid stress dosing during times of illness and emergency [8]. Infants with micropenis can be treated with a short course of testosterone in order to increase penile length. A dosing regimen of 25 mg IM, given every 3 or 4 weeks for three doses, has been successfully implemented [2, 5].

Of note, testosterone therapy has been associated with decreased Sertoli cell function and spermatogenesis [12]. Recombinant FSH therapy during minipuberty, in combination with testosterone therapy, has been shown to improve Sertoli cell function in the short term, although longitudinal data are not available [13]. Topical dihydrotestosterone (DHT) has also been shown to increase penile length in patients with micropenis due to various genetic conditions, with minimal adverse effects. Again, data regarding precise dosing and long-term effects are not available [4, 14].

Patients with cryptorchidism whose testes have not descended by six months of age should undergo orchiopexy within the next year [15].

Patients with SOD should follow with a multidisciplinary team, with management aimed at treating pituitary hormone deficiencies, providing neurodevelopmental support, and monitoring for visual impairment [1].

4. Conclusion

A thorough physical examination is essential in newborn infants as it can reveal signs of a serious underlying condition. The presence of micropenis and bilateral undescended testes in a 46, XY infant should prompt assessment for hypogonadism. In cases of suspected hypogonadotropic hypogonadism, a full pituitary hormone workup should be undertaken along with brain imaging to further clarify the diagnosis. Septo-optic dysplasia is a rare but important cause of hypopituitarism, which necessitates management by a multidisciplinary team of specialists. Patients with SOD should be closely monitored for the potential development of additional pituitary hormone deficiencies over time.

Acknowledgments

The authors would like to thank Dr. Amita De Souza for her contributions to this manuscript.

References

[1] E. A. Webb and M. T. Dattani, "Septo-optic dysplasia," European Journal of Human Genetics, vol. 18, no. 4, pp. 393–397, 2010.

[2] S. Kurtoglu, "Neonatal hypopituitarism: approaches to diagnosis and treatment," J Clin Res Pediatr Endocrinol, vol. 11, no. 1, pp. 4–12, 2019.

[3] L. Bosch i Ara, "Congenital hypopituitarism during the neonatal period: epidemiology, pathogenesis, therapeutic options, and outcome," Front Pediatr, vol. 8, pp. 1–17, 2021.

[4] N. Hatipoğlu and S. Kurtoğlu, "Micropenis: etiology, diagnosis and treatment approaches," Journal of clinical research in pediatric endocrinology, vol. 5, no. 4, pp. 217–223, 2013.

[5] M. M. Grumbach, "A window of opportunity: the diagnosis of gonadotropin deficiency in the male Infant1," The Journal of Clinical Endocrinology & Metabolism, vol. 90, no. 5, pp. 3122–3127, 2005.

[6] W. Rodpraser, "Hypogonadism and cryptorchidism," Frontiers in Endocrinology, vol. 10, no. 906, pp. 1–27, 2020.

[7] A. Grimberg, S. A. DiVall, C. Polychronakos et al., "Guidelines for growth hormone and insulin-like growth factor-I treatment in children and adolescents: growth hormone deficiency, idiopathic short stature, and primary insulin-like growth factor-I deficiency," Hormone Research in Paediatrics, vol. 86, no. 6, pp. 361–397, 2016.

[8] S. A. Bowden and R. Henry, "Pediatric adrenal insufficiency: diagnosis, management, and new therapies," International Journal of Pediatrics, vol. 2018, Article ID 1739831, 8 pages, 2018.

[9] L. Persani, "Central hypothyroidism: pathogenic, diagnostic, and therapeutic challenges," The Journal of Clinical Endocrinology & Metabolism, vol. 97, no. 9, pp. 3068–3078, 2012.

[10] M. B. Abraham, "Efficacy of hydrochlorothiazide and low renal solute feed in neonatal central diabetes insipidus with transition to oral desmopressin in early infancy," *International Journal of Pediatric Endocrinology*, vol. 11, pp. 1–6, 2014.

[11] U. Boehm, P.-M. Bouloux, M. T. Dattani et al., "European Consensus Statement on congenital hypogonadotropic hypogonadism-pathogenesis, diagnosis and treatment," *Nature Reviews Endocrinology*, vol. 11, no. 9, pp. 547–564, 2015.

[12] P. Y. Liu, H. W. G. Baker, V. Jayadev, M. Zacharin, A. J. Conway, and D. J. Handelsman, "Induction of spermatogenesis and fertility during gonadotropin treatment of gonadotropin-deficient infertile men: predictors of fertility outcome," *The Journal of Clinical Endocrinology & Metabolism*, vol. 94, no. 3, pp. 801–808, 2009.

[13] E. Kohva, H. Huopio, J. Hietamäki, M. Hero, P. J. Miettinen, and T. Raivio, "Treatment of gonadotropin deficiency during the first year of life: long-term observation and outcome in five boys," *Human Reproduction*, vol. 34, no. 5, pp. 863–871, 2019.

[14] D. Xu, L Lu, L Xi et al., "Efficacy and safety of percutaneous administration of dihydrotestosterone in children of different genetic backgrounds with micropenis," *Journal of Pediatric Endocrinology & Metabolism: Journal of Pediatric Endocrinology & Metabolism*, vol. 30, no. 12, pp. 1285–1291, 2017.

[15] T. F. Kolon, C. D. A. Herndon, L. A. Baker et al., "Evaluation and treatment of cryptorchidism: AUA guideline," *The Journal of Urology*, vol. 192, no. 2, pp. 337–345, 2014.

48

Combined Staged Surgery and Negative-Pressure Wound Therapy for Closure of a Giant Omphalocele

Vlad Laurentiu David ⓘ,[1] **Mihai Cristian Neagu** ⓘ,[1] **Aurelia Sosoi,**[1]
Maria Corina Stanciulescu ⓘ,[1] **Florin George Horhat** ⓘ,[2] **Ramona Florina Stroescu** ⓘ,[3]
Calin Marius Popoiu ⓘ,[1] **and Eugen Sorin Boia** ⓘ[1]

[1]*Department of Pediatric Surgery and Orthopedics, "Victor Babes" University of Medicine and Pharmacy, Timisoara, Romania*
[2]*Department of Microbiology, "Victor Babes" University of Medicine and Pharmacy, Timisoara, Romania*
[3]*Department of Pediatrics, "Victor Babes" University of Medicine and Pharmacy, Timisoara, Romania*

Correspondence should be addressed to Mihai Cristian Neagu; mihaimng@icloud.com

Academic Editor: Sathyaprasad Burjonrappa

The management of giant omphaloceles had always been a point of interest for the pediatric surgeons. Many surgical techniques were proposed, but none of them succeeded to become the standard procedure in closing the congenital abdominal defect. We present a case of giant omphalocele in which we used staged surgical closure combined with a prosthetic patch, with negative-pressure therapy and, finally, definitive surgical closure. Even though a major complication occurred during the treatment, we were able to close the defect without any prosthetic material left in place.

1. Introduction

Exomphalos (omphalocele) is a congenital defect located at the site of the umbilical cord insertion [1]. Omphalocele is considered a major form when the diameter of the defect is larger than 5 cm [1]. Usually, large defects contain most of the small bowel and/or more than 50% of the liver within the sac [1]. The management of large omphaloceles had always been a point of interest for the pediatric surgeons [2,3]. Even though primary surgical repair is the ideal treatment option, it is not possible in most cases of large defects. Due to lack of content, the abdominal cavity cannot be formed properly. Hence, there is not enough space to accommodate all the herniated organs. So, in this instance, other surgical options have to be considered: staged repair, silobag, prosthetic covers, or conservative management with delayed closure [1–3].

We present a case of giant omphalocele in which we were forced to use a sequence of treatment methods: staged closure using the Fufezan technique [4] followed by a Gore-

Tex patch combined with negative-pressure therapy and, finally, definitive surgical closure.

2. Case Presentation

A male newborn was delivered by C-section at an estimated gestational age of 37 weeks with a birth weight of 2600 g. A large abdominal defect was diagnosed by ultrasound in the 19th week of gestation. The fetal ultrasound revealed a 3.5 cm/2.6 cm mass of bowel loops and the liver contained within a membrane in front of the abdominal wall.

At birth, examination of the abdomen revealed a large omphalocele (app. 8 cm in diameter) with an intact membrane containing part of the liver and small bowel loops (Figure 1). The echocardiogram showed a small ventricular septal defect with patent ductus arteriosus. G-band analysis showed no chromosomal abnormality and normal karyotype. No other congenital abnormalities were detected. Due to the size of the abdominal wall defect, we decided to perform staged closure of the omphalocele using partial

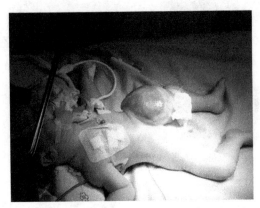

FIGURE 1: Giant omphalocele containing a significant portion of the liver.

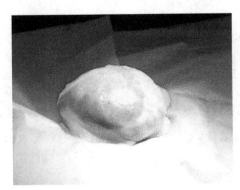

FIGURE 2: The omphalocele after the first stage of the procedure.

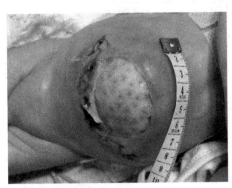

FIGURE 3: Skin necrosis with wound dehiscence and exposure of the Gore-Tex mesh.

resection of the omphalocele membrane (Fufezan technique [4]).

3. Surgical Procedure

The procedure was performed 24 hours after birth. We performed an incision on approximately half of the circumference of the omphalocele membrane near the junction with the normal skin, at the lower pole of the defect. We detached the membrane from the underlying bowel loops and resected a slice of the membrane comprising approximately half of the membrane surface. The content of the sac was gently reduced into the abdominal cavity, and the remaining membrane was reattached using isolated nonabsorbable suture at the abdominal wall (Figure 2). The membrane was dressed with moisture sterile draping.

On the eight day of life, we performed the second stage of the procedure. In the same manner as in the first stage, we detached, partially resected, and reattached the membrane on to the abdominal wall further reducing the content of the omphalocele sack into the abdominal wall. The abdominal cavity was still not large enough to accommodate all the herniated organs.

On day 17 of life, we went into the operating theatre for the third time. We further reduced the herniated organs into the abdominal cavity till the point where all of the organs were inside the cavity. However, the defect could not be closed. We could no longer use the omphalocele membrane to further patch the defect which by now was dry and friable. So, we excised the remaining membrane, and then, we closed the defect using a Gore-Tex mesh. We further mobilized skin flaps and used them to cover the Gore-Tex mesh.

Unfortunately, 5 days later (day 22 of life), the skin overlying the Gore-Tex mesh dehisced and a large portion of the Gore-Tex patch became exposed (Figure 3).

We decided to use a negative-pressure wound therapy (NPWT) combined with an antimicrobial silver dressing. The silver dressing was applied over the Gore-Tex patch and the negative-pressure system over it. We set the pressure at 40 mmHg, continuous negative pressure. The dressing was changed, and the wound was re-evaluated at 4 days of interval. The inflammation decreased, and the necrotic debrides were cleared after the first two dressings. Granulation formed at the edge of the tegument, and the wall defect became progressively smaller from approximately 7 cm to 3 cm diameter. At day 50 (28 days of NPWT), we were able to remove the Gore-Tex mesh and closed the wound (Figure 4). The patient was discharged 10 days later (Figure 5).

4. Discussion

The management of giant omphalocele is still debated among various methods of treatment, in using both surgical and nonsurgical approaches. The mainstay of treatment of such anterior abdominal wall defects is to reduce the herniated viscera into the abdomen and to close with the fascia and skin to create a solid abdominal wall. It is unanimously accepted that surgical closure of the defect should be the first choice and the conservative methods should be reserved for those cases where the patient is not able to sustain a major surgical procedure (associated malformations, shock, etc.) [1]. With regards to the surgical procedure, it is up to the surgeon to make the choice how to close the defect and in how many steps. However, with large defects and large visceral abdominal disproportion, primary closure should not even be attempted [5].

In our case, we preferred to use a staged closure of the defect. The child was well enough at birth to undergo the surgical procedure. We used the membrane omphalocele as a temporary cover of the herniated viscera as described by Fufezan et al. [4]. This method is similar with the use silobag

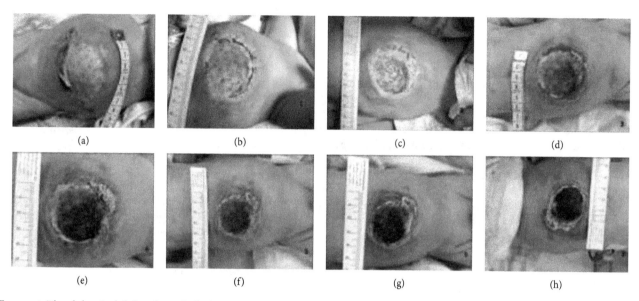

(a)   (b)   (c)   (d)

(e)   (f)   (g)   (h)

FIGURE 4: The abdominal defect through the NPWT. Initial aspect after the wound dehiscence (a) and after each of the 7 dressings (b–h).

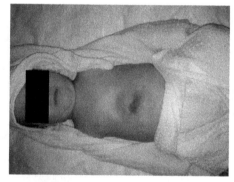

FIGURE 5: The wound at the time of discharge from the hospital. The abdominal wall was closed with only a small skin defect covered by granulation.

temporary containers for the herniated viscera except that it uses the omphalocele membrane as a temporary cover. The method was validated decades ago in an era when silobags were not yet available [4]. We were able to progressively reduce the content of the sac into the abdominal cavity in 2 steps, and in the 3rd, we closed the remaining wall defect using a Gore-Tex patch, without inducing a compartment syndrome. The use of the Gore-Tex patches is a not a novelty in treating abdominal wall defects such as omphaloceles [1]. However, their use is not without risks. In our case, the skin-covering patch became necrotic and ruptured five days after surgery. This happened due to excess tension and lack of underlying vascular support.

Complications due to primary closure of giant omphaloceles are alarming [6,7]. In a survey conducted in 2011, a review by van Eijck et al. showed that the mean postoperative herniation rates were the highest in primary closure of large omphaloceles (58%) and the lowest in nonoperative delayed closure (9%) [3]. This means that an alternative strategy is necessary in GO cases with large tissue defects and large visceral abdominal disproportion, and in

such cases, primary closure should not even be attempted [8–10]. Nowadays, most of the surgeons use temporary covers such as silobags, with good outcomes [8]. The use of conservative treatment that results in early skin cover by secondary wound healing is not without drawbacks. The re-epithelization time on the omphalocele sac can take 2-3 months, and the remaining eventration has to be closed later on [11].

The two main complications possible after closure of the congenital abdominal defects are compartment syndrome, due to excessive intra-abdominal pressure and wound dehiscence with visceral exposure [12,13]. Even though we were able to avoid abdominal hypertension by using stage repair and the Gore-Tex patch, rupture of the skin occurred after a few days after the definitive closure attempt. We were then forced to find a solution to cover the skin defect and protect the abdominal viscera from external exposure. The Gore-Tex patch was in place and was ensuring structural strength to the fascial sheet of the abdominal wall. So, in the absence of the compartment syndrome, we considered it is not wise to remove it. However, the Gore-Tex patch does not have insulation proprieties, so the abdominal cavity was not insulated from the external environment. The solution we found was to use a negative-pressure wound therapy system (NPWT) to temporarily close the skin defect. NPWTs are long used in the treatment of large or complicated skin wounds, infected wounds, etc. [14]. NPWT is seldom used also for congenital or acquired abdominal wall defects [15–18]. NPWT was applied directly over the omphalocele membrane to reduce the size of the defect and promote the reintegration of the herniated viscera [16]. In other instances, it was used for complicated omphalocele with a ruptured membrane and the NPWT dressing was applied directly over the exposed viscera [17]. In both instances, the NPWT was effective in cleaning the wound and promoting the defect reduction and viscera reintegration [16–18]. In our case, even though it took 28 days and 7 consecutive dressings, NPWT proved to be useful. There were several facts we had to consider when setting the NPWT system over the abdominal defect. First, we placed the vacuum dressing over the Gore-Tex patch, which acted as a protective barrier for the intra-abdominal organs. Direct suction pressure over the abdominal organs and contact with the silver dressing would have induced severe lesions. Previous studies' recommendations are to set the vacuum system over a protective mesh when use over and abdominal defect [15]. Secondly, we had to assess which is the optimum interval between dressing changes. Most of the dressings were changed in the operating theatre under sedation, so we prolonged the interval between dressings as much as possible. Last, since there are no clear recommendations, we set the pressure to the minimum of the device, −40 mmHg. We do not know if higher pressure would have a negative (or positive) impact, but since it was effective, we kept it as it is. The wound was cleaned from necrosis debridement, granulation tissue formed at the ages of the hound, the abdominal cavity was protected from external exposure, and the wound decreased in size till we were able to safely close the defect.

5. Conclusions

Delayed closure should be the preferred treatment method in giant omphaloceles. Various methods are available, and with this case presentation, we remind one of the old but useful techniques, the Fufezan technique. Negative-pressure wound therapy is effective in the treatment of congenital abdominal defects and should be considered as a temporary closure and to promote wound healing and shrinking of the abdominal wall defect.

Consent

Written informed consent was obtained from the patient's legal guardian to publish this paper.

Acknowledgments

The authors wish to express their gratitude to Mr. Cristian Tecu Ph.D., a professional photographer and visual artist, for technical support in preparing the figures.

References

[1] D. J. Ledbetter, "Gastroschisis and omphalocele," *Surgical Clinics of North America*, vol. 86, no. 2, pp. 249–260, 2006.

[2] X. Huang, H. Huang, Y. Liang et al., "Modified sequential sac ligation and staged closure technique for the management of giant omphalocele," *Journal of Pediatric Surgery*, 2020.

[3] F. C. Van Eijck, D. A. Aronson, Y. L. Hoogeveen, and R. M. H. Wijnen, "Past and current surgical treatment of giant omphalocele: outcome of a questionnaire sent to authors," *Journal of Pediatric Surgery*, vol. 46, no. 3, pp. 482–488, 2011.

[4] V. Fufezan, "A new concept and surgical technic in treating omphalocele," *Revista de Chirurgie, Oncologie, Radiologie, O.R.L. Oftalmol Stomatol Chir*, vol. 39, no. 1, pp. 37–43, 1990.

[5] B. Bauman, D. Stephens, H. Gershone et al., "Management of giant omphaloceles: a systematic review of methods of staged surgical vs. nonoperative delayed closure," *Journal of Pediatric Surgery*, vol. 51, no. 10, pp. 1725–1730, 2016.

[6] A. C. Akinkuotu, F. Sheikh, O. O. Olutoye et al., "Giant omphaloceles: surgical management and perinatal outcomes," *Journal of Surgical Research*, vol. 198, no. 2, pp. 388–392, 2015.

[7] K. W. Gonzalez and N. M. Chandler, "Ruptured omphalocele: diagnosis and management," *Seminars in Pediatric Surgery*, vol. 28, no. 2, pp. 101–105, 2019.

[8] A. J. Mack and B. Rofdo, "Giant omphalocele: current perspectives," *Research and Reports in Neonatology*, vol. 6, pp. 33–39, 2016.

[9] C. Floortje, F. C. van Eijck, I. de Blaauw et al., "Closure of giant omphaloceles by the abdominal wall component separation technique in infants," *Journal of Pediatric Surgery*, vol. 43, no. 1, pp. 246–250, 2008.

[10] M. Pacilli, L. Spitz, E. M. Kiely, J. Curry, and A. Pierro, "Staged repair of giant omphalocele in the neonatal period," *Journal of Pediatric Surgery*, vol. 40, no. 5, pp. 785–788, 2005.

[11] E. A. Ekot, V. C. Emordi, and D. O. Osifo, "Does omphalocele major undergo spontaneous closure?" *Journal of Surgical Case Reports*, vol. 2017, no. 8, 2017.

[12] F. C. Thabet and J. C. Ejike, "Intra-abdominal hypertension and abdominal compartment syndrome in pediatrics. A review," *Journal of Critical Care*, vol. 41, pp. 275–282, 2017.

[13] V. L. David, A. Pal, M. C. Popoiu, E. R. Iacob, M. C. Stănciulescu, and E. S. Boia, "Prognostic factors for congenital abdominal wall defects," *Jurnalul Pediatrului*, vol. 19, no. 75-76, pp. 85–89, 2016.

[14] S. Mendez-Eastman, "Negative pressure wound therapy," *Plastic Surgical Nursing*, vol. 18, no. 1, pp. 27–37, 1998.

[15] C. A. Bertelsen and J. G. Hillingsø, "The use of topical negative pressure in an open abdomen," *Ugeskr Laeger*, vol. 169, no. 21, pp. 1991–1996, 2007.

[16] K. E. Kilbride, D. R. Cooney, and M. D. Custer, "Vacuum-assisted closure: a new method for treating patients with giant omphalocele," *Journal of Pediatric Surgery*, vol. 41, no. 1, pp. 212–215, 2006.

[17] B. Aldridge, A. P. Ladd, J. Kepple, T. Wingle, C. Ring, and E. R. Kokoska, "Negative pressure wound therapy for initial management of giant omphalocele," *The American Journal of Surgery*, vol. 211, no. 3, pp. 605–609, 2016.

[18] C. A. McBride, K. Stockton, K. Storey, and R. M. Kimble, "Negative pressure wound therapy facilitates closure of large congenital abdominal wall defects," *Pediatric Surgery International*, vol. 30, no. 11, pp. 1163–1168, 2014.

49

Arrested Puberty in an Adolescent Male with Anorexia Nervosa Successfully Resumed with Multidisciplinary Care

Diana Simão Raimundo (ID),[1] **Carolina Figueiredo** (ID),[1] **Ana Raposo** (ID),[1] and **Bernardo Dias Pereira** (ID)[2]

[1]*Department of Pediatrics, Hospital Divino Espírito Santo de Ponta Delgada, Ponta Delgada, Portugal*
[2]*Department of Endocrinology and Nutrition, Hospital Divino Espírito Santo de Ponta Delgada, Ponta Delgada, Portugal*

Correspondence should be addressed to Diana Simão Raimundo; d.simaoraimundo@gmail.com

Academic Editor: Ozgur Kasapcopur

The normal development of puberty depends on the specific pulsatility of gonadorelin, which is finely regulated by genetic and environmental factors. In the published literature, eating disorders figure as a cause of pubertal delay/arrest in females but are rarely considered in males with disordered puberty. A 16.7-year-old male was referred to the Department of Pediatrics with arrested puberty due to severe malnutrition in the context of food restriction. Past medical history was relevant for asthma. Generalized cachexia, facial lanugo hair, cutaneous xerosis, and Russell's sign were noted; he had a height of 155.5 cm (−2.5 SD; target height: 168 cm, −1.1 SD) and a BMI of 12.4 kg/m^2 (−6.8 SD); left and right testicular volumes were 8 mL and 10 mL, respectively. He had a twin brother who had normal auxological/pubertal development (height: 167 cm, −1.05 SD; testicular volumes: 20 mL). Anorexia nervosa was diagnosed, and he was enrolled in a personalized treatment and surveillance program. "Nonthyroid illness" resembling secondary hypothyroidism was noted, as was low bone mineral density. Clinical and biochemical follow-up showed significant improvements in BMI (16.2 kg/m^2, −2.55 SD), completion of puberty (testicular volumes: 25 mL), and reversion of main neuroendocrine abnormalities. Herein, we present an adolescent male with arrested puberty in the context of anorexia nervosa. The recognition of this rare condition in males allows a personalized approach to disordered puberty, with resumption of normal function of the hypothalamic-pituitary-gonadal axis and achievement of pubertal milestones.

1. Introduction

Puberty is the process of maturation of the hypothalamic-pituitary-gonadal (HPG) axis that culminates in the full achievement of final height, secondary sexual features, and fertility capacity [1]. This normal development depends on a specific pulsatility of gonadorelin (GnRH), finely regulated by genetic, hormonal, and environmental factors [1]. When pubertal development is absent or delayed, it may include normal variants or pathologic processes of the HPG axis, whereas if puberty is arrested, pathology is likely. The growth spurt may also be compromised in arrested puberty if not treated as the priming of the growth hormone (GH) axis by pubertal sex steroids is halted [2]. The most frequent cause of disordered puberty is constitutional delay of growth and

puberty (53%), followed by functional hypogonadotropic hypogonadism (19%)—systemic diseases and psychological and nutritional causes—permanent hypergonadotropic hypogonadism (13%), and hypogonadotropic hypogonadism (12%) [3]. Among nutritional causes of disordered puberty, eating disorders should be considered; anorexia nervosa (AN) is an infrequent eating disorder with a lifetime prevalence of 0.6–2.2% [4, 5]. It is rare in adolescents (0.3%) [6], and as a cause of disordered puberty, it accounts for 0.9% of cases in one of the largest cross-sectional studies of adolescents with pubertal delay, where no males were reported [3]. In the Diagnostic and Statistical Manual of Mental Disorders (DSM) V criteria, AN is diagnosed if a person (1) restricts energy intake that leads to underweight, (2) has an intense fear of gaining weight or becoming overweight or has a persistent behaviour that prevents weight gain, despite being underweight, and (3) has a distorted perception of body weight and shape, has an inadequate influence of weight and shape on self-esteem, or denies the medical seriousness of underweight [7]. AN was classically a stereotyped diagnosis of females, clearly illustrated in the previous DSM IV criteria, which included amenorrhea as an obligatory feature to consider the diagnosis [8]. This entity is frequently overlooked in the differential diagnosis of an underweight male due to the rarity of the diagnosis in this gender, although males may represent a nonnegligible 25% of all AN cases [9]; noteworthy, males with AN have greater morbidity and mortality [10]. Due to very small sample sizes of adolescent males with AN in studies published to date [11], there is a paucity of data regarding the systemic impact of this eating disorder in this gender at younger ages, namely, in terms of neuroendocrinology [12]. We present a case of an adolescent male with arrested puberty due to severe undernutrition associated with AN. We also review the impact of AN and its treatment on the neuroendocrine axis, growth, and puberty.

2. Case Presentation

A 16.7-year-old Caucasian male was referred to Endocrinology due to nonfamilial short stature. He referred a weight loss of 13 kg in the last 6 months due to dietary restriction of carbohydrates and fat. He also referred decreased libido, asthenia, and decreased tolerance to physical efforts in the last month. He denied purgative behaviour and judged underweight as normal. He also denied any symptoms suggestive of an intracranial lesion. He had a personal history of asthma controlled with inhaled fluticasone and oral desloratadine. Family history was unremarkable. On physical examination, the patient had normal vital signs; generalized cachexia, facial lanugo hair, and cutaneous xerosis; Russell's sign was noted in his third left finger; height was 155.5 cm (−2.5 SD; target height: 168.9 cm, −1.1 SD), weight was 30.2 kg, and BMI was 12.5 kg/m^2 (−6.8 SD); his height chart showed a progressive decrease in his linear growth, markedly (height velocity: 2.7 cm/year) after an age of 13 years (see Figure 1(a)); his BMI chart paralleled the height chart (see Figure 1(b)); the left and right testis measured 8 mL and 10 mL, respectively (Tanner stage: G3P3). He had a dizygotic twin with a height of 167 cm (−1.05 SD), normal BMI, and testicular volumes of 20 mL. A presumptive diagnosis of arrested puberty associated with an eating disorder was assumed, and the patient was referred to the Pediatrics Department, where he was admitted to the ward and enrolled in a multidisciplinary team approach, including Pediatrics, Psychiatry, Psychology, Endocrinology, and Nutrition. General biochemical evaluation is resumed in Table 1. An abdominal ultrasound excluded steatosis and other hepatobiliary diseases, the electrocardiogram was unremarkable, and chest radiography grossly excluded organic pathologies as causes of weight loss. Psychiatric evaluation suggested an atypical case of AN. A personality with perfectionist traits was revealed, encouraged by a central role played in his family. He also showed fusional relationship with his mother and lack of autonomy for his age. Unlike his

twin, he received many family expectations regarding school performance and admission to a reputable university. Neither body image distortion nor anxiety disorder was perceived. The calorie counting was attributed to a need for control due to his perfectionist personality and obsessive personality traits. He was discharged with a weight of 34 kg, 14 days after initiation of a dietary plan and multidisciplinary support, which included family therapy. He was readmitted 3 months later due to a loss of 1.4 kg, and with further multidisciplinary support plus olanzapine 1.25 mg/day (maintained after discharge), his weight improved to 34.6 kg at discharge from the ward. After 6 months of follow-up, he had relatively unchanged height (156.5 cm, −2.5 SD) but improved in terms of BMI (15.6 kg/m^2, −3.27 SD) and resumed puberty (testicular volumes: 12 mL). General biochemistry showed correction of initially abnormal parameters (Table 1); basal endocrine evaluation revealed normal gonadotropins and total testosterone for his evolving Tanner stage and "nonthyroid illness" resembling secondary hypothyroidism (Table 2). Dual-energy X-ray absorptiometry revealed low bone mineral density (BMD; Z-score lumbar spine: −3.4 SD; Z-score hip: −3.2 SD; lumbar spine BMD adjusted for height: −1.50 SD; hip BMD adjusted for height: −1.58 SD; reference/expected BMD adjusted for height: 0 SD), without imaging evidence of vertebral fractures. Bone age was estimated to be delayed by 8 months relative to chronological age. Currently, at 17.6 years old, he maintains his follow-up with a multidisciplinary team and his personalized nutritional plan, including daily supplementation with vitamin D (800 UI/day) and calcium (1200 mg/day). His height had a slight increase to 157.4 cm (−2.2 SD), as was his BMI to 16.2 kg/m^2 (−2.55 SD). Testicular volumes increased to adult size (25 mL). Basal endocrine reevaluation showed increased total testosterone levels and correction of "nonthyroid illness"; high late-night salivary cortisol was noted (Table 2).

3. Discussion

Herein, we present a rare case of an adolescent male with arrested puberty due to severe undernutrition in the context of AN, which, with personalized treatment, could successfully resume his puberty. Data are lacking regarding the pubertal status (Tanner stage) of patients with AN, both at diagnosis and following treatment institution [11]. Available studies include mostly females and report the age of menarche as a marker of puberty. Premenarchal females with AN have invariably delayed menarche at diagnosis, but noteworthy, weight restoration allows its development in some but not all cases; males with AN have lower testicular volumes compared with age- and gender-matched controls, but pubertal growth spurt is usually able to be attained upon treatment initiation [11, 13–15]. In patients with AN, the LH pulse frequency resembles that of a prepubertal stage [16, 17]. The low levels of leptin that parallel the loss of adipose tissue in AN appear to be a crucial link between starvation and a disrupted reproductive system. Leptin acts on the hypothalamic arcuate nucleus upregulating the expression of kiss-1 and its protein (kisspeptin), a stimulator of GnRH neurons, and downregulating the expression of

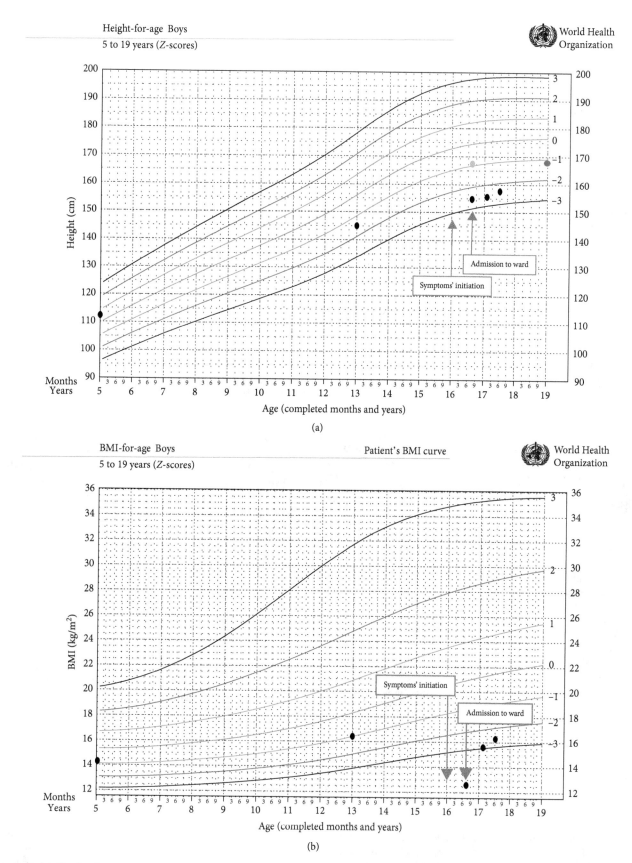

FIGURE 1: (a) Height chart (red dot: target height; green dot: twin's height; black dots: patient's height curve). (b) BMI chart (black dots: patient's BMI curve) of the patient showing shifting of Z-scores after an age of 13 years.

TABLE 1: General biochemical surveys since presentation to the last follow-up visit.

Parameter (units)	Presentation	Follow-up period 6 months	15 months	Reference
Hemoglobin (g/dL)	17.8	13.9	14.2	14–18
Hematocrit (%)	51.1	41.7	41.5	37–49
Creatinine (mg/dL)	0.87	—	0.79	0.7–1.3
AST (U/L)	378	34	24	<34
ALT (U/L)	532	39	23	10–49
GGT (U/L)	75	—	22	<73
Total/direct bilirubin (mg/dL)	0.66/0.16	—	0.32/0.13	0.3–1.2/<0.3
Albumin (g/dL)	4.1	—	—	3.5–5
INR	1.01	—	—	0.75–1.22
Glucose (mg/dL)	47	—	68	70–110
Total cholesterol (mg/dL)	235	—	—	<190
LDL cholesterol (mg/dL)	98	—	—	<130
Sodium (mmol/L)	144	—	143	135–145
Potassium (mmol/L)	4.07	—	4.6	3.5–5.5
Corrected calcium (mg/dL)	9.3	—	10	8.3–10.6
Phosphorus (mg/dL)	2	—	4.5	2.5–4.9
Magnesium (mg/dL)	2.2	—	—	1.6–2.4
25-Hydroxyvitamin D (ng/mL)	11.7	—	—	>30
Antitransglutaminase IgA (U/mL)	0.5	—	—	<7
Antitransglutaminase IgG (U/mL)	<0.5	—	—	—
Total IgA (mg/dL)	389	—	—	70–400
Erythrocyte sedimentation rate (mm)	2	—	—	<15

ALT: alanine transaminase; AST: aspartate transaminase; GGT: gamma-glutamyl transpeptidase; IgA: immunoglobulin A; IgG: immunoglobulin G; INR: international normalized ratio.

TABLE 2: Basal endocrine surveys from 6 months after presentation to the last follow-up visit.

Parameter (units)	Follow-up period 6 months	15 months	Reference
FSH (mUI/L)	3.4	3.4	1.5–12.4
LH (mUI/L)	4.11	4.8	1.7–8.6
Total testosterone (ng/dL)‡	317.7	651	249–836
TSH (UI/mL)	2.06	2.9	0.5–3.4
Free T4 (ng/dL)	0.79	1	0.85–1.37
Free T3 (ng/dL)	—	3	2–4.5
Prolactin (ng/mL)	10.6	—	4–15.2
IGF-1 (ug/L)¥	—	271	126–429
ACTH (ng/L)	—	23.1	7–63
Late-night salivary cortisol (nmol/L)±	—	14.4	<7

ACTH: adrenocorticotropic hormone; FSH: follicle-stimulating hormone; IGF-1: insulin-like growth factor-1; LH: luteinizing hormone; TSH: thyroid-stimulating hormone; T4: thyroxine; T3: triiodothyronine. ‡Collected at 08:30. ¥IGF-1 adjusted for age, in standard deviation (SD) score: −1.17 SD. ±Collected at 23:00.

neuropeptide Y (a GnRH neuron inhibitor) [18]. Thus, hypoleptinemia is linked to an inhibitory drive to GnRH pulsatility. Ghrelin is a stomach-derived peptide that is elevated in AN; it stimulates appetite partially through neuropeptide Y activation, and this may be the link between increased levels of ghrelin and low levels of LH in females, as well as low levels of testosterone and testicular volumes in males with AN [13, 19]. The stressful mental milieu of patients with AN is linked to hyperactivity of the hypothalamic-pituitary-adrenal axis, which is driven by high

levels of CRH [20]. Indeed, higher anxiety and depression scores obtained from women with AN correlate with serum cortisol [21]. Patients with AN maintain their circadian rhythm of cortisol, although at a higher set point [17, 21], and a significant proportion fails to suppress cortisol after low-dose dexamethasone tests [22]. Hypercortisolemia in patients with AN is linked to low GnRH drive and LH pulsatility, although the mechanisms behind this association are not fully clarified [23]. Normal levels of cortisol are usually achieved with weight recovery, although some patients remain hypercortisolemic despite an increase in BMI—as shown in our case—and other psychobiological factors may play a role in maintaining this overactive state [23]. Hypercortisolemia may also contribute to the biochemical pattern of "nonthyroid illness" that resembles central hypothyroidism [24], where starvation plays a major role in eliciting this dysfunction of the pituitary-thyroid axis [12, 17]. This abnormality is regarded as adaptive to spare energy for vital functions [15] but usually resumes with weight recovery [25], as shown in our case. Although our patient had a 33% increase in weight after 1 year of follow-up, he did not show catch-up growth. Studies that focused on the growth of paediatric patients with AN have shown no difference in final height between cases and age- and gender-matched controls, with catch-up growth seen on average at 1 year of follow-up [11]. However, some surveys have shown a failure to catch-up growth, even after weight restoration [11, 26]. The largest study that focused on the growth of young males with AN evidenced that catch-up growth was only attained in patients that had the diagnosis of AN before their pubertal growth spurt [26]. Additionally, although starvation and low BMI are sufficient to impede height and puberty to evolve, bone maturation is not delayed in proportion, and the epiphyseal growth plates continue to close [13, 26]. Considering that our patient had testicular volumes of 10 mL at diagnosis of AN and that pubertal growth spurt is expected to supervene from this Tanner stage onwards, we speculate that the failure to catch-up growth seen in our patient may have been related to a diagnosis of AN close to his pubertal growth spurt initiation, and the delay in recognizing and addressing AN until his 16 years old allowed a bone maturation that impeded the attainment of his target height. The growth failure seen in untreated patients with AN is also related to the disordered GH axis. GH levels are elevated in patients with AN due to low feedback control by IGF-1 and high levels of GH secretagogue ghrelin; IGF-1 is decreased due to hepatic GH resistance, evidenced by the low levels of its plasma binding protein, which constitutes the extracellular domain of the GH receptor [15, 19].

Malnutrition-induced hepatitis is common among individuals with AN [27, 28] as a likely explanation to elevations in aminotransferases seen in our patient. Less commonly, as part of the refeeding process, liver enzymes may also increase due to hepatic steatosis and can be distinguished from malnutrition-induced hepatitis by the finding of a fatty liver on ultrasonography [27]. Individuals with AN and malnutrition-induced hepatitis are also at an increased risk of hypoglycemia due to depleted glycogen stores and impaired hepatic gluconeogenesis [29]. Dyslipidemia is common in patients with AN, but its mechanisms remain unclear. A recent multicenter study showed evidence of elevated lipid concentrations in acutely ill patients with AN compared with healthy controls (HC), some of which persisted after partial weight restoration [30].

Our patient had low BMD. Adolescence is a period of increased bone accrual towards the attainment of peak bone mass, which is markedly impaired in adolescents with AN [13, 31], and earlier age at diagnosis of AN is related to higher severity of decreased BMD [31]. Consequently, individuals with AN at younger ages have a significantly higher risk of fractures (31–57%) when compared with age-matched controls and population-based incidence [31, 32]. Low BMD in AN is multifactorial: low testosterone in males impairs bone formation directly by reduced activation of osteoblasts (through the androgen receptor) and indirectly by low aromatization in adipose tissue to oestrogen, which acts on the osteoclast to reduce its mass (impairing responsiveness of osteoclast progenitor cells to RANKL and inducing apoptosis) and bone resorption [33]; low IGF-1 is also a critical determinant of BMD in patients with AN. Its levels directly correlate with bone turnover markers in adolescent males [13], and recombinant IGF-1 yielded significant improvements in BMD of patients with AN [15]; high cortisol levels are a strong predictor of low BMD in AN, and the well-known bone detrimental effects of hypercortisolemia may explain the lack of efficacy of oestrogen therapy for low BMD in patients with AN [21]; reduced lean mass directly correlates with BMD in males with AN [13], probably due to less stimulatory effects of muscular biomechanical forces on bone formation [13, 15]; BMI at diagnosis of AN directly correlates with the severity of BMD,

and the magnitude of weight restoration is higher, so the best outcomes are achieved in terms of BMD [13, 15, 34]. There is a paucity of data regarding the benefits of pharmacologic options to increase BMD in adolescents with AN. The only small study in this age range included exclusively females and showed that alendronate increased BMD relative to placebo, although statistically nonsignificant; weight restoration was a significant predictor of bone mass accrual, emphasizing the importance of instituting a personalized treatment plan for patients with AN to restore weight and improve long-term bone health [34]. There are no published trials or recommendations to guide the treatment of hypogonadal adolescents with AN and osteoporosis (defined as BMD Z-scores <-2 SD and bone fractures) [15].

In conclusion, the presented case illustrates the importance of identifying the underlying aetiology of arrested puberty and a focused multidisciplinary approach to revert functional abnormalities of the HPG axis that allow pubertal resumption and completion. Early diagnosis and treatment are crucial to blunt the drivers of neuroendocrine abnormalities characteristics of AN, which may lead to suboptimal height gain, unachieved pubertal milestones, and a BMD prone to fractures.

Consent

Written informed consent was obtained from the patient, who is currently 18 years old.

Acknowledgments

The authors acknowledge Dr. Daniel Rego, from the Department of Psychiatry of Hospital Divino Espírito Santo de Ponta Delgada, for his contribution in the review of the psychiatric evaluation.

References

[1] B. Bordini and R. L. Rosenfield, "Normal pubertal development: Part I: the endocrine basis of puberty," *Pediatrics in Review*, vol. 32, no. 6, pp. 223–229, 2011.

[2] M. T. Muñoz-Calvo and J. Argente, "Nutritional and pubertal disorders," *Endocrine Development*, vol. 29, pp. 153–173, 2016.

[3] I. L. Sedlmeyer, M. R. Palmert, and C. N. S. Hospital, "Delayed puberty: analysis of a large case series from an academic center," *The Journal of Clinical Endocrinology & Metabolism*, vol. 87, no. 4, pp. 1613–1620, 2002.

[4] J. I. Hudson, E. Hiripi, H. G. Pope, and R. C. Kessler, "The prevalence and correlates of eating disorders in the national comorbidity survey replication," *Biological Psychiatry*, vol. 61, no. 3, pp. 348–358, 2007.

[5] P. Södersten, C. Bergh, and M. Björnström, "Prevalence and recovery from anorexia nervosa," *American Journal of Psychiatry*, vol. 165, no. 2, pp. 264-265, 2008.

[6] S. A. Swanson, S. J. Crow, D. Le Grange, J. Swendsen, and K. R. Merikangas, "Prevalence and correlates of eating disorders in adolescents," *Archives of General Psychiatry*, vol. 68, no. 7, pp. 714–723, 2011.

[7] American Psychiatric Association, *Diagnostic and Statistical Manual of Mental Disorders*, American Psychiatric Association, Washington, DC, USA, 2013.

[8] American Psychiatric Association, *Diagnostic and Statistical Manual of Mental Disorders*, American Psychiatric Association, Washington, DC, USA, 2000.

[9] T. Wooldridge and P. P. Lytle, "An overview of anorexia nervosa in males," *Eating Disorders*, vol. 20, no. 5, pp. 368–378, 2012.

[10] S. Edakubo and K. Fushimi, "Mortality and risk assessment for anorexia nervosa in acute-care hospitals: a nationwide administrative database analysis," *BMC Psychiatry*, vol. 20, no. 1, p. 19, 2020.

[11] J. Neale, S. M. A. Pais, D. Nicholls, S. Chapman, and L. D. Hudson, "What are the effects of restrictive eating disorders on growth and puberty and are effects permanent? A systematic review and meta-analysis," *Journal of Adolescent Health*, vol. 66, no. 2, pp. 144–156, 2020.

[12] A. Skolnick, R. C. Schulman, R. J. Galindo, and J. I. Mechanick, "The endocrinopathies of male anorexia nervosa: case series," *AACE Clinical Case Reports*, vol. 2, no. 4, pp. e351–e357, 2016.

[13] M. Misra, D. K. Katzman, J. Cord et al., "Bone metabolism in adolescent boys with anorexia nervosa," *The Journal of Clinical Endocrinology & Metabolism*, vol. 93, no. 8, pp. 3029–3036, 2008.

[14] D. Modan-Moses, A. Yaroslavsky, I. Novikov et al., "Stunting of growth as a major feature of anorexia nervosa in male adolescents," *Pediatrics*, vol. 111, no. 2, pp. 270–276, 2003.

[15] M. Misra and A. Klibanski, "Anorexia nervosa and its associated endocrinopathy in young people," *Hormone Research in Paediatrics*, vol. 85, no. 3, pp. 147–157, 2016.

[16] M. Misra, K. K. Miller, K. Kuo et al., "Secretory dynamics of leptin in adolescent girls with anorexia nervosa and healthy adolescents," *American Journal of Physiology-Endocrinology and Metabolism*, vol. 289, no. 3, pp. E373–E381, 2005.

[17] A. B. Loucks and J. R. Thuma, "Luteinizing hormone pulsatility is disrupted at a threshold of energy availability in regularly menstruating women," *The Journal of Clinical Endocrinology & Metabolism*, vol. 88, no. 1, pp. 297–311, 2003.

[18] S. Kumar and G. Kaur, "Intermittent fasting dietary restriction regimen negatively influences reproduction in young rats: a study of hypothalamo-hypophysial-gonadal axis," *PLoS One*, vol. 8, no. 1, Article ID e52416, 2013.

[19] M. Misra, K. K. Miller, K. Kuo et al., "Secretory dynamics of ghrelin in adolescent girls with anorexia nervosa and healthy adolescents," *American Journal of Physiology-Endocrinology and Metabolism*, vol. 289, no. 2, pp. E347–E356, 2005.

[20] W. H. Kaye, "Neuropeptide abnormalities in anorexia nervosa," *Psychiatry Research*, vol. 62, no. 1, pp. 65–74, 1996.

[21] E. A. Lawson, D. Donoho, K. K. Miller et al., "Hypercortisolemia is associated with severity of bone loss and depression in hypothalamic amenorrhea and anorexia nervosa," *The Journal of Clinical Endocrinology & Metabolism*, vol. 94, no. 12, pp. 4710–4716, 2009.

[22] M. Duclos, J.-B. Corcuff, P. Roger, and A. Tabarin, "The dexamethasone-suppressed corticotrophin-releasing hormone stimulation test in anorexia nervosa," *Clinical Endocrinology*, vol. 51, no. 6, pp. 725–731, 1999.

[23] M. Misra, R. Prabhakaran, K. K. Miller et al., "Role of cortisol in menstrual recovery in adolescent girls with anorexia nervosa," *Pediatric Research*, vol. 59, no. 4 Pt 1, pp. 598–603, 2006.

[24] S. L. Berga, T. L. Daniels, and D. E. Giles, "Women with functional hypothalamic amenorrhea but not other forms of anovulation display amplified cortisol concentrations," *Fertility and Sterility*, vol. 67, no. 6, pp. 1024–1030, 1997.

[25] J. E. Schebendach, N. H. Golden, M. S. Jacobson, S. Hertz, and I. R. Shenker, "The metabolic responses to starvation and refeeding in adolescents with anorexia nervosa," *Annals of the New York Academy of Sciences*, vol. 817, no. 1, pp. 110–119, 1997.

[26] I. Swenne, "Poor catch-up growth in late adolescent boys with eating disorders, weight loss and stunting of growth," *European Eating Disorders Review*, vol. 21, no. 5, pp. 395–398, 2013.

[27] E. Rosen, N. Bakshi, A. Watters, H. R. Rosen, and P. S. Mehler, "Hepatic complications of anorexia nervosa," *Digestive Diseases and Sciences*, vol. 62, no. 11, pp. 2977–2981, 2017.

[28] V. Narayanan, J. L. Gaudiani, R. H. Harris, and P. S. Mehler, "Liver function test abnormalities in anorexia nervosa-cause or effect," *The International Journal of Eating Disorders*, vol. 43, no. 4, pp. 378–381, 2010.

[29] R. Ohwada, M. Hotta, S. Oikawa, and K. Takano, "Etiology of hypercholesterolemia in patients with anorexia nervosa," *International Journal of Eating Disorders*, vol. 39, no. 7, pp. 598–601, 2006.

[30] A. A. Hussain, C. Hübel, M. Hindborg et al., "Increased lipid and lipoprotein concentrations in anorexia nervosa: a systematic review and meta-analysis," *The International Journal of Eating Disorders*, vol. 52, no. 6, pp. 611–629, 2019.

[31] A. T. Faje, P. K. Fazeli, K. K. Miller et al., "Fracture risk and areal bone mineral density in adolescent females with anorexia nervosa," *International Journal of Eating Disorders*, vol. 47, no. 5, pp. 458–466, 2014.

[32] A. R. Lucas, L. J. Melton, C. S. Crowson, and W. M. O'Fallon, "Long-term fracture risk among women with anorexia nervosa: a population-based cohort study," *Mayo Clinic Proceedings*, vol. 74, no. 10, pp. 972–977, 1999.

[33] C. Maes and H. M. Kronenberg, "Bone development and remodeling," *Endocrinology: Adult and Pediatric*, vol. 1, pp. 1038–1062, 2016.

[34] N. H. Golden, E. A. Iglesias, M. S. Jacobson et al., "Alendronate for the treatment of osteopenia in anorexia nervosa: a randomized, double-blind, placebo-controlled trial," *The Journal of Clinical Endocrinology & Metabolism*, vol. 90, no. 6, pp. 3179–3185, 2005.

Permissions

List of Contributors

Hina Emanuel, Kimberly Rennie, Aravind Yadav and Ricardo A. Mosquera
Department of Pediatrics, e University of Texas Health Science Center at Houston, McGovern Medical School, Houston, TX, USA

Kelly Macdonald
University of Houston, Texas Institute for Measurement, Evaluation, and Statistics, Department of Psychology, Houston, TX, USA

D. Hettiaracchchi, N. Neththikumara, B. A. P. S. Pathirana and V. H. W. Dissanayake
Human Genetics Unit, Faculty of Medicine, University of Colombo, Colombo, Sri Lanka

A. Padeniya
National Hospital of Sri Lanka, Colombo, Sri Lanka

Dionna M. Mathews
Our Lady of the Lake Children's Hospital, Baton Rouge, LA, USA

Katie M. Vance and Pamela M. McMahon
Division of Academic Affairs, Our Lady of the Lake Regional Medical Center, Baton Rouge, LA, USA

Catherine Boston
Pediatric Hematology/Oncology, Our Lady of the Lake Children's Hospital/St. Jude Affiliate Baton Rouge, Baton Rouge, LA, USA

Michael T. Bolton
Pediatric Infectious Diseases, Our Lady of the Lake Children's Hospital, Baton Rouge, LA, USA

Cláudia Patraquim
Pediatrics Department, Hospital de Braga, Sete Fontes, S˜ao Victor, 4710-243 Braga, Portugal

Vera Fernandes
Endocrinology Department, Hospital de Braga, Sete Fontes, São Victor, 4710-243 Braga, Portugal
Life and Health Sciences Research Institute (ICVS), School of Health Sciences, University of Minho, Braga, Portugal
ICVS/3B's-PT Government Associate Laboratory, Braga, Guimarães, Portugal

Jorge Correia-Pinto
Life and Health Sciences Research Institute (ICVS), School of Health Sciences, University of Minho, Braga, Portugal
ICVS/3B's-PT Government Associate Laboratory, Braga, Guimarães, Portugal
Pediatric Surgical Department, Hospital de Braga, Sete Fontes, São Victor, 4710-243 Braga, Portugal

Olinda Marques
Endocrinology Department, Hospital de Braga, Sete Fontes, São Victor, 4710-243 Braga, Portugal

Sofia Martins and Ana Antunes
Pediatric Endocrinology Department, Hospital de Braga, Sete Fontes, São Victor, 4710-243 Braga, Portugal

José Luís Carvalho
Pediatric Surgical Department, Hospital de Braga, Sete Fontes, São Victor, 4710-243 Braga, Portugal

Carla Meireles
Pediatrics Department, Hospital da Senhora daOliveira, Creixomil, 4835-044 Guimarães, Portugal

Ana Margarida Ferreira
Anatomic Pathology Department, Hospital de Braga, Sete Fontes, São Victor, 4710-243 Braga, Portugal

Gianluigi Ardissino, Michela Perrone, Francesca Tel and Sara Testa
Center for HUS Prevention Control and Management, Fondazione IRCCS Ca' Granda Osp. Maggiore Policlinico, Milan, Italy

Amelia Morrone
Paediatric Neurology Unit and Laboratories, Neuroscience Department, Meyer Children's Hospital, Florence, Italy
Neuroscience, Psychology, Pharmacology and Child Health Department, University of Florence, Florence, Italy

Ilaria Possenti
Pediatric Unit, Pediatric Hospital C. Arrigo, Alessandria, Italy

Francesco Tagliaferri and Francesca Menni
Pediatric Unit, Fondazione IRCCS Ca' Granda Osp. Maggiore Policlinico, Milan, Italy

Robertino Dilena
UOC Neurophysiology, Fondazione IRCCS Ca' Granda Osp. Maggiore Policlinico, Milan, Italy

Tham Thi Tran, Quang Van Vu and Sang Ngoc Nguyen
Department of Pediatrics, Haiphong University of Medicine and Pharmacy, Haiphong, Vietnam

Taizo Wada and Akihiro Yachie
Department of Pediatrics, Institute of Medical, Pharmaceutical and Health Science, Kanazawa University, Kanazawa, Japan

Huong Le Thi Minh
National Hospital of Pediatrics, Hanoi, Vietnam

Leah S. Heidenreich
Mayo Clinic Children's Center, Mayo Clinic, Rochester, Minnesota, USA

Peter J. Holmberg
Mayo Clinic Children's Center, Mayo Clinic, Rochester, Minnesota, USA
Division of General Pediatric and Adolescent Medicine, Mayo Clinic, Rochester, Minnesota, USA

Vilmarie Rodriguez
Mayo Clinic Children's Center, Mayo Clinic, Rochester, Minnesota, USA
Division of Pediatric Hematology/Oncology, Mayo Clinic, Rochester, Minnesota, USA

Jennifer L. Oliveira
Division of Hematopathology, Mayo Clinic, Rochester, Minnesota, USA

Mario Briceno-Medina and Ronak Naik
Division of Cardiology, Le Bonheur Children's Hospital, University of Tennessee Health Science Center, Memphis, TN, USA

Michael Perez
Division of Cardiology, Le Bonheur Children's Hospital, University of Tennessee Health Science Center, Memphis, TN, USA
Division of Pediatric Cardiology, Ann & Robert H. Lurie Children's Hospital of Chicago, Northwestern University, Chicago, IL, USA

Jie Zhang
Department of Pathology, Le Bonheur Children's Hospital, University of Tennessee Health Science Center, Memphis, TN, USA

Samir Shah and Dai Kimura
Division of Critical Care Medicine, Le Bonheur Children's Hospital, University of Tennessee Health Science Center, Memphis, TN, USA

Dimitrios Stoimenis, Nikolaos Petridis and Nikos Papaioannou
Department of Internal Medicine, General Hospital G. Papanikolaou, essaloniki, Greece

Christina Spyridonidou
Intensive Care Unit, General Hospital Papageorgiou, essaloniki, Greece

Sofia Theofanidou
Department of Internal Medicine, General Hospital G. Gennimatas, Athens, Greece

Christina Iasonidou and Nikolaos Kapravelos
Intensive Care Unit, General Hospital G. Papanikolaou, essaloniki, Greece

Shinya Tomori, Seigo Korematsu, Taichi Momose, Yasuko Urushihara and Koichi Moriwaki
Department of Pediatrics, Saitama Medical Center Saitama Medical University, Kamoda, Kawagoe Saitama 350-8550, Japan

Shuji Momose
Department of Pathology, Saitama Medical Center, Saitama Medical University, Kamoda, Kawagoe Saitama 350-8550, Japan

Radhika Maddali and Lily Q. Lew
Department of Pediatrics, Flushing Hospital Medical Center, Flushing, NY 11355, USA

Kelly L. Cervellione
Department of Clinical Research, Medisys Health Network, Jamaica, NY 11418, USA

Lamidi Audu, Amina Gambo and Bilkisu Farouk
Department of Paediatrics and Child Health, Barau Dikko Teaching Hospital, Kaduna State University, Kaduna, Nigeria

Anisa Yahaya and Kefas Jacob
Department of Radiology, Barau Dikko Teaching Hospital, Kaduna State University, Kaduna, Nigeria

Adityanarayan Rao and Joshua Pryor
University of Florida College of Medicine, Gainesville, FL 32610, USA

Jaclyn Otero and Molly Posa
University of Florida-Pediatrics Department, Gainesville, FL 32610, USA

Yasuaki Matsumoto, Junko Yamanaka, Yukari Atsumi, Shinji Mochizuki and Hiroyuki Shichino
Department of Pediatrics, National Center for Global Health and Medicine Hospital, 1-21-1 Toyama, Shinjuku-ku, Tokyo 162-8655, Japan

Katsuyoshi Shimozawa
Department of Pediatrics, National Center for Global Health and Medicine Hospital, 1-21-1 Toyama, Shinjuku-ku, Tokyo 162-8655, Japan
Department of Pediatrics and Child Health, Nihon University School of Medicine, 30-1 Oyaguchikami-cho, Itabashi-ku, Tokyo 173-8610, Japan

Tomomi Ota
Department of Pediatrics, National Center for Global Health and Medicine Hospital, 1-21-1 Toyama, Shinjuku-ku, Tokyo 162-8655, Japan
Division of Neonatology, Nagano Children's Hospital, 3100 Toyoshina, Azumino-shi, Nagano 399-8288, Japan

Takayuki Fujii, Ryuichi Shimono, Aya Tanaka and Hiroto Katami
Department of Pediatric Surgery, Faculty of Medicine, Kagawa University, 1750-1 Ikenobe, Mikicho, Kitagun, Kagawa 761-0793, Japan

Alexander K. C. Leung
Clinical Professor of Pediatrics at e University of Calgary, Calgary, Alberta, Canada T2M 0H5
Pediatric Consultant at e Alberta Children's Hospital, Calgary, Alberta, Canada T2M 0H5

Kin Fon Leong
Consultant Pediatric Dermatologist at the Pediatric Institute, Kuala Lumpur General Hospital, Kuala Lumpur, Malaysia

Joseph M. Lam
Clinical Associate Professor of Pediatrics and Associate Member at the Department of Dermatology and Skin Sciences, University of British Columbia, Vancouver, Canada

Toshihiko Okumura, Makoto Yamaguchi, Takako Suzuki, Yuka Torii, Jun-ichi Kawada and Yoshinori Ito
Department of Pediatrics, Nagoya University Graduate School of Medicine, 65 Tsurumai-cho, Showa-ku, Nagoya 466-8550, Japan

Nobuyuki Tetsuka
Department of Infectious Disease, Nagoya University Hospital, 65 Tsurumai-cho, Showa-ku, Nagoya 466-8550, Japan

Andrea Guala, Micaela Silvestri, Michelangelo Barbaglia
SOC Pediatrics, Castelli Hospital, Verbania, Italy

Benjamin Z. Koplewitz
Department of Radiology, Hadassah-Hebrew University Medical Center, Jerusalem, Israel

Giulia Folgori
SOC Pediatrics, Castelli Hospital, Verbania, Italy
Post-graduate School in Pediatrics, University "Piemonte Orientale", Novara, Italy

Cesare Danesino
Department of Molecular Medicine, University of Pavia, Pavia, Italy

Kasra Zarei, John A. Bernat, Yutaka Sato, Rachel Segal and Guru Bhoojhawon
University of Iowa, Carver College of Medicine, 200 Hawkins Drive, Iowa City, IA 52242, USA

Avigdor Hevroni, Chaim Springer, Oren Wasser and Avraham Avital
Institute of Pulmonology, Hadassah-Hebrew University Medical Center, Jerusalem, Israel

Shreeja Shikhrakar, Pradeep Sharma and Sneha Shrestha
Department of Pediatrics, Kathmandu University School of Medical Sciences, Dhulikhel, Nepal

Sujit Kumar Mandal
Kakani Primary Health Center, Nuwakot, Nepal

Sanket Bhattarai
Paanchkhal Primary Health Center, Kavre, Nepal

Abdullah Alhaizaey and Ahmed Azazy
Division of Vascular Surgery, Aseer Central Hospital, Abha Maternity and Children Hospital, Abha, Saudi Arabia

Ibrahim Alhelali
Pediatric Intensive Care, Abha Maternity and Children Hospital, Abha, Saudi Arabia

Musaed Alghamdi
Department of Pediatrics, Menoufia University, Menoufia, Shibin Al Kawm, Egypt

Mohammed A. Samir
Aseer Central Hospital, Abha, Saudi Arabia

Georg Singer, Christoph Castellani and Holger Till
Department of Paediatric and Adolescent Surgery, Medical University of Graz, Graz, Austria

Karl Kashofer
Institute of Pathology, Medical University of Graz, Graz, Austria

Osama Hamdoun, Asia Al Mulla and Shamma Al Zaabi
Department of Academic Affairs, Tawam Hospital, Al-Ain, UAE

Hiba Shendi, Sharifa Al Ghamdi, Jozef Hertecant and Amar Al-Shibli
Department of Pediatrics, Tawam Hospital, Al-Ain, UAE

Monica Aldulescu
Ann & Robert H. Lurie Children's Hospital, Chicago, Illinois, USA

Farooq Shahzad
Ann & Robert H. Lurie Children's Hospital, Chicago, Illinois, USA
Northwestern University Feinberg School of Medicine, Chicago, Illinois, USA

Ava G. Chappell and Chad A. Purnell
Northwestern University Feinberg School of Medicine, Chicago, Illinois, USA

Sarah Chamlin
Ann & Robert H. Lurie Children's Hospital, Chicago, Illinois, USA
Northwestern University Feinberg School of Medicine, Chicago, Illinois, USA

Sheema Gaffar
Department of Pediatrics, Eastern Virginia Medical School, 700 West Olney Road, Norfolk, VA 23507, USA

John K. Birknes
Division of Pediatric Neurosurgery, Children's Hospital of the King's Daughters, 601 Children's Lane, Norfolk, VA 23507, USA

Kenji M. Cunnion
Department of Pediatrics, Eastern Virginia Medical School, 700 West Olney Road, Norfolk, VA 23507, USA
Division of Infectious Diseases, Children's Hospital of the King's Daughters, 601 Children's Lane, Norfolk, VA 23507, USA
Children's Specialty Group, 811 Redgate Avenue, Norfolk, VA 23507, USA

Nadia K. Rafiq and Paul A. Brogan
Infection and Inflammation and Rheumatology Section, University College London Great Ormond Street Institute of Child Health, 30 Guilford Street, London WC1 E1H, UK

Helen Lachmann
National Amyloidosis Centre, University College London Division of Medicine, London, UK

Frodi Joensen
National Hospital of the Faroe Islands, J. C. Svabos Gøta, T´orshavn 100, Faroe Islands

Troels Herlin
Department of Paediatrics, Pediatric Rheumatology Clinic, Palle Juul-Jensens Boulevard 99, 8200 Aarhus N, Denmark

Anna Lin, Lawrence Chi Ngong Chan, Kam Lun Ellis Hon and Hon Ming Cheung
Department of Paediatrics, The Chinese University of Hong Kong, Hong Kong

Siu Yan Bess Tsui
Department of Surgery, The Chinese University of Hong Kong, Hong Kong

Kristine Kit Yi Pang
Department of Surgery, The Hong Kong Children's Hospital, Kowloon, Hong Kong
Department of Surgery, The Chinese University of Hong Kong, Hong Kong

Gurleen Kaur Kahlon, Anna Zylak, Patrick Leblanc and Noah Kondamudi
Department of Pediatrics, The Brooklyn Hospital Center, 121 Dekalb Avenue, Brooklyn, NY 11201, USA

Ahmad J. Alzahrani and Tariq Alhazmi
Pediatric Endocrine Department, (A.J.A, T.A), Maternity Children Hospital, Makkah, Saudi Arabia

Azzam Ahmad and Lujin Ahmad
Umm Al-Qura University, Medical College, (A.A, L.A), Makkah, Saudi Arabia

Fahd Refai
Department of Pathology, Faculty of Medicine, King Abdulaziz University, Jeddah, Saudi Arabia

Jaudah Al-Maghrabi
Department of Pathology, Faculty of Medicine, King Abdulaziz University, Jeddah, Saudi Arabia
Department of Pathology, King Faisal Specialist Hospital and Research Centre, Jeddah, Saudi Arabia

Haneen Al-Maghrabi
Department of Pathology, King Faisal Specialist Hospital and Research Centre, Jeddah, Saudi Arabia

Hassan Al Trabolsi
Oncology Department, King Faisal Specialist Hospital and Research Centre, Jeddah, Saudi Arabia

Emily Schildt
Ann & Robert H. Lurie Children's Hospital of Chicago, Chicago, IL, USA

Robyn Bockrath
Northwestern University Feinberg School of Medicine, Chicago, IL, USA

Marie K. White
Neonatal Intensive Care Centre, Kings College Hospital NHS Foundation Trust, Denmark Hill, London SE5 9RS, UK

Ravindra Bhat
Neonatal Intensive Care Centre, Kings College Hospital NHS Foundation Trust, Denmark Hill, London SE5 9RS, UK
Department of Women and Children's Health, School of Life Course Sciences, Faculty of Life Sciences and Medicine, King's College London, London SE5 9RS, UK

Anne Greenough
Neonatal Intensive Care Centre, Kings College Hospital NHS Foundation Trust, Denmark Hill, London SE5 9RS, UK
Department of Women and Children's Health, School of Life Course Sciences, Faculty of Life Sciences and Medicine, King's College London, London SE5 9RS, UK Asthma UK Centre for Allergic Mechanisms in Asthma, King's College London, London SE5 9RS, UK NIHR Biomedical Research Centre at Guy's and St. 0omas' NHS Foundation Trust and King's College London, Guy's Hospital, Great Maze Pond, London SE1 9RT, UK

R. Elqadiry, O. Louachama, N. Rada, G. Draiss and M. Bouskraoui
Pediatric   A   Department,   Mother-Child   Pole, Mohammed VI University Hospital, Marrakesh, Morocco

Maurike de Groot-van der Mooren, Sabine Quint and Mirjam van Weissenbruch
Department   of   Neonatology,   Emma   Children's Hospital and VU University Medical Center, Boelelaan 111, Amsterdam 1081 HV, Netherlands

Ingmar Knobbe
Department of Pediatric Cardiology, Emma Children's Hospital and VU University Medical Center, Boelelaan 1117, Amsterdam 1081 HV, Netherlands

Doug Cronie
Department of Obstetrics and Gynaecology, Onze Lieve Vrouwe Gasthuis, Jan Tooropstraat 164, Amsterdam 1061 AE, Netherlands

Gloria Pelizzo and Giovanni Battista Mura
Pediatric   Surgery   Unit,   Pediatric   Surgery   Unit, Children's Hospital "G. Di Cristina", ARNAS "Civico-Di Cristina-Benfratelli", Palermo, Italy

Megan B. Coriell
University of Louisville School of Medicine, Louisville, KY, USA

Aurora Puglisi, Maria Lapi and Giuseppe Re
Pediatric   Anesthesiology   and   Intensive   Care   Unit, Pediatric   Anesthesiology   and   Intensive   Care   Unit, Children's Hospital "G. Di Cristina", ARNAS "Civico-Di Cristina-Benfratelli", Palermo, Italy

Maria Piccione and Martina Busè
Department of Sciences for Health Promotion and Mother   and   Child   Care   "Giuseppe   D'Alessandro", University of Palermo, Palermo, Italy

Federico Matina
Neonatal Intensive Care Unit, A.O.U.P. "P. Giaccone", Department of Sciences for Health Promotion and Mother and Child Care "G. D'Alessandro", Palermo, Italy

Valeria Calcaterra
Pediatrics and Adolescentology Unit, Department of Internal Medicine University of Pavia and Fondazione IRCCS Policlinico San Matteo, Pavia, Italy

Prasanthi Gandham, Kupper Wintergerst and Bradly Thrasher
University of Louisville School of Medicine, Louisville, KY, USA
Norton Children's Hospital, Louisville, KY, USA

Shraddha Siwakoti, Rinku Sah and Basudha Khanal
Department of Microbiology, B.P. Koirala Institute of Health Sciences, Dharan, Nepal

Rupa Singh Rajbhandari
Department of Pediatrics, B.P. Koirala Institute of Health Sciences, Dharan, Nepal

Shuk Ching Chong
Department of Paediatrics, The Chinese University of Hong Kong, Prince of Wales Hospital, Shatin, Hong Kong
The Chinese University of Hong Kong, Baylor College of Medicine Joint Center for Medical Genetics, Prince of Wales Hospital, Shatin, Hong Kong

Chung Mo Chow
Department of Paediatrics, The Chinese University of Hong Kong, Prince of Wales Hospital, Shatin, Hong Kong

Kam Lun Hon
Department of Paediatrics and Adolescent Medicine, The Hong Kong Children's Hospital, Kowloon, Hong Kong
Department of Paediatrics, The Chinese University of Hong Kong, Prince of Wales Hospital, Shatin, Hong Kong

Fernando Scaglia
The Chinese University of Hong Kong, Baylor College of Medicine Joint Center for Medical Genetics, Prince of Wales Hospital, Shatin, Hong Kong
Department of Molecular and Human Genetics, Baylor College of Medicine, Houston, Texas, USA
Texas Children's Hospital, Houston, Texas, USA

Yu Ming Fu
Department of Paediatrics and Adolescent Medicine, Princess Margaret Hospital, Kwai Chung, Hong Kong

Tor Wo Chiu
Division of Plastic Reconstructive and Aesthetic Surgery, The Chinese University of Hong Kong, Prince of Wales Hospital, Shatin, Hong Kong

Tracey Dyer, Paul Dancey, John Martin and Suryakant Shah
Department of Pediatrics, Memorial University, 300 Prince Phillip Drive, St. John's, NL, Canada

Wun Fung Hui
Department of Paediatrics and Adolescent Medicine, The Hong Kong Children's Hospital, Kowloon, Hong Kong

Michael Wai Yip Leung
Department of Surgery, The Hong Kong Children's Hospital, Kowloon, Hong Kong

Ankur Rughani, Monica Marin, Jonathan Meyer and Jeanie B. Tryggestad
Department of Pediatrics, Section of Diabetes and Endocrinology, University of Oklahoma Health Sciences Center, Oklahoma City, Okla, USA

Kenneth Blick
Department of Pathology, University of Oklahoma Health Sciences Center, Oklahoma City, Okla, USA

Hui Pang
Department of Pediatrics, Section of Genetics, University of Oklahoma Health Sciences Center, Oklahoma City, Okla, USA

Jun Kido, Shirou Matsumoto and Kimitoshi Nakamura
Department of Pediatrics, Graduate School of Medical Sciences, Kumamoto University, Kumamoto, Japan

Hannah F Chong
Memorial Hermann Hospital, Houston, TX, USA

Roukaya Al Hammoud and Michael L Chang
The University of Texas Health Science Center, McGovern Medical School, Pediatric Infectious Diseases Division, 6431 Fannin, MSB 3.126, Houston, TX 77030, USA

Hemali P. Shah, Richard Frye, Sunny Chang, Erin Faherty, Jeremy Steele and Ruchika Karnik
Department of Pediatrics, Section of Pediatric Cardiology, Yale University School of Medicine, New Haven, CT, USA

Alexander Lyons
Children's Hospital of Michigan, Detroit, MI, USA

Jamie Lee and Kristen Cares
Division of Pediatric Gastroenterology, Children's Hospital of Michigan, Detroit, MI, USA

Aishwarya Palorath
Department of Pediatric Gastroenterology, University of Miami-Jackson Health System, 1601 NW 12th Ave, Miami, FL 33137, USA

Ishita Kharode
Department of Pediatrics, Division of Pediatric Endocrinology, Richmond University Medical Center, 355 Bard Ave, Staten Island, New York, NY 10310, USA

Vlad Laurentiu David, Mihai Cristian Neagu, Aurelia Sosoi, Maria Corina Stanciulescu, Calin Marius Popoiu and Eugen Sorin Boia
Department of Pediatric Surgery and Orthopedics, "Victor Babes" University of Medicine and Pharmacy, Timisoara, Romania

Florin George Horhat
Department of Microbiology, "Victor Babes" University of Medicine and Pharmacy, Timisoara, Romania

Ramona Florina Stroescu
Department of Pediatrics, "Victor Babes" University of Medicine and Pharmacy, Timisoara, Romania

Diana Simão Raimundo, Carolina Figueiredo and Ana Raposo
Department of Pediatrics, Hospital Divino Esp'ırito Santo de Ponta Delgada, Ponta Delgada, Portugal

Bernardo Dias Pereira
Department of Endocrinology and Nutrition, Hospital Divino Esp'ırito Santo de Ponta Delgada, Ponta Delgada, Portugal

Index

Printed in the USA
CPSIA information can be obtained
at www.ICGtesting.com
JSHW052111140524
63116JS00005B/99

9 798887 406145